Breaking the Walls of Silence

Breaking the Walls of Silence

AIDS and Women in a New York State Maximum-Security Prison

by
The Women of the ACE Program
of the Bedford Hills Correctional Facility

THE OVERLOOK PRESS
WOODSTOCK & NEW YORK

First published in the United States in 1998 by
The Overlook Press, Peter Mayer Publishers, Inc.
Lewis Hollow Road
Woodstock, New York 12498

Library of Congress Cataloging-in-Publications Data

Breaking the walls of silence: AIDS and women in a New York State
maximum security prison / the members of the ACE (Aids Counseling and Education)
Program of the Bedford Hills Correctional Facility.
p. cm.
1. Bedford Hills Correctional Facility (N.Y.). ACE (Aids Counseling
and Education) Program. 2. Women prisoners—New York (State)—
Health and hygiene. 3. Health education of women. 4. AIDS
(Disease)—Prevention. 5. Women prisoners—Counseling of.
6. Health counseling. I. Bedford Hills Correctional Facility (N.Y.).
ACE (Aids Counseling and Education) Program
RA644.A25B74   1993   362.1'9697'920082—dc20   92-35997

BOOK DESIGN AND FORMATTING BY BERNARD SCHLEIFER

Manufactured in the United States of America

ISBN 0-87951-500-7
First Edition
1 3 5 7 9 10 8 6 4 2

Contents

Note to the Reader

Medical breakthroughs and scientific advances in the areas of medical treatment for adults and children, testing and scientific understandings about the HIV virus have occurred since this book went to press. We urge the reader, when using the curriculum materials in the second half of *Breaking the Walls of Silence*, to utilize current HIV/AIDS monthly journals to supplement and update the information presented here.

The most exciting and noteworthy of the advances are the medical treatments. *Combination* anti-HIV treatments, now the preferred therapy, combine earlier drugs such as AZT with the new class of drugs—protease inhibitors. In February 1997, the U.S. Centers for Disease Control and Prevention (CDC) announced an overall 12% decrease in AIDS deaths in the United States in 1996. This represents the first annual decline in AIDS deaths in the history of the epidemic. The CDC report also noted a slowing trend in the number of Americans diagnosed with AIDS in 1996. This decline in AIDS-related deaths is the basis for renewed hope in the effectiveness of anti-HIV treatments for prolonging and enhancing life for PWA's. Yet, many questions and issues remain.

Unfortunately, not all groups of people benefit equally from these advances:

. . . deaths declined 21% for whites, but only 2% for African Americans and 10% for Hispanics;
. . . deaths of men declined by 15%, but increased among women by 3%;
. . . deaths declined among men who have sex with men by 18%, but increased 3% among heterosexuals;
. . . the proportion of female AIDS cases continued to increase, from 18% in 1994 to 20% of newly reported AIDS cases in 1996.

These statistics reflect a wide range of social problems, including unequal access to care, as well as the inability to pay for these expensive, new medications.

Throughout this book we use the term "PWA." The letters "PWA" stand for Person With AIDS. The term came into use when people who were HIV-positive began to challenge the notion that they were "victims" or solely "people to be helped"—suggesting a passive role. Instead they wanted to help themselves through support and education to "survive and thrive," and to become an active voice to improve social conditions affecting the epidemic. By speaking openly about being HIV positive, they educated others as they affirmed their own humanity and dignity. In light of this awareness of self-empowerment and accountability toward one's own health, we celebrate the new term, "PLWA," People Living With AIDS.

Preface
by Whoopi Goldberg

For the most part, when someone asks you to write a preface to a book, it's a pretty straight-forward (forgive the pun) thing. So when I sat down to do it, I found that the words were not coming easily. I thought to myself "Just say why people should read this book!" This proved to be hard too because each reason became a dissertation on AIDS, AIDS and women, AIDS, women and the justice system, etc. I realized that's what the book is about. Duh! So I threw it out. It was then I decided to write about the effect this book had on me when I read it. So again I wrote. Well, by the time I finished writing, re-writing, cleaning up the language, then cleaning up the thoughts so they would be coherent to someone other than myself, I was bored, bummed and pissed. "What's going on?" I thought. "I've done this before. I know how I feel. Why can't I get it down on paper?" Then I came upon the thought that in this book lives facets of my life that were too close to share with other people. I finally understood what I wanted to say to you who is reading this preface.

Everything in the book is applicable to you or someone you know. You will be disturbed by the feelings that are stirred when you read any given page. You'll be glad it wasn't you and sad that others have had to live this so that you might read and learn from it and, perhaps, slow the mighty flow of AIDS. You will come to see courage in some and cowardice in others. You'll understand how programs like ACE can help and why we need them in the big picture. You'll understand the gift you've got in your life when you read about life with AIDS, life in prison and life as a woman in prison.

You'll know that your perception about a lot of things will change when you read this. Not gigantically, but in small ways. You may want to kiss your kids, you may want to help, you may even become a better person in some unfathomable way. But I don't promise. I do promise you'll not be quite the same. So that's my preface, and I thank Glenn Close for writing me about these folks. She's around a lot for these women.

Take this journey, because honey, this is part of our world...

Welcome to it.

—Whoopi Goldberg, 1997

Foreword
by Elaine A. Lord,
Superintendent

A prison is a community, a microcosm of our society. This community is made up of inmates who live there, staff who work there, visitors and volunteers. Since prisons are small self-contained communities, what any of these groups believes or thinks is important and contributes to the feel of a prison. When the headlines worrying most Americans in the mid-80s dealt with a new disease called AIDS, it was no different in prison. When children weren't allowed to go to school because of widespread fear of contagion, the same fears were running rampant in prison. When people were stigmatized and isolated if anyone thought they had AIDS, the same stigma was felt by inmates in prison. Staff, inmates, visitors—everyone was impacted. To this day, I remember Rene explaining that finding out you have AIDS is like falling on the dance floor—the room becomes totally silent, everything stops, the people, the music. Everyone is watching, looking, silent.

In the earliest days, women who had AIDS were isolated in the infirmary. There was little understanding of this illness, and it brought stigma and isolation, lack of understanding—fear—on everyone's part. I can still remember receiving that first letter from a few inmates requesting a chance to visit with those women in the infirmary—to play cards, teach knitting and crocheting, talk. They reminded me that you can't even have a decent game of spades without four people. A little room outside of the infirmary became a place for just sitting down and talking, then doing little things together to pass the time. TIME—the central entity around which all prisons revolve.

Those inmates who first reached out were initially treated terribly by everyone, just as if they, themselves, carried the plague. Other staff and inmates thought that maybe they were HIV-positive, but weren't telling. The small group of women who had initially intervened to help those early patients made a tentative proposal to develop a program to address the bad feelings and hurtfulness inmates with AIDS, or those thought to have AIDS, experienced in prison. We sat down and these inmates became the pivot point for identifying the need, developing the policies and helping to work out the program that became ACE, AIDS Counseling and Education. Together we came to the same conclusions about the need for education to address the misconceptions that led to negative feelings and stigma, and the need for strong peer support and leadership. Working through the early issues in the development of the ACE program was difficult and painful for both staff and inmates. As professionals, we struggled to face our own limitations in terms of training, perceptions and cultural competencies and in our inability to control the sickness and death that were becoming too routine. Developing programs in conjunction with the inmates who will be the main deliverers as well as users is a personally challenging process since it pushes the inmates toward understanding the limits on any prison administrator's powers and raises necessarily difficult questions for everyone involved. It is basically an attempt to develop consensus between two groups that often see themselves at cross-purposes. Yet, inmates have a broad array of relevant experiences that we can draw on and together work toward change in the prison community. When we fail to work together in this manner, our efforts are weak and insubstantial because they are not only one dimensional, but they also fail to recognize that most of the power for change comes from within the person who is changing. Of course, there were hesitations. We had developed other significant programs, like the Children's Center, using inmates as co-developers, but was AIDS going to be different? We were concerned that the AIDS issue would prove too volatile and emotionally laden to be able to work out and develop a program strategy over time. Even if everyone in a prison knows that inmates talk to other inmates and seek their advice and assistance, would we be able to successfully use peer counselors to teach inmates about risk behaviors, and then on top of that, actually convince staff and inmates to call for another, albeit trained, inmate to assist with crises? There were also concerns about inmates being able to move around to other housing units. These issues were discussed with the initial group of inmates over and over again in an attempt to get clear agreement on what expectations would be placed on these peer counselors. One time, a session ended in angry disagreement, and I shut the program down. I asked a friend active in AIDS issues to come in and attend the next session to give me some advice. After the meeting, she suggested I stop and think about what was making me so angry because it wasn't the women I was dealing with, but the inability to control the deaths, the wasting of these lives, the lack of power. So, be angry with them, not at them, she said. I went to Katrina who was a core person in the group and we had a long chat about anger and power. From that time on we kept each other focused on the real issue, helping women incarcerated at Bedford Hills be able to live in the best way possible.

We began this century in corrections with a significant reform movement which saw inmates as having a tremendous ability to change. Sadly, we seem to be ending this century with cynicism, almost having thrown our hands up on any efforts to rehabilitate and restore an offender to society. I believe that programs such as ACE provide the vehicle through which rehabilitation is made possible. Through accepting responsibility both for oneself and for others, positive growth and change takes place among inmates. My hope is that we come around again and begin to recognize that successful communities must be built upon shared values. Implicit to shared values is the value which we place upon each and every individual that is a part of a community—for communities are only successful if they can stay ahead of their problems.

—SUPERINTENDENT ELAINE A. LORD

Foreword
Katrina Haslip
1959-1991

I often ask myself how it is that I came to be open about my status. For me, AIDS had been one of my best-kept secrets. It took me approximately fifteen months to discuss this issue openly. I could not bring myself to say it out loud. As if not saying it would make it go away. I watched other people with AIDS, who were much more open than I was at the time, reveal to audiences their status and their vulnerability. I wanted to be a part of what they were building, what they were doing, their statement, 'I am a person with AIDS," "a PWA," because I was.

Somewhere behind a prison wall in Bedford Hills a movement or community was being built. It was a diverse group of women teaming together to meet the needs and fears that had developed with this new epidemic, AIDS. These women believed that none of their peers should be discriminated against, isolated, or treated cruelly merely because they were ill. They believed that it was necessary for this prison to build an environment of support, comfort, education, and trust. I was a part of this process. In the center of its establishment I stood, struggling with my own personal issues of HIV infection.

While held in some sort of limbo, I felt as if the women of ACE had built a cocoon around me, for me. I felt warmed by them and so totally understood. These were the women who understood my silence and yet felt my need to be heard. They gave me comfort when I needed it and an ear when I needed a listener. They helped me to grow stronger with hopes that one day I would be able to stand alone and still feel as safe. Empowered! I took from them all that they were capable of putting out. I gave back to them what I was given. It was as if I mirrored back what they put out. I had never before noticed in my peers this ability to care so deeply. For I too had labeled them prisoners, cold and uncaring. Yet they had managed to build a community of women: black, white, Hispanic, learned, illiterate, robbers, murderers, forgers, rich, poor, Christian, Muslim, Jewish, bisexual, gay, heterosexual—all putting aside their differences and egos for a collective cause, to help themselves. I could not believe my eyes. Right before me lay a model of how we, as a whole, needed to combat all the issues AIDS brought, and we were building it from behind a wall, from prison. We were the community that no one thought would help itself. Social outcasts, because of our crimes against society, in spite of what society inflicted upon some of us.

We emerged from the nothingness with a need to build consciousness and to save lives. We made a difference in our community behind the wall, and that difference has allowed me to survive and thrive as a person with AIDS. To my peers in Bedford Hills Correctional Facility, you have truly made a difference. I can now go anywhere, and stand openly, alone without the silence.

—KATRINA HASLIP, 1990

We dedicate
this book...

....To Superintendent Elaine A. Lord for her belief that
    incarcerated women can make a difference

....To all our sisters who have passed but are not forgotten

...To all incarcerated women and men who deal with
    HIV/AIDS

...For our sisters and brothers throughout the world where
    the epidemic is raging

We give this book in memory

of our sisters from Bedford Hills Correctional Facility
who have died from HIV/AIDS.

Sonia Perez	Yvonne	Debra
Carmen Royster	Inez	Nancy
Blackie	Sandy	Juanita
Rosa Barbot	Adream	Cynthia
Katrina Haslip	Carrie	Miriam
Jane Davis	Gladys	Ace
Renee Scott	Diane	Rhonda
Doris Moices	Mildred J.	Mildred W.
Xiomara Rubin	Lynn	Black
Nancy Ayala	Ebony	Susan S.
Angelina S.	Peaches	Debroah Williams
Jeweline	Debbie	Angelina Figueroa
Carmen Rivera	Savage	Diane E.
Gladys Howard (Nay Nay)	Jeannie	Jackie C.
Rosa P.	Lafay	Emma
Lye	Star	Tuffy
Milagros	Ro	Nadine S.
Rachel	Tiny	Sharon C.
Frenchie	Luz	Margarita C.
Chino	Cruz	Wanda T.
Nilda	Lettie	Janette Lopez
Fat-Baby	Ramona	Donna Harvey
Linda	Helen	Tiffany Robinson
Cathy	Aurea	
Joann	PeeWee	

The authors of
Breaking the Walls of Silence

We wrote our book over a period of eight years. It has been a collective project. The different periods of writings reflect different stages of the ACE organization and its work.

EDITOR AND PROJECT COORDINATOR: Kathy Boudin

WRITING GROUPS

1988: Rosa Barbot, Kathy Boudin and Carmen Royster completed the first draft of a curriculum for our workshops which laid the basis for the first stage of community education by ACE.

1989: Kathy Boudin, Judith Clark, Katrina Haslip and Carmen Royster finalized the nine workshops which became the foundation for the community education up to the present.

1990: Kathy Boudin, Judith Clark, Katrina Haslip, Maria Hernandez, Aida Rivera, Doris Romeo and Pearl Ward wrote a description of the work, our educational approach and a beginning history of ACE. They sought out voices of the many women to bring the work to life as the curriculum was transformed into a first draft of the book.

1991: Kathy Boudin, Vanita Carrington, B.J. Close, Tiffany Collins, Lisa Osborne, Aida Rivera, Doris Romeo, Ethel Scarpulla and Viniece Walker developed new sections of the curriculum with an emphasis on women's experiences and needs.

1992: Kathy Boudin, Judith Clark, Lisa Finkle, Awilda Gonzalez, Aida Rivera, Ruth Rodriguez and Doris Romeo wrote the present version of the history and the description of the work of ACE.

EDITORIAL ASSISTANT: Judith Clark
ARTISTS/ARTWORK: Arlene Mohammed; Aida Rivera; Ruth Rodriguez
PROOFREADING: Sherri Martindale; Jan Warren.

THE FOLLOWING WOMEN contributed prose pieces and poems expressing their own experiences with the AIDS epidemic:

Carmen Arroyo; Kathy Boudin; Gloria Boyd; Joanne Brown; Toni Bundy; Vanita Carrington; Judith Clark; Linda Gang; Awilda Gonzalez; Debra Gore, Katrina Haslip; Maria Hernandez; Donna Hylton, Debora Irving, Terry Krum; Rachel Luna; Anna Martinez; Doris Moices; Vivian M.; Sandra Ospina; Sonia Perez; Cynthia Rhodes; Aida Rivera; Ruth Rodriguez; Doris Romeo; Carmen Royster; Cathy Salce; Ethel Scarpulla; Renee Scott; Jenny Serrano; Viniece Walker; Leslie Walters; Pearl Ward.

SPECIAL THANKS TO Suzanne Kessler, Debra Levine and Jacquelyn Hawkins ...three civilians who played critical roles at different stages in evaluating, editing and talking with us about the book.

WITH GRATITUDE TO Debra Levine who, as Special Projects Consultant to The Women's Prison Association, coordinated the work between The Overlook Press and the ACE Program and produced and directed the film about ACE, "ACE Against the Odds."

WITH APPRECIATION TO Tracy Carns, Editor of The Overlook Press, who never gave up and persevered to see this book to completion.

Introduction

Perhaps the most dramatic event occurred when we began making quilt squares. Two volunteers from the Mid-Hudson AIDS Task Force who came to the prison infirmary once a week first suggested that we participate in the Names Project, making quilt squares for women who had died from Bedford Hills, adding them to the thousands that were being made nationwide.[1]

I remember the first quilt squares I made. As I was about to paint it I remember saying to myself, "My God, it's the size of a real grave." The sadness I felt within myself as I made this one quilt was unspoken. As I looked around the room at the others, I knew that I wasn't alone in what I was feeling. We all understood that though the making of these quilts would mean sadness to all, it was also a way of letting our sisters know that they will always be in our hearts. For those who remain, how do we grieve the losses which keep happening and remain able to move forward in our own lives? Slowly a culture of survival is growing among us.

The quilts were laid out, fifteen of them, on the floor of the school building corridor. They stayed there for a week. Day after day, women passed through looking at the names, unable to turn away from the reality. Women among us were dying of AIDS. We then brought the quilts to the living units. The women laid them down on the corridor in front of our cells on the floor where we lived. It was so hard reading the names of so many of the women that I lived with. There were about fifteen of them.

It was shocking; it made me realize that one of those names could have been me. It was sad, and that is an understatement—it was overwhelming. Seeing all the names of women who had walked those same corridors was an eye opener. That was the one time that I felt a sense of community.

---

1. The two volunteers from the Mid-Hudson AIDS Task Force were Norma Hill and John King. The Mid-Hudson AIDS Task Force changed its name to AIDS Related Community Services (ARCS) when it became clear that there was a need to establish a permanent organization to cope with the AIDS epidemic.

There was silence as we walked around the quilts. We didn't know that the quilts were coming up, and suddenly they were there.

The quilts captured the people. For Sandy, there was a baseball diamond and her favorite song, "Do Me Baby." Fat Baby had her Newports; Diane loved horses and her quilt was a big horse. I had given the glitter to be put on the quilt for Sandy, and that made me feel good, like I was a part of that. I guess that's what making quilts does for us, it lets us feel connected to the people who died. One of the things that makes our world different from outside the prison is that we can't share the end. We can't go to the outside hospital and we can't go to the funerals. Making these quilts gave us a way to have closure and a way to feel connected to the women we loved or knew as friends and who had died.

These quilts made us face our reality. The quilt project was the final and maybe necessary step before the actual formation of ACE. Our consciousness was raised. Now enough women were ready and willing to act.

Winter, 1988

PART I
THE ACE STORY

I
Who We Are

We are women in prison, incarcerated in Bedford Hills Correctional Facility, a New York State maximum-security prison. AIDS is having a devastating effect on our lives. We are women struggling with the AIDS epidemic.

There are approximately 3500 women in seven prisons throughout New York State. The population of Bedford Hills is close to 750. In 1992, one out of every five women entering the New York State prison system tested positive for the HIV virus.[1] Hundreds more have family members or friends who are sick or have died. Many women have used IV drugs, while others have had multiple sex partners, and some have had lovers or spouses who are HIV-infected. Before we started the ACE (AIDS Counseling and Education) Program in 1988, we lived in a state of constant anxiety over whether or not we would test positive for HIV. Locked up with one another, sharing the same showers, kitchen, and living space, we felt panic: What was AIDS? Where did it come from and how did you get it? We lived with fear: fear of one another and fear for our lives.

We knew that we would have to help ourselves and each other. We started ACE because we felt that as prisoners, we would be the most effective in educating, counseling, and building a community of support. We stated four main goals: to save lives through preventing the spread of

---

1. New York State Department of Health AIDS Institute, *Focus on AIDS in New York State AIDS in Prison Project Fact Sheet* (April 1994), edited by Miki Conn (newsletter) ([Albany, NY]: New York State Department of Health AIDS Institute 1994) 3.

HIV; to create more humane conditions for those who are HIV-positive; to give support and education to women with fears, questions, and needs related to HIV/AIDS; to act as a bridge to community groups to help women who are HIV-positive reenter the outside community.

While some of us were friends when we first came together, most of us knew each other only in passing. What united us was that we were all affected by AIDS. We shared a need to survive the epidemic. If you had used the word "community" about life in prison, we would have laughed. But in the end, we came together with a common goal and created a community, which gives us strength. Community isn't something that exists just because we live together. It is something that we build, something that is fragile, that we have to constantly nourish.

Our story is not about perfect people who created a perfect program. We are women, convicted of crimes, who, in spite of it all, created something that is making a difference in many people's lives. Out of tragedy came one of the most positive experiences in our lives.

This book is our story: the story of a group of women and our struggle to transcend the tragedy of AIDS. We begin with the history of ACE: how we developed the program, working with the prison administration, outside agencies, and one another. We describe the different aspects of our work. We include voices from the women, some who have left the prison, others who have died, and some who are still here. Our voices are diverse, as varied as the women in Bedford. From the beginning, the women in ACE have been black, white, and Latin; street-educated and college-educated; HIV-positive or not, drug users and non-drug-users, gay and straight, in our twenties, in our fifties, from many religions and many different backgrounds. This diversity has been a critical strength, for it has made us richer as a group and it has allowed us to speak to the many different women in Bedford.

The second half of this book is a curriculum of nine education workshops. They contain basic information about AIDS and techniques for teaching. They can be used by any individual or group that wants to learn or teach about the AIDS epidemic.

This book is a tool for organizers, prisoners, men as well as women, teachers, counselors, for anyone who feels the impact of HIV/AIDS and wants to do something about it. We know what it is like to face the problem of life and death without the necessary resources.

The basic underlying concept of ACE and this book is peer education and participation. It is only when people become involved and work together that profound change can occur and a supportive foundation can be built. In our experience, people's capacity to learn to help one another is vast. This book is designed to facilitate the process.

WOMEN AND AIDS

We are women. Today women are 13 percent of those with AIDS in the United States, but the World Health Organization estimates that women are being infected with HIV about as often as men and that by the year 2000 most new infections will be among women; heterosexual transmission of HIV infection is steadily increasing, and 70 to 80 percent of the people becoming infected in this way are women; women die faster than men from AIDS. Yet, women's issues in the AIDS epidemic are still not getting the attention they need.[2]

For many years, the federal government Centers for Disease Control and Prevention (CDC) did not include in its definition of AIDS many life-threatening conditions that women who are HIV-positive often get. Only recently, as a result of enormous pressure by women, did the CDC finally add three of the more common illnesses that women who are HIV-positive get—cervical cancer, bacterial pneumonia, and pulmonary tuberculosis. Doctors often see our illnesses as "women's problems" instead of HIV-related. An HIV/AIDS diagnosis requires timely necessary medical intervention. A classification of "AIDS" as opposed to just "HIV-symptomatic" means an increase in financial support from the government for such things as housing, day care, and nutritional benefits. Until recently, most drug trials—the prescribing of medicines still being tested—have not been open to women. Thus, women did not have access to newly developing medicines that might help them.

For women the issue of safe sex with men is more complicated than just having the knowledge that it is important to use a condom. As women, we confront resistance from men in the form of attitudes, financial dependency, or physical force—all of which can make it hard to get a man to use a condom. And for many of us, condoms were not part

---

2. Federal Centers for Disease Control, *HIV/AIDS Surveillance Report (October 1994),* ([Atlanta, GA]: Federal Centers for Disease Control, 1994); World Health Organization, United Nations Development Program, *Women and AIDS Agenda for Action* (January 1995) ([New York]: World Health Organization, 1995); Lawrence K. Altman, "AIDS Cases Increase Among Heterosexuals," March 11, 1994, *New York Times;* Risa Denenberg, "What the Numbers Mean," in *Women, AIDS, & Activism,* edited by The ACT UP/New York Women and AIDS Book Group (Boston: South End Press, 1990) 1–4; "H.I.V. Found to Kill Women Faster than Men," December 28, 1994, *The New York Times,* p. C10.

of our lives prior to the existence of the HIV virus, because we, too, did not like them and did not feel them to be necessary. We, as well as men, are faced with the need to change. Some women have to worry about their husbands or boyfriends and wonder if they're being faithful, and if not, are they practicing safe sex? This can be even more of a worry for us in prison, separated from our men.

Some of us are lesbians, who, like lesbians on the outside, are anxious about our vulnerability to infection through woman-to-woman sex, and we have lobbied for more scientific studies on this question. Moreover, we know many self-identified lesbians who were infected through sharing needles or through unsafe sex with men. In ACE, we have nurtured a respect for communication and learning between homosexual and hetero-sexual women, drawing on our common bond.

As women, we worry about our families and women's issues. AIDS is the fourth leading killer of women twenty-five to forty-four in the United States; and in New York and New Jersey, it has been the leading cause of death among African-American women since 1988. While AIDS is a grave concern for all women, it disproportionately affects black and Hispanic women and their children. In New York City the overwhelming majority— 86 percent—of the women with AIDS are black (53 percent) and Hispanic (33 percent); 13 percent are white. And in New York City, 91 percent of the children with AIDS are black (55 percent) or Hispanic (36 percent); 8 percent are white. Women enter the crisis of AIDS already vulnerable, carrying the burdens of the social, economic, or political obstacles that they already face.[3]

And if this vulnerability is true in the United States, it is even more true in the worldwide context of AIDS. AIDS is spreading most rapidly in Asia; the overwhelming majority of the 7 million to 8 million women infected throughout the world live in Africa, and AIDS is the leading cause of death for women of childbearing age in most central African cities. There are approximately 1.5 million infants infected with the virus world-wide, and the World Health Organization estimates that by the year 2000, 10 to 15 million children under age ten in Africa will be orphaned as a result of AIDS.[4]

---

3. Federal Centers for Disease Control, *HIV/AIDS Surveillance Report* (October 1994); *World* (January 1994), a newsletter by, for, and about women facing HIV disease, (Oakland, CA: 1994) 1; New York City Department of Health, *AIDS Surveillance Update* (October 1994).

4. Darlene Weide and Rebecca Denison, "Women and AIDS: A Global Problem," *WORLD,* December 1993, 2; World Health Organization, United Nations Development Program, *Women and AIDS Agenda for Action* (January 3, 1995).

We worry about the babies of mothers who are HIV-positive and about the future generations, even when we do not know them. The women of Bedford Hills have "adopted" the Incarnation Children's Center, a residence in New York City for babies with HIV/AIDS. We have raised money in our walkathons for the children who live there, created wall hangings and a memorial quilt for their residence, knitted baby booties, and painted toddler T-shirts as our way to connect, as mothers, to other mothers and their children suffering with HIV/AIDS.

As mothers we worry about our teenage children. We worry about safe-sex issues, rape, and the use of drugs. As mothers in prison we do our best to educate our children on these issues by phone, through letters, and during the occasional visits we have with them, but being in prison makes us feel powerless.

AIDS has affected us as women because we make up the vast majority of the caregivers. We work as nurses, nurses' aides, and home attendants. These are usually low-paying jobs, yet they carry enormous emotional burdens for those caring for people with AIDS. Where is our support?

Today, women entering this prison tell us of spending the last decade caring for and losing children, brothers and sisters, uncles and parents. Some women have literally lost their whole families to this epidemic. Feeling guilty, overburdened, sometimes sick themselves, and rarely enjoying access to needed care and services, women often turn to drugs for relief. But our health, our tragedies, our burdens and responsibilities were—and often still are—rendered unimportant.

Our story is the story of the AIDS epidemic among women.

AIDS IN PRISON

AIDS is the leading cause of death in New York State prisons. New York State prisons contain overwhelming numbers of people who are HIV-positive: an estimated 17 to 20 percent of the 63,000 inmates in the Department of Correctional Services are infected with HIV; 8,000 inmates have been definitively identified as HIV-positive. Among incoming inmates, the HIV infection rate in Hispanics (22.2 percent) is nearly double the infection rate in whites (12.9 percent) or blacks (11.6 percent). Among those diagnosed with AIDS, close to 44 percent were Hispanic, 40 percent were black, and 11.8 percent were white. In the most recent blind study of incoming inmates in New York State Correctional Facilities, the rate of HIV infection among women was twice that of men, 20.3 percent compared with 11.5 percent.[5]

Living with AIDS anywhere is difficult. Being in prison brings added fears and problems. Although the illness is the same, our conditions are different. Perhaps the most important factor that helps people endure HIV/AIDS is love and support, yet in prison we are separated from our friends and families on the outside. ACE has been able to build a supportive environment for women in the prison infirmary, yet many prisons do not have those conditions, and when a prisoner is sick, and most in need of the medicine of love, he or she is alone. In many prisons and jails, health care is a major problem. And in those cases where it is not, there are still limited choices. For example, although doctors stress the importance of nutrition for people with HIV/AIDS, it is not possible in most prisons to have access to the kinds of food and vitamins recommended. Many other holistic alternatives, as well as medicines offered through drug trials, are not available. As prisoners we can get a bed in the city hospital, but as we make the trip in the van or wait for an appointment, we will be chained with leg shackles and handcuffs. Stigma and prejudice affect people in or out of prison, yet in a prison it can be hard to get away from the pressure, because every aspect of life is so connected. In or out of prison, facing death is devastating, yet the one thing most prisoners who are HIV-positive say is, "I just don't want to die in prison."

The close relationship of sex and drugs to AIDS raises yet another issue. Sex and drugs are both prohibited in prison and punishable according to prison rules and regulations. Yet, people must be able to discuss their actual sexual experiences openly, in order to change, if the spread of HIV/AIDS is to be prevented. Drug use also needs to be discussed openly. Thus, prison administrators are faced with a dilemma: How do they balance the need to create a safe atmosphere for open discussion in the interest of public health with the importance of maintaining a prison's rules? How this dilemma is resolved determines how much we as inmates can openly work with one another around these issues.

As prisoners, we cannot do anything as a group unless we have permission. We cannot hold a meeting or teach a workshop or care for women who are sick in the infirmary without permission. This is one of the realities of prison life.

---

5. New York State Department of Health AIDS Institute, *Focus on AIDS in New York State* (April 1994), 1, 3.

While there are limitations to prison life, there are also certain factors that worked in our favor. First, we recognized the problem of AIDS as *our* problem and dedicated ourselves to making a difference. Second, the Superintendent of Bedford Hills was committed to meeting the AIDS crisis in the facility and she was equally committed to the notion that inmates could play a critical part in that process. We were inspired by the example of the gay community coming together to fight AIDS. From publications such as *The PWA Newsline* and *Surviving and Thriving With AIDS,* we learned about PWAs who were fighting to transcend their condition as victims to become survivors and thrivers. The work by men in New York State prisons in building an AIDS peer education and counseling program, PEPA, provided a model for us as well. We received support from women employed by the New York AIDS Institute as well as from those committed to broader women's issues including the Governor's Commission on Women and the ACT UP Women's Caucus.

Holding our program together has not been easy. We have been slowed down on a number of occasions. We have seen many civilian supervisors come and go. The rules and regulations within the prison frequently change. We face positive changes and losses; women leave on parole, women are transferred to other prisons, and women die. We experience the exhaustion, or burnout, that faces everyone doing AIDS work, inside or out of prison. Through it all, we are still here. Looking back we have grown and changed with the experience of dealing with AIDS.

In addition to AIDS, there are other issues that affect us. Most of us are mothers, and when a child dies—from whatever cause—we are sent into turmoil. We have known these children from the visiting room and photos and their mothers' stories. When the eight-year-old daughter of one sister died, we celebrated her life in the tradition of Puerto Rico, with a "Baquine." We all wore white shirts with a pink ribbon and decorated the ACE office with paper balloons and paper birds. Those of us who knew her shared memories of her. Through our tears we played children's games, read children's books, and sang lullabies.

Along with hard times, we have also shared some wonderful times. Some ACE members came to Bedford with little education. We have celebrated the achievement of GEDs, vocational certificates, and associate's and bachelor's degrees. One ACE member, after being paroled, became very sick and was hospitalized. Having completed her work for her four-year bachelor's degree at Bedford, her dream was to come back to march in the graduation procession. She was too sick to travel, so Mercy

College representatives conferred her degree in her hospital room. On her quilt square after she died, we painted a graduation cap and a diploma. We have celebrated Christmas, Thanksgiving, birthdays, and going-home parties. Many of the women cook special dishes representing the different cultures that make up our group.

Many ACE members who have been drafted to other prisons have helped educate or counsel women in the new facilities. Numerous women from ACE who have gone home took what they learned here and found jobs in programs as AIDS counselors or educators, and the work goes on.

WRITING THIS BOOK

We didn't start out to write a book. We started out to build a program—a program of work. But just four months after ACE was born, in the summer of 1988, the superintendent said, "Before you can teach population, you must write down on paper everything you will be teaching so that it can be approved by the Department of Health and Department of Correctional Services of New York State."

We didn't realize at the time how useful this would be. We were just desperately trying to meet whatever demand was made on us. We defined the areas we wanted to teach and talk about, such as transmission, testing, what AIDS is, and women and AIDS. Then one woman spent the summer writing, drawing on information from materials we had received from different organizations.

When ACE was finally given permission to do work among population, the book—which we referred to as "The Manual"—became a tool. The curriculum was our guide for developing seminars we brought to the population. We took the words off the pages and put them into real life. The words suddenly had a new kind of power; no longer was it just a proof of our competence, it was now also our guide for education, community building, and empowering ourselves to fight AIDS.

The experience of our work led us to make changes in the manual. Our struggle within the prison against stigma and prejudice led us to create a new workshop about stigma, drawing on an excellent book called *Blaming Others*. The number and urgency of women's medical questions pushed us to develop an entire workshop about treatment. Our prevention work led to a workshop on sexual transmission.

When ACE became recognized and funded as a model program for prisons, the AIDS Institute urged us to transform our manual into a book to be distributed in other prisons. We expanded and enlivened the curriculum by adding the voices of many more participants.

In 1992, the book was accepted for publication by The Overlook Press. Once again, its purpose was expanded. In addition to writing for other prisoners and AIDS activists, we now had the goal of writing for the general public. This entailed a new period of writing, in which many more women participated. We added the section describing ACE's history and work.

Writing the history of ACE meant looking back into it. This process became a window through which newer members learned about the early struggles, whereas those who had been part of the first period could compare the past with the present and reflect on the changes.

Most of us were never writers. What we had to say was of little or of no importance to anyone. Ironically, it took the tragedy of AIDS and imprisonment for us to be heard. Now our stories matter.

Our definition of "writer" is not the usual one. Everyone here counts. There was intense debate during the writing process. Those who could write with ease tended to do much of the writing, while others resented this because they felt left out. Some didn't feel confident; some felt there were more important priorities than writing. Some just didn't want to write. We learned through our mistakes how to involve more people. Some women like to write in a narrative style; others wrote analytically. Some were more at ease telling their own experiences in their own voice; others preferred to talk while another woman wrote it down. This resulted in a unique end product. Like ACE, this book is a collaboration. Many voices come together as one, but the individual voices also come through.

* * *

Writing this book is a way to share myself, my voice, my work, a way to feel good about myself. I feel that I failed in so many ways, that I'm labeled. This is a way of saying, Look, I can help, I'm more than just a prison number or label.

* * *

From my experience in the 1960s, when something happened in one community that was positive, that worked to help people get together over a problem, if people in other places heard about it, it would inspire them, encourage them, even give concrete methods or inform them how to help themselves, to help organize in their community. I hope that by sharing this experience, it will help other prisons and other people wanting to do something about AIDS.

* * *

The writing helped deal with our losses. It's a form of recognizing our pain, our deaths. I felt defeated when I wrote about the deaths. I'm not much of a crier, but three times I cried. It doesn't ease the pain, but I feel proud of the book—it makes us immortal. Even when we're all gone, this book will live on, and all those who are dead will live on through it.

* * *

We often experience a sense of deep separation and distance when we deal with issues other than those of prison life. We speak of "the street," "the free world," and "outside the walls." Prison life is insulated—we have visits, phone calls, mail, but those bring that other reality closer only for a moment. Now we were writing for a larger world, which seems so far away. Now we were given the opportunity to connect with them.

We would like to give our readers a description of what life in prison is like.

A Day in the Life

Life in prison means living with a lot of other women in a small, confined area.

* * *

Where I live, there are sixty women on one floor, with thirty cell-rooms along one long corridor and thirty on the other. Each floor also has a small rec room with a TV and a kitchen area with hot plates—areas that are empty during part of the day but boisterous with energy and noise in the afternoons and at night.

* * *

It isn't easy to live so close together. That's sixty different personalities, races and nationalities, cultures, backgrounds, religions, with ages ranging from sixteen to seventy-three. There's different musical tastes, TV preferences, personal crises, all sharing the same area, with one TV, two phones, three showers, four hot plates . . . and no partridge in a pear tree!

* * *

Unlike in the prisons you see on television, we do not have bars in front of our cells. We do have a metal door with a small, 5″ by 8″ Plexiglas window. These doors open and close electronically from the officer's station. Our clothing is restricted to solid colors, but no blue, black, gray, or orange; we must wear "prison issue" green pants or skirts.

* * *

My surroundings are pale green cinder blocks. The ceiling is gray with patches of plaster. The door opens and locks from the outside, with keys that only the unsentenced possess.

* * *

The grounds don't look like most people's idea of prison either. There are no high walls surrounding us, like at Attica, and we can see the trees and hills in the distance. But we can't forget for a minute where we are because of the high wire fences with rows and rows of razor wire. The housing units look like small, two-story housing projects. There are two school buildings, a medical building, the administration building and visiting room, a laundry, and a commissary. We walk from building to building on a permission slip— a "pass"—like a hallway pass kids carry in high school.

* * *

When people on the outside think of "doing time," they think of our sentences: 2 to 4, 5 to 15, 10 to 20, 25 to life, life without parole. We do long time. But we also do time every day. Fractured time. Each day is broken up into three three-hour modules—morning, afternoon, and evening. In between we eat and get locked in to be counted: 11:20 A.M. count, 5:30 P.M. count, 10:30 P.M. count. If you are at work, in the middle of a project, you can't just decide to stay an extra hour. You have to go back to your housing unit for count. We do lots of different time and it's all their time. But we also have a choice on how we use our time. In this prison we can get an education: ranging from basic literacy skills to college.[6] There are some vocational classes available: printing, business education, cosmetology. Many women choose to work in programs to better ourselves, and take more responsibility for our families—the Children's Center,

---

6. In June of 1995 the college program was closed down at Bedford Hills, C.F. along with all college programs in New York State Correctional Facilities due to cutbacks in funding.

Family Violence, ACE. So even while we're doing time, we have an important choice: Are we just going to do "their" time, or make our own?

* * *

In addition to security and civilian and administrative staff, the day-to-day functioning of the prison depends on prisoners' work: kitchen workers, laundry workers, cleaners, secretaries, printers, teacher's aides and nurse's aides. Women also work as peer counselors and teachers in the self-development programs.

* * *

Women earn from $5 to $14 every two weeks, depending on their jobs. For a lot of women, this is their sole income. Others knit and make crafts in order to earn money for themselves and to send home to their children.

* * *

At 5:30 A.M., our day begins. The officers wake us with a shouted "Five minutes till count!" Our doors are unlocked at 6:00.

* * *

When I get up at 6:30, I look out the window and see sunlight gleaming on the barbed wire fences. I use the toilet in my cell, sitting directly on the freezing white toilet bowl because our toilets have no toilet seats. Then I go to the shower and wait with all the other women waiting to wash.

* * *

At 8 o'clock, the officer shouts, "School and program line!" and most of us go off to work or school.

* * *

When I am in my program, off the unit, it is somehow easier to deal with prison life. I might be in a classroom or the ACE office, and somehow I can escape my prison reality by getting engrossed in my work. But when I walk back to my unit and hear the officer lock the door behind me, a feeling of being shut off from the rest of the world engulfs me.

* * *

The visiting room is open from 8:30 to 3:30. The visiting room is different from any other place in the prison. It is here where we have direct physical contact with the outside world, keeping us in touch with reality. It's sunny and clean. For many of us, the Children's Center is the main attraction, a colorful playroom where we can hug, roll, and talk quietly with our children. More than 75 percent of us are mothers, and our relationships with our children are sustained, sometimes even built, here.

* * *

At 3:30, the work module ends for most women and a variety of self-development and treatment programs begin. Sometimes participation is by choice; sometimes it's a parole requirement. These programs deal with parenting, violence, drugs, AIDS, inmate-administration liaison, and other issues. The women who are not involved in any programs that day return to their housing units, where they can cook, make phone calls, do their homework, or relax. At about 4, dinner is called for those who go to the mess hall to eat, while others eat their own food on the unit.

* * *

Some women go to school or work in the evening, while others go to the gym or recreation. But many women stay on the floor, to watch TV, cook, use the phone, and hang out in their cell-rooms or the rec room.

* * *

Noise. You can't believe the noise on my unit in the evening. The TV blaring, music, women playing cards or hanging out, swapping stories of the street life—"war stories" as they are called—people yelling down the corridors, keeplocks calling for the officer, women cooking and joking in the kitchen. Sometimes when I'm on the phone with a friend she will say, "God it sounds like there's a riot out there," and I say, "No, it's just a normal evening."

* * *

As 10:30 approaches, the yelling and running around increases. The women realize that they're about to be confined in their cells for the night. They want to say good night to their friends, borrow or return cassette tapes, stamps, something to drink, or a cigarette for the night. At 10:30 is the sound of metal doors clanging shut, one after the other, until all thirty on the corridor have slammed. Then the officer takes the count.

* * *

Lock-ins can bring peace, an ability to concentrate and to feel oneself, which is hard to achieve when the doors are open and there is constant noise and activity. Even though you're locked, you can feel like you have more space, because you can expand your mind's world. But you also know you are locked in, you cannot get out.

* * *

Even at night, your sleep may be interrupted. Sometimes a woman gets sick at night and shouts for an officer. Some of us will wake up and help get the officer's attention. The officer's power is limited. He or she must call the sergeant and get permission to open the cell. Meanwhile, a woman could be having a seizure or asthma attack. It is very scary to hear this happening from behind a locked door, to not be able to help and to know it could be you. Or, on a quiet night, your sleep is still interrupted by an officer's flashlight shining through the window of your door into your face, as the officer counts, even as you sleep. Whether it is night or day, you never forget that you are in prison.

* * *

Prison life is a lot about waiting: waiting for an officer to open the door; waiting on line for a phone, shower, hot plate; waiting at the hospital for a doctor; waiting for a package, waiting for a visit, waiting to get strip-searched at the end of a visit, waiting for the parole board, and then waiting for the letter that tells you whether you're going home or not. "Patience is something you'll learn here" say the old-timers to the new arrivals.

People get upset when they hear that prisoners can go to college, cook our own food, or go to programs that help us. Sure, those things make life more comfortable—and more important, enable us to make something of ourselves, so that we can be something better for our children and in society. And this prison does provide many more opportunities than most. But it doesn't make our time any easier. The pain of prison is not whether or not you can watch TV or lift weights. It's the reality of not being able to watch your child go to sleep at night or take care of her when she's sick. It's being taken outside of life, home, in society for ten, twenty, a lifetime of years. That's our punishment.

It's up to us to take advantage of what is here, to come to terms with what brought us here, with the crimes we've committed, and to rebuild broken lives and families.

2
How ACE Was Conceived

Before ACE was formed, we were in the midst of a crisis. We were faced with an illness, and all we knew about it was its name and the fact that people were getting sick and dying. No one knew how you got it. If a woman was skinny, or went to the doctor too much, people said she had AIDS. Whether it was true or not, some people wouldn't sit near her in the cafeteria, take a shower after her, even breathe the same air. Death from AIDS hadn't hit Bedford yet, but the fear of it had.

On my living unit in 1985 there were two women who kept having appointments to see the nurse. People began whispering about them, saying not to sit next to them while they were watching TV and not to shower after them. I would be in the yard and people from the other housing units would come up to me, telling me that they had heard about these two women and warning me to stay away from them. This wasn't the first time something like this had happened. Prior to this, other incidents had occurred, but this was the straw that broke the camel's back. Several of us talked about doing something about the fear, rejection, and ignorance.

* * *

I remember going to the mess hall and a girl had a plastic bag on her tray. I asked, "Why are you putting a plastic bag on your tray?" and she said, "I don't know who used the tray." I said, "Well, who used the plastic bag? At least you know the tray is washed." She said she just felt that the plastic bag was cleaner, so I let her know that it made no sense. Then she said it was because of AIDS.

In August 1985, a handful of women, responding to incidents such as these, brainstormed about what to do. We decided to write a letter to the superintendent saying that there was a need for more education about AIDS. Some also wanted to be able to give support to those who had AIDS and to protect the well-being of those who didn't. We wanted to begin a dialogue with the administration about those issues.

* * *

Eleven of us signed the letter, including those two women who were being whispered about. We didn't expect to meet with the superintendent ourselves. We suggested that she meet with the formal representatives of inmates, The Inmate Liaison Committee. We didn't expect anything fast, since nothing happens fast in prison. But this time we were surprised. Two days after the letter was sent, all of us who signed were called to a meeting with the superintendent.

* * *

While writing this book, we asked the superintendent what had led her to respond to the letter as quickly as she did. She answered,

I was beginning to get concerned by 1985. I heard that people were saying when they got off the bus, "I came to prison, now I'm going to catch AIDS." Women were talking about whether it was safe to take a shower. I think we were a microcosm of society at that time, with the fears and questions. So it didn't surprise me to receive a letter from inmates around AIDS issues. I, too, was concerned. There was already a strong precedent for inmates' having responsibility here. Sister Elaine, who directs the Children's Center, had refused to take the job here unless inmates would be permitted to take real responsibility. So when I responded to the inmates' concerns by meeting with them, it was not the first time that had happened here.

The meeting was significant, mostly because people were dealing with and talking about the problem instead of avoiding it.

* * *

We really didn't know a lot. We weren't even coming from the same mindset. Some of us leaned toward wanting the administration to be better about isolating people; others were more concerned about supporting people who were sick. But the one thing we all shared was that we knew that our greatest enemy was fear and ignorance. We didn't want to get sick and we wanted to stop the spread of AIDS. We asked such things as was the laundry being separated. There's a laundry where everyone sends their clothes to be washed. Although the clothes are in individual laundry bags, they are all washed together in one machine. One of the fears raised at the meeting was that maybe AIDS spread from clothes to clothes and what could be done about that? We also asked whether the administration notified everyone who was testing positive for AIDS, and could we get some education in here.

* * *

Two concrete decisions came out of the meeting: the superintendent said that she would try to bring in outside experts, such as doctors and AIDS educators, to educate us about AIDS, and she gave everyone at that meeting permission to visit the women who were sick in the prison infirmary, known as IPC (In-Patient Care).

* * *

IPC was known as a dungeon. It was a dreary place where people went when they were sick and then they were forgotten. No one was allowed to visit anyone there prior to the meeting with the superintendent. If you were caught standing by the door that was the entrance to IPC talking to a patient, you would be given a direct order to move and you risked being issued a misbehavior report. Some of the women would be there for days without their personal items, without their mail being delivered, without contact with their friends, and without access to a telephone, which all other living units had. For the superintendent to give women permission to go there was a very big step. Just being there and talking to the women made a big difference—for once the women no longer felt isolated and alone. They felt that someone cared. Many struggled to live fully rather than be buried alive in isolation.

* * *

A few of the eleven women who were at that meeting chose to go.

* * *

I didn't know Petey well when I first started to visit her. I went because I thought that women like myself from population visiting IPC could help break the isolation and challenge stigma and all the unfounded fears of casual contact. But my feelings got much deeper over the time I spent with her. She had such feistiness and spirit, and oftentimes when we were all hanging out, I felt blessed by the chance to be with her, share her energy and struggle.

* * *

In those days there was so much fear that it became a big thing just going to IPC. Then, when I would go to the yard afterward, some people would come up to me and actually whisper, "Hey, I think it's great what you're doing, going to the hospital to see people. I really support that." And others would stay away from me. Even though there was absolutely no danger, people reacted very strongly because of the fears and ignorance. I had my own fears and uncertainties, even though I went to IPC. I knew in my head that AIDS didn't spread through touching, but a part of me was still afraid, so every time I was preparing to leave IPC, I went into the bathroom and washed my hands with detergent. That made me feel that I had taken the necessary health measures, and that I could tell other people that I was safe and that I wouldn't get them sick.

* * *

The others were reluctant to go to IPC out of fear, which further emphasized the necessity for the education we were requesting.

The education sessions that the administration set up for us shortly after that meeting were held in the gym, because it was big enough to hold several hundred people. Although these sessions were a first step in bringing AIDS education into the prison, we needed much more than that and something very different in order to deal with our fears as a whole community. Clearly, we needed more than the large lectures with an outsider. We needed a smaller, more personal and informal setting where people's own experiences could be talked about, without having to worry about the whole population knowing. At the time we didn't know how we were going to deal with this; we just knew we needed something different. Support grew in tiny steps, but the fears increased more rapidly. A church service took place for two women who died: this was the first time we had a church service where it was acknowledged that two of our women died of AIDS. One woman wrote the following poem right after the church service:

A Harsh Poem, an Angry Poem, a Hard Poem

Two sisters died this week . . . of AIDS!
How dare they call it AIDS!
"To aid" is to help, to lend assistance
An aid—someone or thing which helps.
But there is no help, no cure, no vaccine
What a cruel name
Cruel as the name of the town Liberty, Alabama
Where so many black people have been lynched.

Kathy B.

During the next two years it was the courage of the PWAs, the women living in IPC and those who chose to support them, regardless of their status, who made the greatest impact.

* * *

Petey fought to be on the yard crew on days when she felt well enough to work. Before Petey got sick, she used to work on yard crew, mow the lawn, rake leaves, and shovel snow. When Petey was living in IPC, there were many days she felt well enough to work, and she wrote the superintendent, asking her for permission to work. She finally got permission, but it wasn't easy. At first, no one on the yard crew would go near her. She had to work the area around the hospital and work it all alone. They would leave her tractor for her early in the morning and then, after she was done, they would pick it up. With time, more people were willing to work with her. Why? It is our guess that as people saw other women reaching out to Petey, and not getting sick immediately, their fears lessened to some degree—enough to at least know that if they stayed and talked to Petey and others that they wouldn't get sick. Just having people be willing to talk to Petey was a big step. Petey wanted to go to a celebration in the gym held for inmates and their family and friends. She knew that some people would whisper and talk about her. They did and it was hard for her. But she would always push the limits. She wouldn't let people's fears and rejection stop her. There was so much whispering about her that some of us, including the superintendent, sat at a table with her outside, both to talk about what was happening around her and demonstrate our own lack of fear.

* * *

The superintendent remembers,

I began to try to use my own position to make a difference. So when Petey went to family day, I let the supervisors for that day know that Petey would be there. Sergeant Russell was on that day and he said, "Some of the staff are anxious, but I've talked to them." I sat at the picnic table with Petey along with some other women. We talked about whether she should stand in line to get food, how would the outside families react, did she want to take the pressures of dealing with their reactions.

* * *

Sandy was very popular with the in crowd here, she was a long-termer. She had a lot of street knowledge and street ways, which made it easy for her to have a lot of friends. Sandy was athletic and healthy-looking and worked in physical programs such as yard crew and construction here in prison. When Sandy started to have symptoms, it made a lot of us take a look at ourselves, because we lived the same way she did. She forced us to look at healthy people and wonder if they had it too. We knew then that you didn't have to look sick to be sick. That added to the fear. Eventually, the physical transformation that took place with Sandy was very difficult for us to see.

* * *

Before she died, Sandy said,

I dipped and dabbed and here I am. I had to be the one to get caught. I can't blame nobody. These women here have temptation, they been down a long time. They say, "Here, Sandy," and there's only one set of works. I never thought about nobody dying. Then in '82, '83, I heard about AIDS and said, "Oh my God, it won't happen to me," and it did; boy, did I hope I missed it. Look at me. All I can do is tell you what I was and what happened to me. I was 100 percent fit.

* * *

Sandy slowly started deteriorating. She changed completely, it was a drastic change. She yelled at people, and many just didn't want to deal with it, but those of us who were her friends stood by her. Sandy used to be on the softball team. Before she disappeared into IPC, there was a period when she would come to the yard with help from friends to sit in the shade and watch the softball games. She was like an old warrior.

* * *

One person I always think of from that time was Vikki. She fought a losing battle against lung cancer. Even though she didn't have AIDS, she had a terminal illness, was in IPC with many of those women with AIDS, and was one of the women whose courage in the face of death was moving for everyone.

I remember how Vikki took her sheets in IPC and made curtains for different people's rooms; she had a doll named Arnold to keep herself company. Her sense of humor and fun stayed with her throughout her illness. Vikki wrote a letter to me telling me that she had to have chemotherapy and would probably lose her hair, and that if I were a real friend I would shave my head bald as a symbol of our friendship. She never lost her sense of humor. She was the type of person who cared about everyone else's happiness. One Christmas she went around asking each of the sixty women on our housing unit, "If you had a wish, what would you want for Christmas?" She wrote everything down, went through magazines and cut out individual pictures such as a car, a boat, a mink coat, and put them in envelopes. She then gave everyone her present at a Christmas Eve party, when she herself was dying. Her spirit, sense of humor, and love for people moved everyone that knew her in this facility—the inmates, officers, and administration. People loved her. I remember Vikki was given six months to live. Incredibly, the doctors were right. Vikki tried to get released from prison before she died, in order to spend time with her children and to die with dignity. We knew she was dying, and we would have long talks about it. We discussed her coffin in a joking manner. She wanted to wear her red boots and her green vest and have a red coffin. She said that she wanted to go out in style. There was no policy or law that allowed people to leave prison before parole if they were dying. Vikki tried a different approach to getting out—a temporary medical furlough. Finally, ten days before her death, she was released to a cancer hospice. I called her every day, until one day she didn't answer the phone anymore. I'll never forget that day for as long as I live.

We had a memorial service for her in the gym, and we talked about her. We laughed, told stories about her, cried, and remembered Vikki for who she was. There were several women in the memorial service who had AIDS, Sandy being one of them. She came to the service in a wheelchair. We didn't know then whether to continue or to stop because of wanting to protect her feelings, but she was there for Vikki and we continued with the service. This memorial for Vikki paved the way for the kind of memorials we would begin to do when people died of AIDS once ACE started, a memorial in which we, as inmates, talked and sang about our friend who died.

* * *

Ann was healthy-looking, active, the inmate coordinator of the drug program here. She ate health foods and was athletic. Although she helped others here, when she needed help, it was hard for her to ask us for it— maybe because she was a role model or maybe because she wanted to keep her illness a secret, although as time went by everyone eventually knew. She contacted the Mid-Hudson AIDS Task Force in order to reach out and get help. This was an important step, because two buddies from there began to make weekly visits to IPC, something they sustained for a number of years. Not only did this make a difference for the women in IPC, it also brought us in touch with the outside AIDS movement.

* * *

The two buddies from the Mid-Hudson AIDS Task Force—Norma Hill and John—also had an effect on the superintendent. She remembers,

They stopped me in the parking lot one evening after coming from IPC. They were concerned about the stigma they were finding. They said that women told them you could go to IPC with a broken leg and population thought you had AIDS. They pushed me about the doctors not being adequately trained. I arranged for them to bring brochures into the prison with information about AIDS.

* * *

All these people, as well as others, moved us with their courage and spirit of life. By the fall of 1987, even more women at Bedford were directly affected by HIV/AIDS—they themselves were vulnerable and/or they had friends and family members who were sick. You could see this in a number of things that were happening in the prison. You could feel an undercurrent of growing anxiety. Discussions about AIDS were happening throughout the prison: in the cafeteria, in the hospital, in cells, and in the corridors among friends. The school also became a place where the topic of AIDS was discussed: a college psychology class spent many of their classes talking about AIDS, as did the ABE class (Adult Basic Education).

The ABE class began discussing their questions about HIV/AIDS and it led to the writing and producing of a play. It was powerful because it showed very real situations: a woman finding out that she is positive and having to tell her family or her lover, others deciding whether to take the test. The ABE class showed the play to all the other classes and staff counselors. All this helped break the silence.

A key development occurred during that fall of 1987: a small number of women decided to develop a proposal for a peer-education and peer-counseling program around AIDS. They had seen the drawbacks of huge lectures in the gym. Some of the members in this group would change over time, but for the next several years they were known as the "core group" for ACE. Coming from different living units, we met in the yard, which was a common meeting place, and talked and wrote. We presented our proposal to the superintendent and waited for a response.

* * *

I was one of the women who met with the superintendent in 1985 and then spent a lot of time that summer with Petey in IPC. While IPC was like a dungeon in those days, my time with Petey was special. Then, in the fall of 1985, I was put in SHU [Special Housing Unit] — punitive solitary confinement — for two years. Even though I was out of population, the AIDS crisis continued to affect me.

There was a woman in SHU who was very sick and losing weight, and most people assumed she had AIDS. All night long we listened to her wheeze and cough and choke. Women were scared because we were locked into such tight quarters. But mostly it was a nightmare to watch someone deteriorate mentally and physically, until she was often raving and ranting between outbreaks of coughing. Twice a day, a nurse came to give out medication. She handed it through a slot in our doors. But S. had gotten paranoid after being locked down for so long and often she wouldn't swallow her medication. Finally, one day she was released, jubilant, from SHU. But that night she was brought back, because she had not completed her SHU sentence. After that, she got much quieter. She stopped cursing at us and stopped throwing garbage and shit at the officers. That's when we really got worried. Soon after that, she had what seemed like a very bad asthma attack and they took her to the outside hospital, where she died.

We all felt powerless and angry. We heard that they held a church service for her in population, but we weren't allowed to go. I think that someone came up and held a short service with us, but it didn't soothe me at all.

A year later, my codefendant, who was in a men's prison, died of AIDS. If prison is a difficult place in which to deal with loss, SHU is worse. It's like mourning in a tomb.

When I finally got out of SHU in 1987, I had a hard time readjusting to population. But I knew that I wanted to find some way to work with other women to face this crisis that was stalking us. I read a book put out by the People With AIDS Coalition, called *Surviving and Thriving with AIDS* and got a subscription to their *PWA Newsline*. I learned about people who were not just letting themselves be victimized, who were empowering themselves collectively to live and to fight the epidemic. Their boldness, self-affirmation, and community mobilization reminded me of what it was like to be a part of a mass social movement, like the civil rights, antiwar, and women's movements.

Could we in this prison mobilize our own energies and transform our powerlessness into collective efficacy? Could I utilize my skills and experience from the past in new, less confrontational ways, to work with others in solving some of the problems AIDS was presenting? The challenge excited me.

* * *

I was an IV drug user. I worried that I might have the virus. I didn't want to take the test in Bedford, because I was going home in eight months. I wanted to wait. I had too much on my mind to handle a positive test result. But my sister had AIDS. AIDS was on my mind. When I heard about the idea of starting a program about AIDS, it sounded like a good idea to me. I liked writing and I thought maybe I could help. I never dreamed that from our small beginning we would be able to create ACE.

* * *

What led me to work on the proposal for ACE? When I look back, there were many threads that came together. After we got permission from the superintendent to spend time in IPC in 1985, I began going there, and I came to know a number of women with AIDS. I felt the horror of the illness and also the courage of the women. They were struggling to give some meaning to their lives as they faced each day with uncertainty about the next one. I myself was struggling to deal with a long prison sentence, and I learned from them about trying to find meaning in the present, and I could also measure my relative luck, I appreciated my life.

AIDS came closer in 1986, when I heard that my codefendant had gotten sick and was in the hospital. I sent him a get-well card, writing about health food—bulgur wheat, miso soups—and ten days later it was returned, stamped "deceased." His death from PCP was one of the early

AIDS deaths that happened quickly, when there had been no knowledge that he had AIDS and no preventive treatments.

In the fall of 1987, I was teaching a literacy class and we watched a TV show about AIDS. The fears, anxieties, questions, and life stories of the women about AIDS transformed the class from a fairly low-energy classroom into one filled with a drive to learn. As we jumped into learning about AIDS and through that improving basic reading and writing, I felt the need to do something about AIDS in the prison as a whole.

I knew of an AIDS program in a New York State men's prison based on prisoners being peer educators and counselors, and that idea made sense to me. I felt that we, as prisoners, were in the best position to help ourselves. I also had been a community organizer in the sixties, and the notion of a community solving its own problems when people come together was a model for me from the past. I never could have predicted back then all that it would be: the close friendships, the sharing of tears over friends who have died, comforting those friends whose sisters and brothers have also died, the experiencing of stigma and cruelty and trying to turn it around, the massaging away the tensions, the hours in the IPC unit, the laughter, and the courage—even in the face of death—to laugh, the experience of struggling together in this totally tragic situation. Somehow through it we have been able to give ourselves strength to survive and turn the stigma and fear and isolation into a feeling of community.

* * *

It all began with that incessant coughing that would not go away. Night after night, I would lie awake praying for it to stop. "Oh, God," I could hear myself say. "Please help her. She is suffering so much!" I did not know at the time what was wrong with my neighbor. I only knew that she was desperately ill. I found myself visualizing her 100-pound body shaking uncontrollably from these racking coughing spells. After a week of this, I had to do something. I approached NayNay and suggested that she see a doctor. She informed me that she had already done so and was told that she should sign up for Nurse's Screening again and she did. Again, she was told there was nothing wrong, but this time they gave her cough syrup. This procedure was to go on for what seemed like an eternity. Finally, one day, she came to me because she felt she could trust me to confide in me. She told me what we both dreaded. The test results had come back HIV-positive. My heart went immediately out to her, but in my mind there were reservations: Could I catch this from her? Was it a safe distance? The questions were numerous. Then, suddenly, I was jolted to my senses by the reality that if I'm reacting like this, how will others treat her? Women were already being ostracized by the stigma of AIDS. No one wanted to shower or eat with those they thought might have it. It was at that exact moment when I knew I had to find out more about this deadly disease. I could not bring myself to treat her any differently than I had been.

For whatever our personal reasons, five of us eventually came together with a definite goal, which was to make a difference in the prison in regard to AIDS. We witnessed the inhumane ways in which the women were treated by other women, and we vowed to do what we could to change things. We knew that in order to do this, we would have to change the ways in which the medical department, staff, and other inmates viewed AIDS. This, we felt, could be done by educating, but before we could educate others, we first had to be educated. In order to do this, we contacted Montefiore Hospital. They agreed to meet with us and the administrative staff of the prison. Around this time, we became an official prison organization (ACE), recognized by Albany. We were now ready for new members, and about thirty–five new people signed up to join us. The five of us continued to meet with Montefiore staff and the prison superintendent on a regular basis. After several meetings, we began our formal training. This was done by volunteers from Montefiore Hospital staff.

When reading this, it all sounds so easy, but it was far from that. The obstacles were many, but we were determined; our optimism, perseverance, and energy prevailed in overcoming any and all barriers to reaching our goal.

I later left ACE, but I resigned in membership only. Although no longer a member, I would always make myself available whenever and wherever needed for a woman afflicted with HIV or AIDS. My reason for leaving ACE was very personal at the time. I can now speak and write of it. My brother contracted AIDS while I was still an ACE member. I was taken out to see him on a deathbed visit in the hospital. What I saw when I arrived there was a skeleton of who my brother once was. I never knew if he even recognized who I was as I stood there beside him. I like to believe he did know who I was and that he heard my promise to him that I would stay in there, fighting against this deadly disease until the battle was won.

After my brother's death, it became very difficult for me to work closely with the women I originally had vowed to work with. I found I could no longer handle death and dying. All I could see was my brother's suffering. As time passes, I hope this picture will change and that I will once again be able to envision the time when my brother laughed, loved, and enjoyed life and living.

* * *

During January and February 1988, those of us in the core group waited for a response from the superintendent about our proposal to develop a peer education and counseling program. We began to meet once a week in the library. First we decided to begin educating ourselves. We knew almost nothing. Two of us read *And the Band Plays On,* by Randy Shilts, and reported on it to the group. This book gave us an understanding about the beginning of the spread of AIDS and a sense of how the gay movement came together around the epidemic. Their togetherness inspired us, it made us more aware of the different forces—government, medical, and the bureaucracies that, in time, we too would be dealing with. One woman in our group took on the responsibility of writing letters to outside AIDS groups, agencies, and hospitals asking for information. This work put us in touch with the outside world—helped break our isolation—and soon our consciousness about being part of a larger struggle increased. One letter opened up a critical connection: it went to Montefiore Medical Center, to Monnie Callan, a social worker in their AIDS Program, who wrote back and expressed a willingness to help us. Within a few months they would come in and train us. Finally, we talked about organizational details such as a name. One woman came up with the idea of ACE. It stood for AIDS Counseling and Education, but it was also a good luck symbol, the ace card, an ace in the hole, and a person who is your number-one friend.

The final step before the creation of ACE was the making of the first quilt squares. We got a donation from Reverend Benton's church for paints, and for four days during a February school break we set up tables, each covered with a six-foot-by-three-foot piece of cloth for quilts. We tried to remember all the names of the women who had died of AIDS during the past several years. We were finally paying tribute to the many women who died, and from this moment on, we as a community would no longer hide from AIDS.

3
The Birth of ACE

Finally, in March 1988, the superintendent gave her approval for us to create an inmate peer education and counseling program about AIDS. In looking back at this decision, the superintendent said that she had been concerned with the increase of fear and stigma:

> I think the best way to deal with stigma is by building community . . . and I think that women do it easily. Before I came to Bedford, I had been doing program development in sixteen male facilities. Here, there's a different sensibility: women tend to focus a lot of energy on personal relationships and the way they relate to others. I don't think that people necessarily pick up on this or use it as a strength, but it is a strength that makes an important difference in developing programs and in the way institutions run.

First, the core group began looking for people who wanted to do something about the AIDS epidemic—the recruitment of people was critical. We needed to reach out to diverse segments of the population, because that is what we consist of: racially mixed, Spanish-speaking, gays as well as heterosexuals, women who have AIDS as well as women who do not, women who have been involved at one time or another in high-risk activities, women serving long as well as short prison terms. By word of mouth each of us asked women we thought might be interested. By the end of March 1988, when we had found thirty-five women who were interested, we called our first meeting.

* * *

I remember one evening when Blackie and I were hanging around on our unit and Tammy asked if she could speak to us. At first we were a little surprised—we had no idea what she wanted. We went to a corner in order to have privacy. Tammy spoke to us about what they were trying to do around the issue of AIDS and asked us if we were interested in coming to the first meeting. Neither Blackie nor I had ever been approached with anything like this before, so we told her that we would discuss this among ourselves and that we would get back to her. After Blackie and I discussed it, we both admitted to each other that we wanted to say yes to Tammy on the spot, but that we weren't sure how the other would have felt. Although people knew that Blackie and I were close, and that she had AIDS, this meeting would have meant that we were coming out with our issues in public. We felt good, and a sense of relief that after being talked about and put down for so long there were finally people who cared and weren't worried about us infecting them. Although I didn't have AIDS, I was treated as if I did. People thought that because I was close to her that I had it too. Although I have never experienced the actual physical illness, I can honestly say that I have experienced some of the psychological aspects. I now know what it feels like to be rejected and talked about because one has AIDS. After Blackie and I discussed our feelings with each other, we decided to go to the meeting. We had no idea who was going to be there, but we knew that we were finally coming together with people who cared.

* * *

When I first came to Bedford, I had never been around anyone in my life who was infected with HIV, and I was very paranoid. I felt that they should be kept in quarantine. I voiced it, "Why are they back here with us?" I didn't want them sharing my cube, food, shower. I felt it was a violation of my rights and I said it over and over again.

The next thing that happened was that a good friend of mine, Lany, introduced me to Ro, and we all began to hang out together. Then Ro started getting sick, so we helped her, cooked for her, cared for her. You can't tell by looking at someone that she's sick, so I was helping her like I would help anyone who was sick. She was a beautiful person. It never occurred to me that she would have AIDS. I got moved to a regular living area, with my own cell. And then I found out that Ro had AIDS. She knew but she didn't want to tell us. I stopped going near her, but Lannette stuck by her, doing her hair in the yard, just being with her. I was confused. I would send things for her by Lannette, but I wasn't going to see Ro anymore. I told Lany, "You better watch out, you better take care of yourself." I was thinking about my family, my kids. I wanted to get out of here alive. But I also felt bad because I had already gotten to know her and I really liked her, and I watched Lannette waver not at all.

Right at that point, Mo comes to me and asks me if I want to be part of ACE that's going to start up soon. By then I wanted to know more, I needed to know more. So I went to that first meeting. I think if Mo hadn't approached me, though, it would have taken me longer.

* * *

In the beginning of 1988, I made a phone call to my mother, only to find her crying and unable to speak to me. She gave the phone to one of my sisters, who was also crying. In the background, I could hear other members of my family crying. My first thought was that someone had died and no one wanted to tell me. I remember yelling into that phone, asking, "What happened? What is going on over there? Did someone die?" In between sobs, my sister gave me the news that my youngest sister, age twenty-five, and her newborn baby had AIDS. At that time I had no idea what AIDS was, I only knew what I heard on the news or the whispers I heard from other people. All I knew was that many people had died from this illness.

Crazy as it sounds, two days later, as I was coming back from school, a woman named Kathy approached me on the hill and told me about some group they were trying to put together that had to do with AIDS. As Kathy talked to me, I asked myself, "Who told this person about my sister and niece having AIDS? How could she have known?" To get rid of her, I told her that I had to think about this. The reality was that I didn't want to let anyone know about my sister and niece for fear that people would think that I had AIDS too. In the days that followed, I did my best to avoid Kathy. I didn't want to bump into her, for fear that she would ask me again about the AIDS group. As the days turned into a week, I thought more and more about AIDS. Every chance I had, I watched the news for information on this illness my sister and niece had. Then one day, as I walked to my unit, I bumped into Kathy again, and she asked me again. Even though I was still hesitant, I said yes.

Finally, the day of the first ACE meeting came. I almost didn't go to the meeting, but I knew that, for myself, my sister, and my niece, I had to go and find out what this meeting was about. I told myself that I would attend this meeting, I would listen, but I wouldn't talk, let alone mention my sister. I remember walking up the stairs to the meeting and this feeling of anxiety coming over me. I just wanted to turn around and go back to my unit. As I walked into the room and looked around, I found myself face to face with thirty-five other women I knew. This helped me relax a little, but the anxiety was still hanging on to me. As I was sitting in this room, I could feel the tension. Everyone was very tense. We just sat there looking around at one another waiting for someone to say something. Finally, it was decided that everyone would say why she was there. I was glad to be one of the ones that sat at the end of the table. I just knew that by the time they got to me, it would be time to leave, but I was wrong.

As people went around the table talking about why they were there, about the fourth or fifth person there came out and said she had AIDS. The room fell silent. I myself felt my heart and mind stop at that point. I just sat there looking at this woman, or looking for this AIDS she said she had. Before I knew it, another woman came out and said that she had AIDS too. Another one talked about taking the test and being afraid. I couldn't believe what I was hearing—all these women whom I'd known for five years now talking about having AIDS.

I was unable to move, I stopped thinking altogether. Now it was time for me to say why I was there. I was in such a state of shock that I told everyone about my sister and niece and didn't even realize I had said it. Once it was out, I felt this tremendous relief within myself. For some unknown reason, what I felt in this meeting after talking was a newfound bond between these other women and myself. When I left that morning, I left with a sense of relief and peace of mind, knowing that I would be a part of ACE from that day on.

* * *

The first meeting was powerful. People were tense. The room was filled with their own fears of AIDS, and I wanted to be a part of that. It didn't stop people from dying, but it changed the dying process.

* * *

From the beginning of ACE, PWAs have played a key role in giving our program meaning and direction. Their courage gave everyone motivation and strength. At the same time, the existence of a safe place, a group that was supportive, gave them the strength to play their roles. PWAs and the larger ACE group nourished each other.

* * *

When Blackie and I went to that first meeting, we didn't know what to expect. When the meeting was over, we felt a sense of relief, knowing that we weren't alone anymore, and that there were people who accepted and respected us. One of our main concerns was when the next meeting was going to take place.

* * *

Sonia was at the first meeting and spoke openly about being HIV-positive:

I would like to tell you the story of a woman named Sonia, who, when she found out she had AIDS, thought she would die. "No, no!" she screamed. Then she thought of her kids and granddaughter who she'd never see again. "No, I'm not going to die right now," she said. Sonia decided to fight for her life. A brave women. She's fought death three or four times since finding out. In each case, the doctors gave up and expected the worst. The family was notified, and a priest came in to administer the last rites. Sonia would tell the priest not to deliver the last rites: she wasn't going to die. After all these agonies, she decided to enroll in a small group called ACE, which had just formed. She wanted to learn more about AIDS and the treatments. She received training from doctors who came to visit from Montefiore Hospital. The doctors taught these women about AIDS. Sonia, during a period of remission, decided to do more for her companions who were sick and needed help. In her desire to learn and help, she continued to take courses and therapy until she felt comfortable enough to counsel. She did this counseling while she lived in IPC. She helped the women who were sick. She helped bathe them, she cooked for them, and was always there for them when they needed her. But she suffered and cried when some of the women died. They had become part of Sonia's life. At this time, she felt it was time to leave IPC, since while living there she was not allowed to attend school, the Hispanic festivals that took place at Bedford, or any ACE meetings. She fought for these rights and was finally allowed to go. She was transferred to the Honor Floor shortly after. But she still tended to the women in IPC. Sonia was allowed to attend a conference in Albany, a conference that dealt with women's issues. She also attended a few conferences given at Columbia University, and finally she attended a conference at the Westchester County Court House, where ACE was recognized as Program of the Year. ACE was given four plaques of recognition. Today she is still in ACE as a peer counselor for the newly arriving women. To Sonia, there is no race barrier when a woman needs help. If you need her, she is there. She understands your pain.

The Sonia I just spoke to you about is me. I'm very happy to be able to help my companions. God bless you! I love you.

* * *

The first stage of our work involved community building. During the first couple of meetings, we began a process of building trust, support, caring, love, and a commitment among ourselves to do this work. Although we knew that it was crucial for us to support one another, we also knew that we had to educate ourselves in order to be educators in our community. We looked for training from outsiders active in AIDS work, and the earlier contact with Montefiore Hospital was immensely helpful. A social worker, Monnie Callan, from the hospital, organized a team of several doctors, nurses, social workers, and an open PWA to come and educate us. They came for four afternoon sessions.

* * *

The sessions were electric. Nothing like this had ever happened before. For once, we were all treated as equals. Most of our experiences with doctors in and out of prison were not good, but here were doctors and nurses willing to listen and take the time to really explain things to us until we understood. The people from Montefiore were as excited as we were. We were a group of women, in prison. Some of us were PWAs, most of us weren't, but we were all affected in different ways by the epidemic. We were driven to learn and do something about AIDS in our community, and back then there simply weren't women organizing in this way around AIDS.

* * *

We developed the training sessions with them, meeting before and after to plan and evaluate. We said what we needed to learn, they prepared presentations, and we developed role-plays to put information into practice concerning sex, counseling someone about testing, and drugs. These sessions continued our process of building a safe place and a sense of trust. We all used this time to ask questions about health issues. This experience helped us to prepare for similar experiences as we reached out to our population.

* * *

This meeting with Montefiore took place in the Officer's Mess Hall. This was the first time that we were given their dining area for anything. Up to then, the only time you would see an inmate in that building would be when they were serving the officers. Usually, someone from high up in the prison administration attended, giving it their sanction and validation. While we were learning, we were laughing and appreciating one another's company. I remember doing some meditation. A lot of us, as well as civilians, lay on the floor and learned relaxation techniques. For many of us, this was the first time we had done anything like this. It was during this time that we had our theme song, "Sister." The woman who led us in meditation brought the song in, and someone said, after hearing it, "Let's make it our theme song." The song was so powerful that there were no objections. To this day it still makes people cry.

SISTER

Born of the earth, child of God, just one among the family.
And you can count on me to share the load.
And I will always help you hold your burdens.
And I will be the one to help you ease your pain.

Lean on me, I am your sister.
Believe in me, I am your friend.

I will fold you in my arms like a white winged dove.
Shine in your soul; your spirit is crying; spirit is crying;
Born of the earth, child of God, just one among the family.

And you can count on me to share the load.
And I will always help you hold your burdens.
And I will be the one to help you ease your pain.

Lean on me, I am your sister.
Believe in me, I am your friend.
(repeat chorus three more times)

—CHRIS WILLIAMSON[1]

THE PRISON REALITY

Underneath the growing strength and positive developments, the contradictions began to emerge. We inmates were now educated and mobilized to do something about AIDS, but AIDS raises many controversial issues of

---

1. By Chris Williamson, from the album *The Changer and the Changed*, Olivia Records, 1975.

sex, drugs, and medical care, even more intensely in prison than elsewhere. Also, there is an ongoing issue for prison administrators as to how
much cooperation and self-reliance among inmates is permissible and
under what conditions. From this time, in early June of 1988, these issues
emerged in a variety of crises. We began a summer of positive developments, as well as setbacks, culminating in a temporary shutdown of ACE.

Although we were not aware of it at the time, the first crisis occurred
during the training sessions with Montefiore over the issue of condoms and
dental dams. In one of the discussions about safe sex, one of the social
workers asked about the Department of Corrections' policy on condoms
and dental dams in the prison. We explained that they were not permitted.
She made the suggestion that we should write to the commissioner about
changing the policy. As a result of this suggestion, Montefiore was not
allowed to complete the training sessions at Bedford. We did not know at
the time why the Montefiore training was cut off—we had planned several
more of them.

* * *

A lot of times when people come in from the outside, they don't really
grasp our reality. The most natural idea outside of a prison, even one that
is part of the United States Constitution, such as writing your representatives about an issue, can be seen as a major threat by prison authorities.
We in ACE who heard this suggestion knew enough not to write to the
commissioner, even though there were some of us who agreed in principle
with the idea. We knew that as an inmate organization, we would be shut
down completely if we started actively campaigning to change DOCS
policy prohibiting condoms. At the time we were just beginning, there
were almost no other prisoner organizations about AIDS permitted in
New York State. We didn't want to get shut down before we got a chance
to do anything. But we never thought that such a suggestion would lead to
the superintendent's ending the training sessions.

* * *

Looking back, the superintendent says:

The safe-sex issue was an extremely high-profile one, a real point of
contention in the department. I felt very betrayed when she (the social
worker) made that suggestion at the end. It just wasn't necessary, because
we had talked about this issue prior to their coming in. I had no understanding why anyone would do that. If you cover safe sex, why say

everyone should write to the commissioner? If ACE had done that, we wouldn't have had ACE. You see, at that time, the department was really struggling with the issue of condoms in male facilities—it was a very hot issue nationwide. In male facilities, rape is very common, and it is a significant and difficult problem to deal with. And to say that all that heat was coming up to Albany because of something that was happening in ACE would have been very negative. Usually, the explanation for such a foolish move is not connecting to the big picture, the outside. It's just an example of people not knowing about prison realities at all. So that if ACE had written at that point, I would have been very fearful that it all would have gone down the tubes. DOCS would have just come down and said, "No more, no more of this."

We were never formally told that the Montefiore trainings were canceled, but when we asked representatives of the administration when the next date was, we could never get an answer. Yet our progress was not halted, because two civilians—M. Sharon Smolick, the Program Coordinator of the Family Violence Program at Bedford Hills, and Marcy May, Executive Director of the Effective Alternative in Reconciliation Services (EARS), a conflict-resolution training group for teenagers—held two sessions with us on peer counseling. By the end of our six training sessions, we were ready to try a formal outreach to population. We felt strong because of our knowledge, our unity, and our sense of commitment. We had a mission. We developed an outline for work, and some of us met with the superintendent and other high-ranking administrators.

* * *

I remember that day we used the blackboard in the superintendent's meeting room to unfold our plan of action. We opened with one woman from ACE: Blackie. At the time, she was losing her eyesight. She came to speak about what it meant to her that ACE now existed, a place to go, a place to feel safe. Then we went through our vision: to educate population, support, counseling, to have an office that would really be a drop-in center, medical advocacy, caring for people in IPC, a summer concert to raise consciousness, videos of PWAs speaking to others—our list went on and on. We were seven people representing thirty-five, knowing that we were going to make a difference.

* * *

We ended the meeting asking everyone there to hold hands and sing our theme song, "Sister." This was an unusual moment. Everyone sang, some tears fell, and our entire program was approved. Implementation remained to be worked out.

The presence of ACE could already be felt in population.

* * *

Some officers, inmates, and civilians assumed that all of us in ACE had AIDS. They didn't really understand what ACE was about, that people were there for different reasons. At first, this stigma stopped some people from coming to meetings, especially those who were HIV-positive, because they didn't want the focus on them. But people also felt our unity and saw that we were learning about AIDS. Soon everyone began to come up to me and ask me questions.

* * *

There were many individual acts of support and caring that began to take place. The fact that there were now a number of open PWAs began to start a ripple effect of change in others who came into contact with them.

What changed me from that person who felt very negative toward people with AIDS, who wanted to isolate them, was a person named Carmen. I had heard about Carmen. It had been pointed out to me that she had the HIV infection. I would watch her sit in the yard and she would sit by herself. She did not look sick. It didn't correlate with the videos I had seen. Then what did it was being in school with her. I remember going on a cigarette break from class and talking to her. She had disclosed on the first day of class that she was HIV-positive asymptomatic. I didn't know what it was that made me want to go deeper, to tell her how I used to feel. I could feel what was happening to her when she was off-balance. I could tell when her moods were not too nice, when she would be aggravated with something, and it made me know that I could be there. I didn't have to be a problem solver. I had to be a listener. If she hadn't been there, it would have taken me longer to be where I am today.

* * *

Another woman tells about how knowing another Carmen changed her.

* * *

I was one of those people that, once I knew someone had AIDS, I didn't want them around me. That was until Carmen got sick. She was my friend. My first reaction when I found out she was sick was I felt hurt because she didn't have the confidence to tell me. Maybe it was because she knew what my attitude was, and she knew how I felt about her. First, it was a rumor, and I asked her and she said no. Then she was on my unit and I started seeing signs. I questioned her and asked her if she wanted me to go to the hospital, and she didn't want me to go with her. Then she got sicker and went into IPC. And then she sent for me. I went. She told me the rumors were true, but she knew my attitude and didn't want me to turn my back on her. That's when I started researching how you can and can't get the virus and my fear left. ACE also helped me with things I didn't know. Even though Carmen had AIDS and I didn't, I felt that I was living with AIDS through her. I told her that I loved her whether she had AIDS or not.

* * *

The presence of a group that supported people who were HIV-positive began to have an effect on the fears and the stigma that existed.

* * *

When Blackie first moved onto the floor, she could leave her cigarettes on a table and no one would touch them. And you know in here, people take things that are left around, especially cigarettes—you can't ever forget a pack of cigarettes on a table because it won't be there when you go back for it. Then one day Blackie came into the ACE meeting so happy and told us, "They stole my cigarettes, they stole my cigarettes." She was so happy that now she was being treated like anyone else.

* * *

ACE created the possibility for women to help one another, and it brought out this part of our humanity—the part that wants to serve. There were women who supported ACE yet felt they could not become part of it.

* * *

What will my friends think of me if I don't accept the offer of working with the ACE program? Blanche, I thought to myself, just the thought of being allowed to help the women should override the thoughts you have of one day possibly losing them. Why can't you keep that in mind, instead of images of real sickly women on their death beds? Oh, no,

I can't take it. I'll become too involved and do the rest of my years in a total state of depression. I know me, I would make myself sick with depression. I would give all of myself to these ill women, and have no thoughts for me ever again. Blanche, don't do it, your friends, your true friends, will understand, and those that don't, they really don't know you, so why care what they may think about you? You have to do what's best for Blanche.

* * *

The first major role that ACE played in the prison happened when we had a memorial for a woman named Ro. In less than three months, the entire atmosphere around AIDS in the prison had changed enough to have an outpouring of support for a woman who died.

The memorial would not be held in the small white prison church, which was too old to continue being used. A recreation room on the ground floor of one of the housing units was transformed into the place of worship. Filled with wooden pews and an altar with saints, it has served its purpose. In this single place of worship, Protestant, Catholic, and Jewish services are held.

* * *

I wanted to do a real memorial for Ro. Lannette and I had talked about how Ro didn't really have any family out there, no one to grieve her death. She had more friends in here that were going to grieve and miss her than out there.

When Ro died, Lannette was locked in her cell for thirty days (for disobeying a rule). I knew how much Ro's death hurt her. I had watched Lannette, giving Ro ice baths to bring down her sweats, feeding her, dealing with her tantrums and having things thrown at her as Ro was getting sicker.

We wanted to say goodbye with love. That's when we came up with the idea that we should do our own memorial.

We wanted to get flowers to send to the outside funeral service and to have here. We divided ourselves up and made announcements on all the floors that we wanted to do a real memorial if people wanted to contribute. A lot of people gave money through filling out inmate disbursements. People gave like a dollar to three dollars. By the end we had more than $350.

The memorial was beautiful. They let Lannette out of lock for that one day. The Hispanic ladies sang, the black women sang gospel, the chapel was packed. People got up and spoke about her. All the ACE members were there. In the beginning, we sang "That's What Friends Are For," and in the end, we sang "Sister" holding hands. When we left, we all took a flower. It was a good feeling, being there for somebody.

* * *

The change was felt not only among inmates but also among civilians and officers who worked here. Many officers began to offer support through making an extra call to the hospital for a woman who didn't feel well, or giving us a chance to spend some time supporting a woman, even if we were talking in an area where we weren't supposed to be.

* * *

One person I will always remember is Dr. Keats, a psychologist who worked with the Office of Mental Health. She started having a Significant Others Group for those of us who chose to go. We would gather in her office cramped up because of lack of space, and we would talk and share in a more private setting. I remember the day before Blackie was to go home. Dr. Keats gave her a surprise going-home party. This was the first time that anyone had ever done anything like this for Blackie.

* * *

During this period, when ACE was having its training and was beginning to have an effect on the prison, larger political forces were at play, some of which we were not aware of. AIDS was becoming a major problem within all New York State prisons. There was growing publicity about prison conditions and AIDS. Although women were largely still ignored within the AIDS epidemic, a blind study of women entering the New York State prison system in 1988 showed that almost one out of every five women would test positive for the HIV virus, even higher than for men entering the state prison system.

The superintendent of Bedford Hills was part of a network of women who were committed to issues affecting women, including those in prison. Some women who had become concerned worked at state agencies—Linda Loffredo, a program assistant at the New York State Division for Women of the Governor's Women's Commission; Eileen Hogan, Chaplain at the Women's House of Detention on Riker's Island; and Gloria Cuccurullo, Deputy Director of the HIV Healthcare Division at the New York State Department of Health AIDS Institute. There were conversations among them that focused on women in prison and AIDS. The AIDS Institute set aside money for a women-and-AIDS project. This was a chance for the ACE program to be recognized and supported from outside the prison.

THE DEVELOPMENT OF ACE —
AS REMEMBERED BY LINDA LOFFREDO

Bedford Hills Correctional Facility has a history of developing and implementing "cutting edge" programs. Bedford has a children's center, a nursery, and a family violence program; all were the first of their kind in the country, and all are unique.

Sister Elaine Roulet, a legend in her own time, has been a staff member at Bedford for almost twenty years and is the director of the prison's children's center. She set a tone at the facility by implementing new, commonsense programs that were inmate-centered. I still remember walking into the Children's Center, with its huge rainbow hung over the door, emblazoned with the words: "Joy is unbreakable, so it is perfectly safe in the hands of children." The center was alive with children and inmates, and I was invited to participate in the weekly talent show. I could have been in a children's center anywhere in the world.

Elaine Roulet's daring and joy were supported by superintendent Elaine Lord. From the beginning of her tenure at Bedford Hills Correctional Facility in 1982, where she was initially deputy of programs and then superintendent, Elaine Lord was committed to programs that provided the women with avenues for growth and self-esteem. Elaine was smart, caring, and willing to move into uncharted territory.

At the inmate liaison committee meeting in 1985, Ronnie Eldridge, who was then the Director of the New York State Division for Women, suggested to Elaine and the committee members that we hold a public hearing at Bedford to examine the relationship between domestic violence and incarceration. Elaine agreed with the idea and received the support of New York State Department of Corrections Commissioner Thomas Coughlin. The hearing, the first of its kind in the country, was held inside the prison. Attended by New York State commissioners, leaders in the domestic violence field, and representatives from the governor's office (and the Legislature), the hearing revolutionized the ways in which we thought about domestic violence and linked advocates from the battered women's movement to women in prison. Equally important, funding was made available for a family-violence prevention program in the prison. Sharon Smolick, who was selected to direct the program, provided extraordinary leadership in developing a program that reflected the needs of the inmates and helped create a sense of community at Bedford. I believe that the hearing paved the way for ACE.

During this period, the world was struggling with the fear and stigma of AIDS. For several years AIDS had been considered a gay, white male disease, and the notion that women might be affected by this disease had been considered by very few people. In 1986, Lynne McArthur (then at the New York State Division of Substance Abuse Services) and I (then at the New York State Division for Women) formalized the hundreds of hours of discussions we had had with women concerned about the impact of AIDS on women and created the Women and AIDS Project. The Project developed monthly forums and a newsletter that brought women's perspectives to programs, policies, and funding.

During our work with the Project, we met and talked with women who were very concerned about women in prison who were HIV-positive. ACE, by this time, had begun to emerge within the prison. During one of my visits to Bedford, I mentioned to Elaine Lord that Monnie Callan, one of the first people to draw attention to the issue of women and HIV, was working at Montefiore Medical Center and was interested in creating a team of experts who could provide training to the women in ACE on HIV-related issues. This volunteer training effort became a reality and lent formality and legitimacy to the development of ACE as a recognized entity.

Later, I remember receiving a telephone call from Gloria Cuccurullo, a deputy director at the New York State AIDS Institute, who told me that ACE would receive a grant. I don't know exactly how discussions about Bedford and ACE resulted in a grant, but when Gloria called, I was thrilled. ACE now had, I thought, the financial means to develop AIDS-prevention education materials, increase its support for HIV-positive women in the prison, and develop links with outside community groups and resources. I had no idea that the grant and the way in which it was awarded would create problems that became almost insurmountable. There were times when Elaine felt that the necessary layers of approval and politics were not worth the grant. She reminded me often during those early days that her first responsibility was to run a maximum-security prison, and that anyone who worked on the grant needed to understand and respect that basic premise.

As I struggled with Elaine's frustration, I told her that the issue of women and AIDS outside the prison was also rife with doubts, misunderstandings, competition over turf and funding, and giant egos. One had to understand that ACE was the extraordinary product of strong, caring, competent women. Staff at the AIDS Institute were able to develop a framework for granting funds that would have respected the ways in which ACE developed.

During this time, ACE was moving in a variety of ways, and Elaine began to feel uncomfortable with both its direction and the requirements of the grant. I highly respected her opinion and knew that when these issues began to be resolved, Elaine would allow ACE to continue and the grant to proceed. In addition, I had the highest respect for Gloria Cuccurullo, who became a strong and, I think, often lone advocate at the AIDS Institute for the funding of women's programming. Without Gloria's advocacy, I doubt that ACE would have been funded. I knew that if Gloria and Elaine could talk through their concerns and frustrations, the issues related to the grant could be resolved. In time, they were able to do this, and ACE moved forward.

I believe that ACE exists and has flourished because of the many remarkable women who were unafraid of new ideas and, even within the prison walls, viewed all things as being possible. The women in the prison and the superintendent believed that inmates working together could create a community at Bedford that dispelled the fear and stigma of AIDS and provided an atmosphere of respect and healing. I think they have succeeded.

A week following the meeting during which our program was approved, the superintendent called us to her office again and she made an announcement: the AIDS Institute had just given ACE a quarter of a million dollars to develop a model AIDS program for prisons. The money would go to an outside community-based agency, which would hire civilian staff to work with ACE and help develop a program. The superintendent told us that it could be as long as a year and a half before the program was put into effect but it would eventually happen.

Only two months before, we had started with a small group, trying to determine whether population wanted to do anything about AIDS. Now here we were, united, with both a vision and a quarter of a million dollars. It all seemed unreal.

It *was* real, but there was a competing reality: the prison administration was not ready for this level of mobilization of educated and unified inmates, especially around AIDS. The termination of the Montefiore training was not a direct criticism of ACE; the next ordeal, however, which came three weeks after the announcement of the AIDS Institute grant, did focus on us. By the end of June, the first open crisis with the administration occurred: it concerned the issue of drugs.

* * *

I remember the day we were having our regular Monday morning ACE meeting. Everyone arrived bubbling with energy, ready to implement our plan and divide responsibility. When the superintendent arrived, she said that a woman who was HIV-positive from the infirmary (IPC) had taken an overdose of pills, and that ACE members were under suspicion because we had access to IPC. After the overdose occurred, many women in population had to undergo urine analysis, including many ACE members. The superintendent said that we had to get ourselves together and deal with it. There was a sense of disbelief that passed through the room. People tried to explore the matter with her, but she was angry.

* * *

There was one other accusation as well. The superintendent asked whether members of ACE were using the name of ACE to gain access to places in the prison where we were not supposed to be. Since Bedford Hills is a maximum-security facility, movement is restricted. If you live in one housing unit and a good friend of yours lives in another, you cannot visit each other; you can only meet in the yard, on your way to work, or in school. People are always looking for ways to meet, to get around these restrictions.

When the superintendent left, we were stunned. Her entire tone and approach toward us had changed in a matter of weeks. We kept a sense of optimism but decided to focus on the problems she had raised.

The next meeting was intense, as we talked about drugs, ACE, and AIDS. Most of us agreed that ACE as an organization should not preach against drugs, because then we would turn off many of the women who would most need support and education. In years to come, we faced the issue of drugs in our education and counseling work. Some women would choose to argue strongly against drugs, while others were more concerned with educating women about the importance of using clean needles.

We reached a consensus: if women wanted to remain members of ACE, those who had inappropriate behavior should consider changing for the benefit of the group. Inappropriate behavior among our members endangered our relationship with the administration and our own ability to function as a group. People had different reactions.

SOMEONE WHO LEFT

I have something to say. Please hear me out before anyone says anything! This has been the first time that I really enjoy what I am doing. For once I really feel good about myself, because this is something that affects all of us in one way or another. Anyway, I just want to say that I'm leaving. For one thing, I'm not ready to stop what I'm doing, I don't want to jeopardize ACE and the work that everyone is doing. This work is very important, and it is needed because women are dying. You guys can make a difference. I hope that everyone can understand why I'm leaving, and that it's not held against me, but I feel it's the best thing, for me. Well, it's not the best thing, but it's what I want to do. So with that I say, good luck my sisters, and I'll pray that everything goes your way. Bye. . . .

SOMEONE WHO STAYED

Well, I just want to say that I am staying and I do respect those of you who chose to leave at this point for whatever reason you may have. I am willing to change my behavior in any way that I possibly can to stay, because this work is important to me, not only because I need it for myself, but because I feel that it will be important to the women in this facility. Granted, I don't like the idea myself of being under suspicion about IPC, especially when I know that I had nothing to do with what happened. I look at it this way—I'm not about to give up, because it seems to me that this is going to be an ongoing issue between the administration and us. So if we are to do this work, we are going to be faced with many things that might cause us to be under some kind of suspicion.

In addition to the crisis between ourselves and the administration, we in ACE were involved in our first crisis around the issue of confidentiality. It came up in a number of ways.

As a PWA, when I first found out my status, I told someone outside of ACE who I thought I could trust. Unfortunately, I was wrong—she broke my confidentiality. This put me in a very compromised position, because now everyone in population knew of my status before I even had a chance to accept the fact that I was HIV-positive. At this point, my only choice was to become open. As time went on, and with the help of my ACE sisters, I learned not to be ashamed of my HIV status. I found comfort in being open. A person needs their confidentiality to be respected. No one should ever be forced, as I was, to become open before she is ready, because if the person is not mentally ready to deal with a positive test result, there is no telling what may happen—healthwise or mentally.

* * *

One woman who was really important as an open PWA, willing to talk about her health and having AIDS, kept bringing up the names of other women with AIDS in the meeting. She said, "Well, I feel this way. I'm a PWA and I feel that all PWAs should say that they have AIDS if they have it. That's why I said that J.R. had AIDS. Besides, I heard her tell some people the other day." Some other women active in ACE who were HIV-positive threatened to quit if we didn't try to stop this breach of confidentiality.

* * *

The drug issue and the confidentiality issue raised for us the more general problem of inmates telling other inmates what to do. One inmate said:

This place is run by strict rules and regulations. I resent other inmates doing the job of the police, telling me that I can't do something that I want to do, whether it's use drugs or visit a friend, breaking a rule to do that. She wears green, just like I do.

The voice of this one inmate reflects how many inmates feel, including those in ACE. We respected this, but at the same time, our new program was very important to us, and so were the women in population who needed it. So we decided to develop a contract women would have to be willing to abide by as ACE members, not because we were trying to play police but because we had to protect the program and to maintain trust with the prison administration and within ACE itself.

PRINCIPLES OF ACE CONTRACT:

1. Support:
The more support I can give others, the less fear people will have for those in need. People will be able to find help, advice, and friendship and they will be able to develop a supportive way of living with HIV/AIDS. As ACE members, our vision is a community of full support for our peers.

2. Confidentiality:
As an ACE member, I will not reveal any information about another person's situation relating to HIV/AIDS. People will not seek my help or advice unless they are certain that they will be protected. Confidentiality will also protect both the individual and the community as a whole. As an ACE member I shall not discuss matters of ACE business except with

other ACE members, unless it is information of general importance to others, such as HIV/AIDS or ongoing ACE activities.

3. Empowerment/Giving Each Woman Her Own Voice

It is always important to let each individual "as a person" speak about her own situation. This will give each person control over her own situation. If an individual talks about her health issues or HIV status in one meeting, making the information no longer confidential, it is still her right to decide if she wants to talk about herself at another time. Always remember that only she knows how she feels at any given moment, and recognize that the process of empowerment is at an individual's pace.

4. Respect and Protect ACE

As an ACE member I will respect and protect the ACE organization; its name, its space, its access, and its materials. I shall not use ACE's name for my own personal reasons, nor will I use ACE in any illegal manner. I will notify and communicate my whereabouts regarding any ACE activities. Approval should be via memo, with permission from the ACE coordinator.

5. Come to ACE Activities Able to Work

I, as an ACE member, shall come to meetings and counseling, education, and other work sessions totally able to focus on the issues at hand. (This related to the issue of drugs.)

I fully understand and agree to adhere to the above. My failure to do so will result in either counseling and/or removal; to be determined by the ACE Core Group or ACE members, depending on the situation.

This contract came out of the beginning period of ACE, when there was a particularly intense level of commitment. These principles helped us through a crisis and gave us structure and certain ideals. Looking back over the past four years, we can see that a contract cannot in itself define someone's behavior. Those of us in ACE are not angels, and each of us has violated one rule or another at some point, but the rules helped us through some difficult times.

We expected, or at least hoped, that when we sent the contract to the superintendent, we would have her approval and we would begin to do outreach to population. Yet, it was from that time that we were slowly brought to a halt. The administration never said that ACE was being shut down, but instead it put out one new restriction after another until we were unable to function. ACE could no longer meet at the time we had been meeting, and the meeting room was no longer available. We began to meet in small groups in the yard, but never as an entire group. We were told to prepare educational presentations, which we worked on in the yard or rec rooms, but they were not approved for use. ACE could no longer carry on its correspondence with outside AIDS agencies or organizations without going through a long bureaucratic procedure; the superintendent said that we could not refer to ourselves as counselors. When we pointed out that the very name ACE, which she had approved, contained the word "counselor," she still insisted that we could not use the word.

In addition to all these obstacles, the medical department was experiencing its own crisis, of which we were also a part. After the training sessions, there were now enough inmates with confidence to help other inmates who were struggling to understand what was happening to their bodies. Medical advocacy began to take place spontaneously—most often productively but occasionally in a disruptive manner. Often one inmate would be able to help interpret for another what a doctor had said, or give support, or help a friend develop questions before a doctor's appointment. Occasionally, a woman would inappropriately intervene, getting angry at a nurse in a manner that was not useful. But Bedford Hills was not in a position to absorb the added pressure on the medical department from educated and mobilized inmates. Because of the settlement provisions of a 1977 class-action lawsuit—*Todaro v. Ward*—over medical conditions at Bedford Hills, the medical department and care at Bedford are monitored for the court by an outside expert. After a period of assessment ending in January 1987, that expert had issued a report pointing out inadequacies of certain aspects of the medical department, including the inadequacy of meeting women's AIDS-related medical needs. The prison was facing a court hearing. Because of the 1977 lawsuit and its settlement provisions, the crisis of AIDS in Bedford was much more quickly brought into the courts than at other prisons.[2]

During that summer, the administration was involved in negotiations with Prisoners Rights Project of the Legal Aid Society over medical conditions, and the pressure of ACE was not a welcome addition. Although the superintendent continued to allow ACE members to go to the infirmary and care for the women, the court struggle over medical condi-

---

2. *Todaro v. Wara,* 31 F. Supp. 1129 (S.D.N.Y. 1977), aff'd, 565 F.2d 48 (2d Cir. 1977), aff'd without opinion, *Todaro v. Coughlin,* 652 F.2d 54 (2d Cir. 1981); Frank L. Rundle, M.D., "Evaluation of Medical Services at the New York State Correctional Facility, Bedford Hills, New York (1987).

tions was one more pressure that led the superintendent to close down the ACE organization that summer. We didn't give up hope that the superintendent would some day allow us to function as a group.

* * *

We kept talking with one another, sharing what we had learned from our training sessions. We knew we were needed. A lot of people were coming out from all over for counseling and help. I remember going with Carmen to a meeting being held in IPC with buddies from Mid-Hudson AIDS Task Force. They came in every Monday night to talk with women who were HIV-positive. I felt that we could cry together, that we could do everything. We just kept going in spite of the problems.

* * *

I remember in the middle of that summer the administration invited some outside speakers to talk to the women about AIDS in the gym. We were frustrated that we couldn't use our education to speak to our sisters and instead once again there would be outside people in the gym. We attended, partly to see just how much we really knew compared with outside experts. The outside guests introduced themselves and they started their presentation—the same things we had learned: casual contact, who was in the high-risk groups . . . And when the women started asking them questions, the outside speakers had trouble answering some of them, especially the ones about woman-to-woman sex. So we raised our hands and began to answer, and each time we spoke we introduced ourselves, "My name is Toni and I'm from ACE," "My name is Katrina and I'm from ACE," "My name is Carmen and I'm from ACE." We communicated well, we used our own language—a down-to-earth way of talking—and we gave more details and were comfortable answering the questions about sex. Soon the women began directing questions to us as well, and it was a wonderful feeling. Finally we were able to share information with population. After it was over, the officers and inmates alike crowded around us to ask questions. When it was time to leave, we politely went over to the outside speakers and introduced ourselves and thanked them for coming. It turned out to be a good thing, because inmates realized they could really rely on ACE for information and it gave us a chance to see that we really were capable—we had the facts and we could break things down for people. And as we walked up the hill, we slapped one another's hands and said, "ACE is in the House!" It felt so good, because now we knew we were prepared. Whenever the superintendent would let us teach, we were ready.

* * *

In spite of our determination, our ability to feel the strength of community was slowly disappearing, because we were not permitted to meet as an organization. As the summer wore on, it became a summer of death.

Several weeks into the summer, a second woman died. Then several more women died in August. Each memorial was smaller—the second one only had about fifteen women attending. People had been willing to face the deaths of their friends when they felt the strength of a larger community, which had been catalyzed by ACE. By the end of the summer that larger community had disappeared again.

* * *

For me, I guess it started with Lye. I was visiting her in the hospital. I was able to get her to drink broth, juice on ice. At that time she couldn't eat anything solid, and sometimes she wouldn't eat anything unless I came. I couldn't stay away. I could see she was getting in a really bad condition. I kept telling the nurse that she was really sick. Lye cried, "Toni, I don't want to go to the outside hospital, I don't think I'll come back." In the previous weeks, other people had died, and she was really scared. I got her mother to come and see her. They weren't really on good terms, and I don't think her mother knew that her daughter was really sick. And just like she said, when she went out, she did not come back. I couldn't take it. I don't know how many people died. It seems to me that in about five weeks, five people died, mainly of AIDS but not only. It got so that dreaming and waking, I was thinking death all the time, of the ice baths, the final stages. It wasn't something I could leave behind, like an office job. I had to get away from it.

Out of a desperate situation created by AIDS, we had gained hope among ourselves. When we realized we were not going to be allowed to do anything, we felt worse than before we started ACE. Our expectations and hopes had risen, yet there was nowhere to go with them.

* * *

I remember what it did to ourselves, our unity. Some people said it was too much hassle to keep trying to meet—it was hard enough being in prison, but to go up against the superintendent for something, they couldn't take it. Someone else said, "Let's protest." People began arguing with one another. Others said, "Let's just keep trying to meet her requests." I wanted to keep meeting, but I started getting intense nosebleeds every time we would come out of a meeting with the superintendent.

* * *

Adding to the confusion was the fact that the superintendent herself often spoke about the importance of empowering us, as women, even in prison. We had felt, in fact, a sense of empowerment, but now it seemed to have disappeared. There was a gap between the language and the reality. Over the next years, we would ponder the concept of empowerment of prisoners. One woman wrote, several years later, after another crisis with the administration:

I remember one conversation with one of the coordinators. She kept talking about empowerment this and empowerment that. Till finally I said to her once, "Stop using that word to me, it's losing all meaning. Empowerment is not something that people in authority can give to those they control. Empowerment is something people struggle to attain for themselves as a group. There's no such thing as empowerment on a leash. Any one of us can make choices and take responsibility and grow through that. But that's not empowerment." Later I kicked myself for my honesty. . . . My mouth always gets me in trouble.

* * *

The superintendent's final request, which we met, was that before we could do any educational outreach to population, we had to put down on paper everything we would be teaching. Then it would have to be approved by the New York State Department of Corrections. Three women worked to produce what would later be used as part of this book, although significantly revised. It consisted of eight educational workshops, an educational seminar, and an orientation for new inmates. We handed it to the superintendent at the final ACE meeting that summer.

It would be more than three months before the superintendent would finally reconvene ACE and allow us to work again. During that time, three ACE members did have permission to speak with the newly arrived inmates about AIDS, but without a functioning organization or program, there was no way to connect with those inmates after the short orientation. Four years later, in writing this book, we asked the superintendent to reflect on why she had closed ACE down. There were a number of factors that she spoke about, but there was one overall issue: We were building a community organization inside a prison to cope with the crisis of AIDS, and that, in itself, posed a contradiction with what was considered normal in prison: "I like dealing with the women and seeing them as a community, but how can you talk about community organizing in a prison when prison is a community paranoid by definition?"

She also spoke about the health crisis of that summer:

> The deaths happened. I was dealing with medical-care issues, and institutions are not on the cutting edge, they aren't the first to try new things. I was frustrated and discouraged. There is the human part of me and also the superintendent part of me. As a human being, I sometimes lose my personal perspective. I reacted from a power-and-control point of view. Control and rehabilitation do not go hand in hand. In fact, I don't think prisons are in the business of rehabilitating people's self-esteem.

Part of what led the superintendent to call ACE back was that the lawyers representing the prisoners in the class-action law suit and the lawyers representing the administration had been able to agree on changes in the medical department. A new medical director was hired, and so was a specialist in AIDS, to begin a once-a-week HIV clinic. This would make a big difference in beginning to deal with the AIDS crisis and with a group of educated inmates advocating around AIDS.

The superintendent also looked at the counseling issue:

> I am in a position of trying to negotiate between two worlds, and I have to ask, Where does an issue sit in the philosophy or policies of that moment? My views sometimes reflect the department. I don't want them to think that we're in left field. I think that peer counseling is much easier now because the department has shifted its position a great deal and talks about peer counseling in male facilities. You don't see me raise the issue as much, because it's easier system-wide—the focus has changed. And I guess the other concern is trying to make sure that all of us have to be cognizant of the time, education, and degrees necessary to make you counselors. We have to define how much responsibility we have in

the counseling situation and we have to learn how to know what your limits are.

The superintendent spoke about being the superintendent of a woman's prison in a prison context that is largely male:

When you talk about women's issues, there are 3400 women in our [New York State] system, and something like 58,000 men. Women are only 3 percent of the population. So when we're talking about condoms and women's needs, they're talking about rape and suicide in a man's prison. But if you look back over the four years, there has been some significant change in policy. Now at least we can hand out condoms for furloughs, family-reunion programs, and parole. You just have to fight harder when you're only 3 percent of the population. As somebody once told me: Don't worry about rocking the boat, you're not even in it.

Finally, the superintendent spoke about the problems that emerge in creating something new such as ACE:

We talk about what the limits are on a superintendent, and if you know the boundaries, that helps. If it's not clear, you're liable to step over the boundaries and the superintendent is likely to react. Sometimes the anger comes from looking for the boundaries, and if we're doing something new, we may not be real clear on what they are on either side. Back when ACE started, peer counseling was in that kind of area. Could you do pre- and post-test counseling? What kind of issues were appropriate for you to talk about?
     The department has really come full circle, because at that time it was "You can't talk about this and that," but you, ACE, would talk about it in conversations, so you were really testing the boundaries and trying to define the limits.

By the fall of 1988, although the ACE organization was no longer functioning, informally we said among ourselves, "We just have to be patient. The crisis of AIDS is growing, we are educated and able to make a difference, and there is a grant of $250,000. And the superintendent is very committed to doing something about the AIDS crisis. She permitted us to get started." We were hopeful and we waited.

4
ACE Reaches Out

Finally, in November 1988, the superintendent called a meeting and agreed to let us work again. She announced that they had hired a new medical director, Dr. Nereida Ferran, and she was hopeful that it would lead to improvements in medical care. We raised the fact that there was a rise in stigma due to the absence of ACE's presence in population. Several fights had broken out in the back buildings—the large dorms where newly arrived women lived—sparked by fears and stigma over AIDS.

BACK BUILDINGS AND TURNER[1]

These are the waiting places, stops-offs during our entry into Bedford. The reception process that occurs when we first arrive here is really our first glimpse of prison.

When I arrived at Bedford Hills, I came from an upstate jail in a police car. It was January, but I only had the clothes from when I came in—no coat, hat, or boots. Just a pair of gloves that an officer in jail had given me.

The building that is for reception is old-looking and sits on top of a small hill. I was taken inside, uncuffed, and unshackled. The room was small and cold from the door always being opened. It had metal chairs set up in rows. I was the only one there, and I was scared to death of what was

---

1. The Turner Building is no longer being used. It is scheduled to be replaced with a new building for other purposes.

ahead, hoping that what I was seeing wasn't what prison was "really" going to be like.

A few minutes after I arrived, a bus pulled in from Riker's Island. About twenty to thirty women were brought in to begin the reception process. They all seemed to know one another and talked loudly. I felt out of place and alone. I couldn't stand it, I desperately wanted to go unnoticed. Finally, the woman to my right asked me my name. I told her, and for one second I thought I'd found a friend. Then there was her next question: "What are you here for?" I'm here for murder, and it's not easy to say to anyone, not even myself. But I knew I couldn't run or hide from it, not in prison—it's not like that here. So I told her, determined to survive this. I never expected her reaction. She was excited and curious. Immediately, she announced it to everyone she could. That was my first hour in prison, waiting and fearing. Finally, the process began. First the lectures about punishment for misbehavior, then the showers. I've never lost the feeling of that shower, the degrading feeling that all the water in the world won't take away. Reception truly was an insight into being an inmate. The shower room was tiny and a few women were called in at once. There were no shower curtains, and the water was frigid. The guard watching us gave us a liquid shampoo that kills lice, bugs. We weren't there to wash, we were being "debugged." After the guard said I could stop scrubbing, I rinsed and got out naked. Our clothes were replaced with summer nightgowns or pajamas, scuffy slippers, and a robe.

I spent the next half hour trying to untangle my hair with my fingers while we were called one by one for paperwork and to see mental-health representatives. My paperwork was simple to get done; the guard was efficient, never once looking up at me. No one answered your questions. I just sat and waited, and prayed about the terrible reality that nothing in my entire life was useful in coping with that moment. It's terrible when you're in your twenties, in prison, and suddenly longing for your mother, but I was.

The last steps in reception are being fingerprinted and photographed and getting your inmate ID card and your state clothes. The clothes I received left a little to be desired. The waist of my pants was a 36 and my waist was a 21, so the fit was a little off. You don't even feel familiar to yourself by that point, you feel foreign and desperately isolated. It's not so much an entry into anything as it is a stripping down of all that you have inside you when you come in.

After being up since 3:30 to leave the county jail, I was officially a "processed person" by about 10:00 that night. I almost wanted to get to a

cell just to rest, but I'd obviously watched too many movies, because it's
not like that. We were marched two by two to the Turner building in the
green pants that the state issued, which was to be our wardrobe for our
time in prison. I lived on the second floor, which had a shower room and
two sections of beds. There were no private cells. The beds on the left
were separated by metal partitions. The ones on the right were all in the
open. I was on the right.

The recreation room is actually a TV in the basement, several chairs,
and a few small tables. That's also where the two phones are for us to use
to make collect calls. It's a lousy location, because it's the noisiest place in
Turner. The first day we were allowed to use the phones, *everyone* wanted
to use them to inform their families that they'd been taken to prison.
County jails don't let your family know when they ship you out. I had five
minutes on the phone the second night I was there. It was an awful five
minutes. "Hi, I can't talk for long, I just want to let you know that I've
been taken to prison, that I'm doing 'fine,' and that I love you." By the time
you give them your address and number, the next word is "Goodbye."
Letter writing becomes important when you're in prison. While in Turner,
we had no writing paper, but we were desperate to write our families. The
whole time I was there, I tore up envelopes to write my family on. When
envelopes were scarce, I took outdated memos off the corkboard and
wrote on the back of them or any paper that I could find. I always told my
family that it wasn't that bad here, that I had all I needed, and that I was
doing great. I didn't want them to worry or to hurt, but I always wondered
if it occurred to them that prison was a little less than cheery as they read
these letters written on shredded envelopes. Another thing that is difficult
is that inmates who had just arrived didn't have their own personal items.
Nothing was given to us in reception except toothpaste, state soap, a
toothbrush, and a small black comb.

Women have stayed in Turner for various lengths of time. I was there
for half a month. During that time inmates get cleared by the medical
department. Every day we went to the hospital to see different doctors, to
give blood, and to have our teeth checked. The entire first week I spent
from morning to night at the hospital. No one is allowed to get a visit from
her family during that first working week. We also are kept somewhat
isolated from the rest of population. We only went to meals when the rest
of population was locked in for a count. Even then, Turner eats in a small
eating area near the mess hall that's only for reception inmates. When we
walked to the hospital I saw it as a chance to talk to the other inmates we
had to pass, but our officers forbade us to speak to them. My entire stay in

Turner, all I wanted to do was talk to someone. I needed to know if Turner was all there was to being in prison, I wanted to ask what to expect, where to go for different services, and how other women survived living in a prison. The fact that so many of us had needs and fears was compounded by the fact that we were kept away from all the other inmates. The only other women I met at that time were the two women from ACE who did an HIV/AIDS orientation when we arrived. Fear and stigma about AIDS were high among new inmates. They shared dormitory space and bathrooms and had anxiety about so many uncertainties that their fear often focused on AIDS. It was a relief to know that somewhere in the prison were other inmates who were saying, "Reach out, we're here."

The day I left Turner, I waited to hear my name and the back building I would go to. I was nervous, but so excited. Wherever I was going, I just knew it had to be better than where I was.

ACE IN THE BACK BUILDINGS

The four back buildings are dormitory-style buildings, each holding either fifty women, or a hundred women with double-bunked beds. There are no cells. The bed areas are separated by thin metal dividers that are approximately five feet high. Instead of a door, curtains create some amount of privacy. Each of these divided areas is called a cube, or cubicle.

The superintendent asked that we hold our seminars in the back buildings.

The seminar is really a "happening" in which there is a combination of personal testimony about what HIV/AIDS has meant in our lives, information and question-answering on transmission and testing, role-plays, and singing the theme song, "Sister." The primary goal of a seminar is creating a community of support and openness around HIV/AIDS-related issues. It is this kind of community context that is the foundation for education to really take hold and for PWAs to get the necessary support. Seminars also have the goal of communicating information about AIDS, and to make the direct connection between ACE and women who may have personal needs.

About twelve women volunteered to work on producing these seminars. We looked at the educational outline that we had written over the summer, and together we tried to transform it into a dramatic, interactional happening that would not only provide information but inspire women to open up their minds and hearts. Only a few of us had ever done any public speaking, and everyone was nervous about teaching what we had learned—about transmission, casual contact, testing, and what is AIDS. But we were fueled by our sense of mission and knew that this was our chance to prove ourselves and our belief in the power of peer education. Each of us took a section to present, and we practiced our presentations in front of each other. But we really came to life when we started to act out role-plays. Once again, the information came to life in real-life situations. Our laughter and camaraderie helped us overcome our inhibitions.

Finally, we felt ready to go to the back buildings. We had posted announcements. The superintendent had made attendance at the seminars mandatory, so everyone who lived in the back buildings was there. Two teams worked simultaneously in adjoining dorms, sending psychic energy to each other. We needed all we could generate.

* * *

The first time we went to that back building, I was so nervous I had diarrhea. I was yelling at the others and everything. It was the first time in my life that I was going to talk to people publicly, and I was terrified.

* * *

We from ACE gathered with our large easel pad, Magic Markers, and two-by-five cards with the information on the presentation we were making. We moved in twos and threes through the connecting tunnels to the building. When we arrived, some of the women were sitting in the rec room. But many others were in their cubicles/cells. They asked what we were here for. We looked like a traveling troupe—and we felt like it, not knowing what to expect. Some women were excited that we were going to talk about HIV/AIDS. Others said, "Forget it," or "Fuck you, I've heard enough about it. It's depressing."

* * *

People slowly gathered, noisily dragging chairs into the rec room, and we began. As we introduced ourselves, one by one, and said why we joined ACE, the noise and card playing died down.

My name is Maria. Before I came to prison, I was a certified nurse's aide. I was being paid by licensed nurses to give injections and give care to AIDS patients. I started to become scared because I thought of these nurses as professionals and more knowledgeable than me. Yet they were scared of becoming infected. I quit my job, I quit doing nurse's aid work altogether. Then I came to prison. I was petrified! I was scared of being in prison and becoming infected, because I heard in the county jail that more than 33 percent of the women in Bedford Hills were infected with the disease.

As part of orientation, I met one of the many members of ACE, and she spoke about how you don't get AIDS. I asked so many questions, I know I put Renee through the mill. She answered so many questions for me, but I wanted more information. I later participated in a seminar, and I realized that I was living with AIDS, not as someone who is infected with HIV, but as someone who lives in a world where people are infected. I didn't want to be scared any longer, and I didn't want to scare others and instill fear.

I wanted to make a difference, no matter how small the contribution. So I committed myself to a cause of love and nurturing, becoming informed and sharing that with others, and that is why I joined ACE.

* * *

My name is Dee. I'm thirty-seven years old, and am now serving my eighth year in Bedford Hills Correctional Facility for Women. I am a member of AIDS Counseling and Education—ACE. My purpose for joining ACE initially was a need to know what HIV/AIDS meant, but as I learned and became more educated, I realized I needed to join ACE because I felt helpless: not knowing what this illness was, seeing women who were once healthy deteriorating and not being able to help them and, last but not least, realizing that at that time the administration of BHCF was not doing what it should or could do for those who were HIV-positive.

For myself, I needed to do something to help make a change. ACE has allowed me to educate myself on the subject of AIDS/HIV, help my peers who need education and someone to talk to, and have a liaison with the administration, enough so that they are working *with* us now.

* * *

My name is Cathy. I truly didn't know a lot about this virus, except that street junkies and gay men got it. I was certain I was safe. I am a lesbian and not a street junkie. Then I started looking deep within myself. Years ago I slept with men, and I did shoot drugs two years before, but that wasn't what I thought of as a street junkie. Then I thought about my lover at the time of my arrest; she was using IV drugs at the time of my arrest.

So I joined ACE. As a matter of fact, I was at the first group meeting. After being educated by my peers and outside people, I realized that I had lived a high-risk behavior lifestyle. I sought the support of my peers, and I decided to test. My results came back negative. I originally joined ACE for myself. Now I am here for everyone and anyone who wants or needs my support in any way or who just wants to know more about AIDS.

* * *

My name is Aida. As we know by now, living with AIDS has become everyone's nightmare. I never wanted it to be real in my life. But in January 1988, my worst nightmare came true when my sister and niece were diagnosed with AIDS. I couldn't believe it, or should I say that I didn't want to believe?

This was my youngest sister we were talking about, and I didn't want to hear it. I went through lots of changes. I went through the anger, I cried, I even spent many nights asking God not to let them die. Just the thought of it would bring me to tears. I thought of my mother and what this would do to her, and my niece, so young, only four years old and dying! I thought until I couldn't think anymore.

ACE and I have come a long way since that time, and I feel free in saying that though I may not have AIDS, I am one of the many that are living with AIDS.

My sister died on August 23, 1989, at the age of twenty-seven. I went through some hard times after her death, but I also know that she is at peace now. I also have to thank God, because we still have my niece Jennifer, who is seven years old now and beautiful. I don't know how long she will be with us, but I do know that I will love her as my own for as long as we're allowed to keep her. I also know that my fight against AIDS has just begun. I thank the ladies in ACE for their love and support in helping me through hard times, and if I could share what I've learned in ACE with someone else, I will gladly do so.

* * *

The crowd grew quiet. ACE consists of people from all walks of life—poor, middle-class, Latin, black, white, straight, gay, HIV-positive and not HIV-positive, streetwise, formally educated women whose family members are sick, women who want to help their friends—and we had built our teams so that they reflected this diversity. The women listening could find at least one of us with whom to identify.

We worked hard to draw women in, asking them what they knew about HIV, letting them interrupt us with their questions as we talked about how the virus can and cannot be transmitted. Our role-plays recreated situations with which they were familiar.

We asked the women to help us role-play a situation, such as a woman going home from prison and trying to convince her man, who has been taking care of her while she was inside, to use a condom. Then the role-play is analyzed. What problems were encountered and how do we deal with those problems? We try to come up with solutions as we place ourselves in that situation. We talk about the risk of violence.

In another role-play, Toni, who is HIV-positive, is cooking food in the kitchen on her living unit for herself and her friend Linda. Another woman, Pat, says to Linda, "Don't eat her food; she's got AIDS." Linda counters, "That's silly, you don't think about who cooks your food in a restaurant on the streets." She turns to the audience and says, "What do you think?" Together we sort out issues of stigma and fears and questions women raise.

When we did the role-play of three junkies "getting off" together, and one getting mad because the other was taking the time to clean the works, everyone laughed at the sadly familiar scene. We asked, "Do you think that addicts will take the time to clean their needles?" Almost everyone says no, and they talk about their own experiences and state of mind when they are caught up by drugs.

We expected that issues of casual contact and stigma would be hot ones. But we were less prepared for the emotional intensity when we discussed the pros and cons of testing. You could feel people's tension and need. Women had questions and some horror stories of past experiences—no counseling, being told that she was HIV-positive just before getting on the bus at Rikers to come to Bedford. . . . We realized that many women were worried and trying to decide what to do.

Then, one of us, Carmen, stepped forward and looked out at the faces of all the women now sitting in a large circle. She began to speak:

I am HIV-positive. What brought me and ACE together? I tested positive March 8, 1988. While waiting a month for my results, I was able to spend many hours talking with a dear friend and founding member of ACE, Diane. That was really my pre- and post-test counseling, and I thank God that I had her there at that point in my life. After I got my results, we spent days working through the depression, anger, crying, and bargaining, until I finally was able to say, "Okay, so this is the reality; now what am I going to do about it?" She informed me that ACE was having their first meeting of the women who might want to be members of ACE, and with her supportive shoulder I was able to open up to the group and inform them that I had just been diagnosed HIV-positive. That was the beginning of a whole new life for me.

My involvement with ACE was essential for my acceptance and survival with AIDS in my life. ACE and AIDS have enhanced my life. I was able to turn around from self-hate into a positive outlook about myself and about life. Through ACE I have learned the meaning of social conscience and consciousness.

I openly expose my status to the world in hope that I can show other women that having AIDS doesn't make you any less of a person. We should be taken into account when treatments are addressed, because *men* are not the only ones infected with AIDS. And just to give the people a sense of hope that life can be just as good regardless of AIDS in our lives. AIDS doesn't mean the end of the world. We are all born to die, and if it means dying from AIDS, do not die with *shame* but die with *dignity.* Sharing my status makes me feel that in some small way I am able to give back to someone what I have received from the support of my sisters in ACE.

Women listened, cried, and called out words of encouragement. When she finished, we all joined hands in a great big circle and sang "Sister." What a powerful moment!

By the end of that week, we had held seminars in all four dorms in the back buildings. The word was spreading all over that ACE was breaking the silence, talking about living with AIDS, offering support, and challenging stigma. We got together to evaluate. We made note of questions women had raised that we needed to understand more to answer. We evaluated what approaches worked best and what changes to make. But overall, we felt exhilarated. We were finally doing what we felt was our mission: community building, peer education, and reaching out to break the barriers of ignorance, fear, and apathy.

Thus opened a year of intense work for ACE. Over the next months, we conducted seminars in all the classes and vocational programs. We met regularly and invited people from outside who were involved in AIDS work. Several times, reporters came to interview us as a group. Some people working in other prisons came to learn about ACE. We felt that our success would encourage administrators and policy makers to use the ACE model in other prisons.

PWAs in ACE, by speaking openly, encouraged other PWAs, who then participated in support groups and other activities. Renee was someone who spoke out:

I found I was HIV-positive in June 1990. At the time, I had been in a relationship with a woman for two months. I think I was more afraid of losing her than of dying from AIDS. When I first told her, she was supportive and understanding, but after about a week she ran.

1. I am black.
2. I am a female.
3. I am a lesbian.
4. I am in prison.
5. I have the AIDS virus.

This last statement I wrote and I still say to myself, "This can't be happening to me—no, not me. Not the fly girl, not Renee." But it is me and I have to deal with it. Okay, so, so I'm dealing with it, thanks to ACE, but what about my family? How do I tell them? How do I say, "I need your support?" and then . . . suppose they [my family] reject me, eat out of paper plates and such?

I have two adult children. My son will be twenty-five and my daughter will be twenty-three. My daughter lives in North Carolina, and we talk constantly about my illness, my plans, my hopes, my dreams. My son, on the other hand, does not want to talk about it at all. Whenever I bring up the discussion, he changes the subject. Or for instance, Sunday, on a visit with my mother, oldest brother, nephew, niece, and son, I was discussing what my being HIV-positive meant. Peanut got up and went into the Children's Center to play with Special (my niece). I've tried every way that I could to talk to my son about this, but to no avail. I can imagine what's going through his mind, but he doesn't verbalize it to me or anyone that I know of.

What is my child thinking? I say "child" because even though he's twenty-four going on twenty-five, he is still a child. When I look at him, he's my baby boy. How can I help him understand that Mommy's not dying, not yet anyway, and that I'm the same person I was when I left home?

These are just a few of the problems PWAs have in prison and out, but fortunately for me, I have ACE. Imagine me, riding the rapids in a rubber raft with pointed rocks all around in the water. Well, every time I've found myself in that rubber raft and a pointed rock just punctured my raft, ACE has been there to mend the punctures and/or throw me a lifeline.

* * *

We met with doctors and nurses from the medical staff, advocating and negotiating for a more humane, interactive relationship between doctors and patients. And we learned more about the medical issues and new treatments. We shared articles in *PWA Newsline* and *Treatment News* and became more knowledgeable.

While every day we faced the ever-widening impact of the epidemic, it was in many ways a time of hope.

* * *

I first got to know Sonia in IPC, where she lived in between periodic trips to the hospital. She was very frail and thin, and she kept getting PCP pneumonia, each time worse. One time, when she went out, they said that they didn't expect her to come back alive. But they didn't know Sonia! That was right about when aerosolized pentamidine had been discovered as an effective treatment against PCP; it worked for Sonia. But she told the story differently. She said that there were always guys in the hospital who were more sick than she was, and she'd get so involved with caring for—and flirting with—them, that she'd end up getting better. Whatever was her secret for surviving and thriving, it worked. Sonia came back from the hospital alive and got stronger in the following months, until Dr. Ferran finally ordered her to leave IPC and move to a regular housing unit. At first, Sonia kicked up quite a fuss—what a scene she made! But finally, people gave her an argument she couldn't ignore. She had to set an example of hope for others. That's what Sonia became: someone who had gone to the brink and made it back. She moved out of IPC and became one of the most active and outspoken PWAs in ACE.

* * *

One aspect of our work in the first year involved talking to outside groups and the media about the ACE model. We held several group interviews with reporters. Individuals in ACE went out on trips with the superintendent and others to speak at conferences. We came back excited at the positive response we got and the growing respect for ACE "on the outside." In the summer of 1989, we received the Project of the Year Award from the Coalition of Westchester Women's Organization and an award from the New York State Legislature.

We also experienced plenty of growing pains and problems. We were meeting weekly, but fewer members were coming to meetings. While some women were excited about their work, others were frustrated that their ideas were not listened to by the group. The core group tried to provide leadership and give direction, but others felt that there was an inner elite and that they did not have an equal voice. Some members felt that while they worked hard every day, others only showed up at meetings when the superintendent came. Some women left the group in frustration.

While the administration encouraged some of our work, there were still frustrating limits placed on other areas of work, especially peer counseling. Many women approached us after seminars with problems and issues they wanted to discuss privately. We had always felt that we had to follow up our educational outreach with supportive peer counseling. But the administration was reluctant to grant us that responsibility. We proceeded on an informal basis, meeting with women in the yard and rec room. Sometimes, staff people called one of us to a living unit to help in a crisis. But other times, we were blocked from doing what we felt was needed. One time, we got the go-ahead to put up a list of peer counselors who were available to population. The next week, we were told it was not properly authorized and it had to come down. While we were informally involved in buddy work with women in and out of IPC, we couldn't get permission for any kind of buddy training, such as that provided by Gay Men's Health Crisis.

Meanwhile, some of us were beginning to feel the stress of working with women who were very ill and of suffering the loss of loved ones. A counselor, Barbara Simmons, facilitated a stress group for ACE members in which we got to talk about some of the emotional toll of our work. We watched videos about working with people who are dying. For the first time, we shared our feelings and questions about working with friends who were dying—how to let go, how to allow people to live and die on their own terms, and how to cope with our own survivor's guilt.

ACE wasn't just encountering women who needed help and support. More and more women wanted to get involved, become better-educated, and join ACE. We decided to organize a workshop series, along the lines of the workshops that Montefiore had done with us. We already had our curriculum, written during the summer shutdown. We put up an announcement and asked women to sign up if they were interested. The response was tremendous; we had more names than we could handle.

The workshops presented us with new challenges and questions. Should they be available to everyone, or should there be criteria? What if someone came just to snoop and gather gossip about who was HIV-positive? How could we encourage women to be open and yet protect their confidentiality? How could we teach the more technical aspects of AIDS without losing some of our participants who might not have the educational background to understand? How could we go beyond sharing information to communicate the spirit and ethos of ACE? What did we as peer educators have to learn from the participants in the workshops?

We interviewed every woman who signed up and discussed any individual about whom there were misgivings. We made sure everyone knew that there was no certificate offered for those who completed the workshops. The only reward was what each woman gained from her participation. We decided that while we would argue strongly for the principle of confidentiality, we could not expect the same standards of adherence as we demanded from ACE members. So we warned everyone that the workshops were public events and that therefore each woman had to decide what she felt comfortable saying. Within that, we worked hard to create an atmosphere in which women were comfortable to ask questions and explore feelings.

The workshops provided us with an opportunity to explore specific issues more deeply and thus expand ACE's analysis and understandings. During the first series, in the spring of 1989, this was particularly true in the workshop on women and AIDS.

* * *

We began the women's workshop with some statistics and ideas about ways that women are affected by the epidemic differently because we are women. Then we asked the participants to brainstorm on this issue.

- "Women are more vulnerable because we don't control the terms of our lovemaking. We can't get men to use condoms."
- "What about being raped?"
- "We don't just have to worry about ourselves, we have our children to worry about."
- "We have no access to health care."
- "Women with AIDS are doubly stigmatized. They assume we're sluts if we have the virus, but men who are HIV-positive aren't viewed that way."
- "Our communities are already under siege. We have no health care. We can't afford one more problem like AIDS."

- "I don't believe all these statistics that show the prevalence of AIDS in our communities. I think that white people are getting AIDS at just as high rates, but these statistics are used to stigmatize black and Hispanic communities."

We generated more than a list. As we discussed each of these issues, we began to see ourselves as women in a new light. Many of us usually see things in individual and private terms. Now we were thinking in social and political terms. It made us angry and emboldened. We wanted to act. Our collectively forged women's consciousness united us and moved us to create a women's voice for women who bore so much of the burden of this epidemic. We also became more aware and articulate about our diversity and the different ways that the epidemic affected each of our communities.

* * *

At the end of the workshop series, a number of women wanted to join ACE. This was the first large group of new members since the early days of ACE. We had to figure out how to bring new members in, train them, and involve them in work. Final decisions about membership were made by the superintendent. Then we met as a group and talked about ACE's principles and why they were important. Everyone signed a contract and then decided what areas of work they wanted to get involved in.

The infusion of energy that came from the new members was great. Once again, we were thinking up new role-plays and coming up with new ideas. Several of the new members were open PWAs, who strengthened the PWA voice in ACE. But the very growth of ACE brought us up against the limitations of being prisoners. We didn't have a meeting place. We didn't have permission to do counseling. We didn't have any place to talk with women in need. As prisoners we could not run an office or make a telephone call for a woman in need to come for counseling. Rose Palladino, the librarian, had volunteered to help ACE, and the library became a center for us during that time, but we needed a full-time civilian staff in order for the program of ACE to be carried out.

Once again, we were waiting endlessly for permission to do things and never getting it. We felt as though the only time we saw anyone with authority was when some media people came to interview us, or we received some public awards or recognition. As we pushed to do the educating and counseling, our relationship with the administration once again became strained. The superintendent, for her part, was in a quandary, because she could not just keep allowing us to function without supervision. But the negotiations for the AIDS Institute grant, which was to provide funds for civilian supervision, were tied up in red tape and politics.

* * *

It was the fall of '89. We had had a pretty good year. But now things were stuck again. We couldn't do our work. One day, we were invited to a meeting with a group of women from the outside who were involved in AIDS work or in local government. This group, chaired by Linda Loffredo, wanted to hear all about ACE and to talk about our putting on a public conference to project ACE. We listened and we went through our stock raps, but our hearts weren't in it. Finally, one of them asked us if there was a problem. We exploded with our frustrations—our inability to hold meetings, educate, counsel, support, get buddy training—all of it. What good was it for us to talk and talk and talk with people like them when we couldn't do our real work, when we weren't serving our own community?

* * *

As wary as we were about what would happen if the grant came through and civilian staff and supervisors came in, we realized it was the only way that we would be granted permission to continue our work. The women at that meeting pledged to help get the grant for ACE through the bureaucracy. And they succeeded!

It was a few months later that one day, ACE members were notified that they were to report to the administration building immediately. Many of us arrived completely stressed out, because usually an inmate is called to Traffic to see their counselor to be told about a death in the family. (I wish Renee were still alive to tell this story, because she was really livid that day!) Others had been threatened with charge sheets if they did not report immediately. So all together, we were not a very friendly crew as we gathered in the board room under the auspices of the deputy superintendent, who introduced us to our new director, Marie St. Cyr, and temporary coordinator, Suzanne Kessler. The grant had finally come through, and ACE was now a project of WARN-Women and AIDS Resource Network and the Columbia University School of Public Health.

5
ACE: A Funded Project

I remember the day the administration gave us a space to work out of. It was a large empty room. We hugged one another, we yelled, and we started roaming around the facility, trying to find furniture wherever we could. We looked in empty offices and classrooms, begged a bookshelf, a desk, and chairs. It was the excitement of a dream long waited for finally come true.

* * *

Since the beginning of ACE, one of our dreams was to have an ACE drop-in center. We felt that having a room would make our work easier. It would give the women in population easy access to us whenever they had a crisis. We would be able to utilize the office to do more educational work. Our workshops, seminars, counseling, and memorial services could all be done in our office. Having a space would mean a place to call our own.

Once the grant came through, we began asking the superintendent for space from which to work. Within a month, we were given a room, which we turned into our long-awaited ACE center.

With our new room came the agency that was handling the grant, civilian staff, and ACE inmate staff. The ACE inmate staff were self-chosen: anyone who wanted to be a staff member out of the experienced ACE members could do so. Twelve people chose to become ACE staff, and we divided ourselves up. Six of us would work program modules in the morning and six in the afternoon.

Now we had a room, and we had twelve inmates whose assignment was to actually do ACE work. It would no longer have to be squeezed in during free time, and we had a civilian whose job was to help ACE. Everything seemed ready to take a wonderful leap. But instead, we stumbled.

* * *

Almost immediately upon getting the new space, we began to face a series of problems and differences among ourselves. We faced the question of how to spend our time. What were our priorities? We began to paint the office. But some people were more willing to paint than others, and right from the start, resentment developed. Then, after the painting, some women moved ahead on setting up the center, getting a clipping file together, setting up a library. Some women didn't show up. And others moved ahead with writing. The grant from the AIDS Institute required that the ACE program print its educational curriculum so that it could be used by other prisons. Now that there was a room and a computer and we had the time, such a project was possible. There was pressure on us to get that project done. At the same time, ACE was offered the possibility of writing a chapter about ACE for a book on women and AIDS. Both these writing projects required an enormous amount of time.

I remember the arguments. Some of us wanted to do the writing. It was a chance for ACE to help other prisons as well as make an impact on society around women-and-AIDS and prison-and-AIDS issues. Others of us felt that we needed to get the office together and set ourselves up to do the work that we wanted, and there was criticism of the writers for doing it in an exclusive manner.

We all had dreamed of doing counseling, but in the past we did counseling wherever we were—in the yard, on our living units, in school. Now we wanted to do counseling in the office. Yet we were spending so much time in the office dealing with ourselves, and we didn't have a plan of how to get people to begin to come to the office. I remember not long after we got the office, we used to laugh through our tensions and frustration saying, "This office is like a prison."

* * *

How did we now determine priorities of work? How did we deal with the priorities set by outside agencies and with the differences among ourselves? We were now faced with an entirely new structure for decision making, which we didn't know how to work with.

* * *

It was confusing. For two years, we had functioned with a fairly simple structure: a core group of about five, from which some people left on parole and new people joined. And an organization of about twenty-five to thirty people, which met on a regular basis. Now, suddenly, we were responsible to an outside agency, which was responsible to the AIDS Institute, and we were all responsible to the conditions of a grant. Several civilian staff members, an ACE staff, a core group, an organization—how did all these things fit together? Who set priorities? The role of the organization began to disappear during that early period, as the office and twelve staff and civilians became an intense world of its own, occupying a lot of our energy. It took time to realize that the staff was going to replace the core group as a day-to-day decision-making body, but half the staff worked in the morning and the other half in the afternoon, and it was hard to ever all meet together. This caused divisions and friction.

* * *

And how were we going to build accountability among one another around our work? And how did we resolve differences? Was the civilian coordinator or outside agency director now going to begin to make decisions that we once had made as inmates? Where did that kind of power reside? Before the grant, the core group members were people who were willing to use a lot of their free time, including Saturday nights, to work. Although at times over the two-year period there had been complaints of exclusiveness or elitism, by and large it worked as a form. Now, being on staff was a formal prison job, and there were twelve of us. A few people never showed up for work, but who was going to hold them accountable?

Before the grant, a person chose to work with ACE knowing it was an organization led by inmates only. The people who made decisions about the work were other inmates. Now, suddenly, inmates weren't sure they wanted other inmates telling them what to do. Was the new coordinator going to do that? Yet there was, on all of our parts, a reluctance to lose our own control over ourselves. We didn't want a civilian to have that kind of power, and yet the old way of functioning also wasn't working.

* * *

I remember one day realizing that some sort of shift was happening. I overheard one ACE staff member tell the civilian that she was going to switch her module from morning to afternoon. As a staff we had organized the morning and afternoon staffs according to ethnic backgrounds, different strengths, and individual schedules. It had been decided by us carefully at that point. I was amazed that the staff member was telling the civilian and not the rest of us as staff about her decision. She and I talked about it. She hadn't done anything wrong, yet I realized that something was changing.

* * *

Just as we were grappling with our role, so was the new coordinator, Suzanne Kessler, who remembers,

With some ambivalence, I agreed to temporarily fill the position of coordinator of ACE. Although I was eager to work with and learn from women who were at the forefront of AIDS education, I recognized that these women in no way needed to be "coordinated." In spite of my experience as an educator and administrator, I had to stifle my impulse to educate and administrate and, instead, just let the work begun long before I got there continue. From my journal, one note illustrates the spirit of the group and the tightrope I walked: "Today Katrina criticized me for handing out sign-up sheets at the last general meeting of ACE members. She couldn't say exactly what bothered her about what I had done. Other women agreed that something was wrong with it, and suggested that perhaps it was that I did this first thing, without the meeting having been opened by Pearl. Apparently, I had acted exactly like a staff person— taking over. Their worst nightmare."

* * *

Slowly, we began to move into doing work with population, and one of the key areas that we focused on was counseling. A civilian, Linda Malmberg, was hired as a counselor. She counseled women in population, served as a counselor for some ACE members and staff, and began a much needed death-and-dying bereavement group for ACE and other people in population.

For the ACE staff, an office was a prerequisite for pursuing the goal of counseling. We now had the office, and were inspired by the idea of becoming skilled, even professional, counselors. We knew we were going to get the training by the New York State AIDS Institute to become certified HIV pre- and post-test counselors within a few months. This concept of ourselves as "professionals" was different from how we previously had seen ourselves, as simply sisters supporting sisters.

The issue of how we saw ourselves related to how we conceptualized the office. Was the office going to be a drop-in center, or was it going to be used as a place to provide more structured services to the women? This related to how we set it up in terms of use of space.

How did we deal with the different levels of knowledge and experience among ACE staff and ACE members, as well as among women arriving from Riker's Island, who were educated from the Riker's Empowerment program? Before the office, anyone who wanted to work, anyone who had anything to contribute would find her role. We tended in this early period of the office to develop more of a hierarchy among ourselves. Newer members criticized staff members for not allowing them to participate fully. And when the certification process developed and we had to decide who would participate, a struggle emerged among the staff as to how much time and experience an ACE member had to have in order to participate.

We spent the first few months after getting the office tied up in tensions around the different issues, but we also slowly began to learn to use the office for our work.

* * *

It was sinking in my hard head that ACE was changing and had to change and that if I was going to be useful and happy, then I needed to change my approach to my work. Peer counseling was a new and needed skill that I wanted to master. I developed a new routine. Twice a week I went to orientation with a few other members. We always met new women who were in crisis. We encouraged everyone to come to the office, and many signed up for counseling or for group discussions. Then, on the days I was in the office, I'd call women who had signed up. I was blown away by how many women were coming in to Bedford who were HIV-positive, many for years already, and even more, how many women had lost family members—mothers, brothers, cousins. A lot of times, a woman would come in, saying she wanted to talk because she was considering getting tested, but had hesitations. She'd start out pretty tense and nervous. Eventually, she'd open up about having watched her brother, or whoever, slowly die of AIDS right before she got busted. Or she'd spill her grief and guilt because she was in jail when her sister died and couldn't be there. I realized that women were so full of unresolved grief that they couldn't make the choices they needed to for their own personal and health needs.

* * *

Women came in to talk who had been living with AIDS for quite a while on the street. They were often well informed and experienced. But coming into prison brought new problems. Most of them were living in the back buildings and worried about others finding out their status. Some had experienced taunts and gossip already. They would come day after day to ACE. At first they wanted individual counseling, which they could get either from us or from Linda Malmberg. But often they would soon want to get involved in work. Because it would be several months before they could go to a workshop series and join ACE, we were pushed to figure out ways to involve nonmembers in ACE. With all the problems, we slowly began to learn to use the office.

In the spring of '90, the medical department shifted its policy from providing the antibody test to anyone who asked for it to strongly encouraging women to take the test. This, along with other developments, led to many women coming to ACE because they wanted to test and needed support, information, and counseling. The waiting period at that time was one to two months, so the whole process—from having to decide, through getting the results—was painfully protracted. Often, the only thing that made it surviv-able was having someone from ACE there at each step of the way.

* * *

I saw Rosa one day when I went to talk at the orientation. She'd been here once before several years ago. It's always sad to see someone come back. She didn't look too good, but often people look pretty bedraggled when they first come in and start looking healthier and more put together within weeks. She came up to me and asked if I would call her to the ACE office. I said sure. When she came the next day, she told me that she'd gotten back into drugs; that her man had died of AIDS and she was very worried about herself but didn't know if she was ready to face finding out bad news, on top of the blows she'd already had. She looked scared and defeated. She came in almost every day for about two weeks and talked and talked. At first, it was a lot about her husband and her family, then she wound back to thinking about herself. By the end of the second week, she was thinking less about how she had messed up and more about what she could do now to take some control of her life. She decided to take the test.

The weeks of waiting seemed endless to me—so I can imagine how they felt to her! At first, she spent a lot of time in the ACE office, reading and educating herself about AIDS. But after a point, she said she didn't want to keep coming there—it made her feel as if she already knew she was positive. So we'd get together in the yard and just hang out and talk about everything except AIDS. I didn't think of myself as a counselor with a client. We were just friends, sharing sunshine and quiet intimacy in the middle of the storm.

I was on a visit when she got called to get her test results. We'd agreed that she could get me to go with her when she got her test results. But the day she was called, I was on a visit and she didn't want to wait. That evening, she came to the quiet yard to tell me: she was positive. She was very quiet and calm. I encouraged her to let it out a little and finally she cried. We sat comfortably in silence for a while, then she pointed to the sunset, which was turning the sky a golden crimson. I pointed to a flock of geese flying overhead. She said, playfully, "Let's count our blessings." And that's what we did, starting with the trees and grass and nature around us and then naming our children and loved ones, people and places and memories.

She wasn't ready to come back to the ACE office, but she planned to take the workshop series that was soon coming up. But right before then, she was transferred to another prison. What a kick to the gut, when that happens.

* * *

There was some debate among ACE staff about how to involve these new women. Some got upset when nonmembers ended up finding out confidential information—"other people's business"—and were included in discussion and work that were supposed to be only for members. At least one breach of confidentiality resulted from such a situation. But on the other hand, more and more women were coming into the office who had been living with AIDS for a long time, who wanted counseling. They also wanted to get involved.

We began holding open meetings and rap groups almost every week. We put out announcements, and anyone in population who was interested could sign up. Sometimes we had a particular theme, like talking to your children about AIDS, or new information on medical treatments. We had a Black Awareness Rap Group and a Hispanic Awareness Rap Group about AIDS. Often they became more general open forums for women to talk, learn, and teach. Quite often, a PWA who had been coming to the office and talking privately with ACE members would take the opportunity of a rap group to speak publicly for the first time about being HIV-positive. Sometimes, when one woman would do so, another would follow, and others would be moved to talk about their issues and questions. It was exciting, in the way that the early ACE meetings had been for us originally.

* * *

I had been counseling Jay for about a month. She had been HIV-positive for several years before coming to prison, but this was the first situation where she had to struggle with her fears about other people finding out. She was in the back buildings. Most women didn't know, but she had told one friend, who was very supportive and had encouraged her to come to the ACE office. She came almost every day, to talk, to read, to watch videos—just to be in a supportive place where she could relax and be open. She was pretty shy and seemed fragile.

Then, one time, she came to an open meeting. When we broke up into small groups, she was in my group. As we were going around the group, each woman speaking, Jay came out and said that she was a PWA. Then she just kept talking, answering other women's questions and sharing her wealth of experiences and hard times. I watched her get stronger before my very eyes. She sat up taller and spoke louder. And other women listened and learned from her. Afterward, she came up to me and gave me a big bear hug and said, "I feel wonderful. And proud. Funny, huh? I've been so fearful and ashamed, and now I feel so proud."

* * *

Katrina organized a PWA empowerment group. While there had been support groups for a long time, which offered a safe and confidential space for women, the empowerment group was a more open meeting that enabled PWAs to develop their collective knowledge, voice, and political power.

The empowerment group helped to create a strong PWA voice in ACE in that period that carried over into all our activities—from PWAs breaking the silence in orientation meetings and seminars, in living units and classrooms, to very active medical advocacy, to creating an environment that encouraged others to come to ACE and to be open about their status. Women who were HIV-positive knew that there were PWAs to whom they could come for support.

* * *

In 1989, I was called from work to go see the doctor. I started wondering why the doctor wanted to see me. When I arrived at the hospital, Dr. Ferran told me, "We have to talk." I sat down and listened to what she had to say. The first thing she said was "You are HIV-positive." I went into shock, my mind was blank. I knew she was talking, asking me if I knew anything about this disease. The only thing that came out of my mouth was "no." She kept talking to me, but I did not hear a word she said. When I finally came out of her office my mind was blank. My attitude changed, I was not myself. I tried to tell myself that this was just a bad dream.

A few weeks later one of my girlfriends noticed my change and she approached me about it. I could not hold any more; at that point I needed someone I could talk to and with whom I could let out all my confusion and pain. I told her, "I am HIV-positive," and I could not accept it. She recommended that I talk to Katrina Haslip about it, that she would help me. I met Katrina and she explained to me everything that I needed to know. Katrina also introduced me to the ACE program. I feel good because all the ladies working in the ACE program were inmates like me. My sisters in ACE have always been there for me. They share with me new information about the HIV virus, they offer me support, when I need to cry we do it together, and whenever I need a hug their arms are open for me. The ACE program offers rap sessions, counseling, video showings, and support groups for PWAs. In addition, they offer support to the women in IPC that are extremely sick and that are not capable of taking care of themselves. I love the girls that work in ACE, they have hearts of gold.

When a woman makes the choice to be an open PWA, she takes on special burdens. One woman who is an open PWA speaks about this:

Outside of the group I find that people often look to me for strength to tell them what's going on with them. But because I'm always smiling and seem to handle things so well, it's rare that anyone ever asks me, "Viniece, how are you doing?" Everyone always assumes that Niecie is all right. And sometimes that gets hard, because sometimes when I'm not all right, I don't want to say it because I feel like people look up to me, so I isolate myself. There are a few people who ask how I am, but most people come to me and say, "I have the name of someone who is HIV-positive I want you to see" or "I need to know this," or "How's so-and-so doing," but they don't ask me.

I still get strength from ACE and my sisters in ACE and sometimes it feels good just to be treated as Niecie, the Niecie I was before, but sometimes I'd like people to remember that I do have a positive test result and that some days are harder than others and that some days they could give me the same encouragement and support that everyone gives their clients. I guess maybe it's easier for my sisters in ACE to remember me as Niecie before the positive test result. That way they don't have to think that one day I may be one of the names of the people on the quilt. It seems like the only time somebody will ask me how I'm doing is after somebody else has died. Overall, I love my sisters in ACE and I love the women in my support group. And together we will beat this epidemic.

Our connections to the outside AIDS struggle grew during that period. Suzanne arranged for many outside guests to visit and talk with ACE. This included people involved in exploring alternative treatments and opening up access to treatment trials; people from the Human Rights Commission AIDS Discrimination Unit, women involved in film and media work, others dealing with the women's health problems from HEAL. And Agness Alvarez, the administrative assistant, connected us through subscriptions to many AIDS publications, found videos, and built our library. We learned a lot, and we were also energized by being plugged in to people and activities outside the walls.

We got a copy of a film about Philly Lutayya, the Ugandan singer who was one of the first African celebrities to come out in the open as a PWA and who toured his country to break the silence about the devastation of the epidemic throughout Africa. We loved his music and decided to learn his song and add it to "Sister" as our second ACE song.

* * *

In that period I remember we used to sing in the office. Kathy brought her guitar down and we learned Philly Lutayya's song and sang other songs as well. Some people groaned at the off-key voices, but we really enjoyed ourselves.

ALONE

Out there somewhere; alone and frightened
Of the darkness; the days are long.
Life in hiding; no more making new contacts.
No more loving arms going around my neck.

Take my hand now; I'm tired and lonely.
Give me love; give me hope.
Don't reject me; don't desert me.
All I need is love and understanding.

Today it's me, tomorrow someone else.
It's me and you, we have to stand up and fight.
We share a light in the fight against AIDS.
Let's come around; let's stand together and fight AIDS.

In times of joy; in times of sorrow.
Let's take a stand and fight up to the end.
We open up and stand out and speak out to the world.
We'll save some lives; save the children of the world.

Let's be open; advise the young ones.
A new generation to protect and love.

Hear them singing, playing lovely.
Let's give them everything, in truth and love.

Take the message; confront the frontier.
Break the barriers; fight together.
Doors are open; we lead the struggle.
For hope and life, and peace, truth, and joy.

Today it's me, tomorrow someone else.
It's me and you we have to stand up and fight.
We share a light in the fight against AIDS.
Let's come around; let's stand together and fight AIDS.

—Philly Lutayya

We watched another film called *As Is,* which was about two gay men who were ex-lovers when one of them finds out he has AIDs. We showed these over and over to new women, who were always moved and able to reach past the cultural differences to our shared human frailty.

In this period, we were able to focus on deepening our roots within the Hispanic community at Bedford Hills. The percentage of Hispanic people in New York State prisons has been steadily rising—it is now 40 percent. And in New York State as a whole the rate of HIV infection for Hispanic people coming into the prison is 22.2 percent, nearly double the infection rate of whites (12.9 percent) or Afro-Americans (11.6 percent). But we didn't need those statistics to know that there was an urgency in reaching our Hispanic sisters. We were meeting woman after woman who was HIV-positive and hearing stories of families who were suffering one death after another.

First Carmen buried her eight-month-old son; then Carmen's mother buried Carmen and continued on to visit Carmen's brother at Riker's Island, who was also HIV-infected.

First my sister Yvette died; then two years later her daughter—my niece Jennifer—died; now I'm just praying for my nephew. He's made it until he is eleven. They just started giving him AZT.

From the beginning Latina women have been a strong force in the creation of ACE, and throughout its history these women have felt a deep commitment to reaching Latina women in Bedford. Many women in Bedford speak Spanish as their first language, and without a bilingual

AIDS program, there will be no way to meet their needs. Beyond language is the issue of culture, which affects how HIV/AIDS can be talked about and what will bring people together to help one another.

* * *

I began to feel that the workshops didn't deal enough with ethnic differences. To me, being Puerto Rican and half-Indian, some of the ways people were talking about sex wouldn't work, don't apply in a traditional Hispanic family.

* * *

There has been steady progress as we have overcome obstacles. Some of the limitations have been our own:

In 1990, some of us in ACE who are Latina began to conduct some seminars in Spanish and hold open meetings for the population to foster Spanish awareness of HIV/AIDS issues. At first, we found it hard to start the Hispanic sector of ACE, mainly because most of us in ACE are what some would call Spanish-Americans or New Yoricans, and though we know the language we were intimidated to use it in a large group of Hispanic women.

* * *

Beyond our own limitations, there is a severe lack of Hispanic materials about HIV/AIDS, both written in Spanish and with an understanding of Hispanic cultural issues. Additionally, we do not have enough outside Hispanic resources, such as speakers coming to prison. One woman said, "Some Hispanic people that get trained and educated, they move to another place and they forget where they come from, that their culture needs them, we need them."

Perhaps the most striking evidence of the lack of materials and educators for Hispanic people was the fact that as of 1992, the New York State Department of Health AIDS Institute, responsible for training HIV/AIDS pre- and post-test counselors throughout New York State, did not have either materials in Spanish or bilingual trainers. When they came to Bedford Hills in that year, we had both English-speaking and Spanish-speaking members ready to receive certification and training. But the certification was not offered in Spanish. The AIDS Institute trainers recognized the problem and were willing for us to create special accommodations.

* * *

I remember Windy and Aida sat with the ten Hispanic women at separate tables, and for three days, eight hours a day, they sat and translated the training into Spanish that the AIDS Institute trainers conducted in English. They were exhausted but committed.

* * *

By now our Hispanic ACE members are from many places — Puerto Rico, Colombia, Dominican Republic, New York City. We have a staff member who is the Hispanic Sector coordinator and a workshop series that is conducted in Spanish. We collect materials in Spanish and reach Latina women in a variety of activities. As Sandra describes it, it takes trial and error:

Sometimes we have an organizational meeting and I sit with the Hispanic women and translate what is being said and what they want to say. The noise in the room gets crazy. In a way being present at the organizational meetings helps us feel part of the whole program, but having everything translated also makes us feel more passive. So recently we decided to have the Hispanic sector's meeting on a separate day, and this seems to work better now. We will do a separate Hispanic project for making quilt squares for babies from the Incarnation Children's Center, and we will also have a joint project — English and Spanish — when we do our quilt project for friends and family members.

The commitment to have a truly bilingual, bicultural program continues; we maintain flexibility and creativity in order to do so.

With the office giving us a stronger base, we began to also have greater interaction with the correctional officers. COs have a lot of power over us. They search our cells; they give us direct orders, which, if disobeyed, result in a charge sheet; they take us handcuffed and shackled to the outside hospital — in sum, they are the security and control personnel in the prison. Their attitudes toward AIDS have always been part of our reality. When they are afraid or just mean, their negative attitudes can harm an individual and generally increase fear. And when they are educated about AIDS and care, they can be of enormous support and help.

* * *

I remember often seeing a scene after a woman who was HIV-positive vacated her cell to go to the hospital. Several guards would pack up her cell, and they would be wearing rubber gloves, even masks. Everybody would watch them. Ten minutes later, a new inmate, arriving from the reception area with all her belongings in plastic garbage bags, would be moved into her room.

What was the message? First, that HIV infection can be spread by casual contact and is even airborne — neither of which is true — and second, that inmates' lives are not important, only the officers need protection.

* * *

ACE tried to take on attitudes like this. ACE members talked with individual COs, sharing their education, and COs got to know PWAs living on their units or at their workplace. More and more COs expressed interest and support.

* * *

One CO worked in commissary. ACE had placed a large wooden donation box — with the ACE logo painted on it — right by the commissary window for the women in population to give donations to the women in IPC. The CO wouldn't let any of us out the door until we gave something for the IPC box. She would stand there and yell at people if they were leaving without putting something in it. "I don't care what you put in it, even if it's a lollipop." And if she was on the telephone and saw someone leaving without putting in something, she put the phone down and would call the person, embarrassing them until they put something in that box. She protected it too. You couldn't sit on it, you couldn't steal from it. Even if you were pretending to steal from it, she would say, "Get away from that box." And if she knew you had money and saw you put a bag of chips in there, she would say, "Don't be cheap. Put more."

* * *

At one point during the next year, the administration at Bedford took an unusual step. It was running a mandatory training in the gym for all civilians and officers, and ACE members did the training on the topic of AIDS. One officer who has been supportive of both ACE and women who are HIV-positive over the past four years had this to say about ACE:

As a whole, the project is really needed here, where so many people are HIV-positive or whose lives have put them in a position where they could have it. It gives support, a place where they can feel comfortable, where they feel accepted, even if their family on the outside still is afraid of them.

I see ACE as a connecting thing, like you have people who don't really like each other, but if they see someone who has a family member who's sick, they'll put that aside and help one another.

There's not as much negative feeling among the women now as there was. I think that's from the education and from the girls' seeing their friends get sick. And there is an admiration shown toward the girls who say out loud, "I'm HIV-positive," because it takes strength to say it out loud, because the person never knows when it's going to get thrown back in her face. The support doesn't take away the pain, but it eases the pain.

The memorials are good. They give people a chance to admire, to show their last respect and acknowledgment to a friend, to say, "Even though you were sick, I still love you."

Among the officers, there is a change. It used to be more that we'd whisper, "She's got AIDS" like a gossip, like a put-down. Now we still tell each other, but it's more to just let one another know, maybe as a way of saying the person needs support or we need to take precautions. Still, among the officers there's a bad feeling around confidentiality. I feel like I have a right to know, say, if I'm taking someone out on a trip, so I can take precautions, like wear gloves in case they have body sores.

ACE takes the pressure off, helps us as COs. If you have someone who's HIV-positive on your unit and you don't feel comfortable talking to them, you know there's an ACE member who can talk to them. That helps.

* * *

Also that spring, after we had our certification training, we held another workshop series, which brought many new women who wanted to join ACE. Learning from past mistakes, we developed a more systematic process of training and involvement in work so that new members could more fully take their place and make their contribution to ACE. The superintendent would always review the list of women who wished to become members, and occasionally she would not allow a woman to join ACE:

ACE, ACE ACE, ACE ACE! In the beginning that's all you heard on the campus. Not because it was a new program but because of the fears it instilled. Many of us knew that we needed ACE, but we were still not ready to face what it stood for. I didn't want to be a part of ACE in the beginning, but yet I would listen to the women and sometimes throw out ideas. I didn't want anyone hearing or seeing me involve myself with the program. I was afraid of the stigma.

There were so many mixed emotions about it. Some felt that ACE consisted of the superintendent's pets, and others felt that anyone affiliated with the program had AIDS. Little did I know that for a number of different reasons, the administration would not have permitted me to be a member of ACE at that time.

There were so many different functions of the program, and I wasn't prepared for any of it. In 1989, something happened that changed my whole outlook on ACE. A very dear friend of mine was dying before my eyes with the virus. I felt angry. I even hated the virus for making Helen sick. I knew it was only a matter of time before it took her from me. From then on, I knew and felt in my heart that I had to contribute something to the program, to the women. I guess I had known this from the beginning. But ignorant, like some of the other women, I refused to see it. Now, five years later, I am an ACE member and volunteer my services when needed. It took a lot to get here, years of proving to the superintendent and the women that I could belong and contribute. Sometimes I wonder if it was worth it, but when I remember Helen, I know that I'm not just doing it for me, but for those who have been infected by the virus.

* * *

The result of all these activities was that during the late spring and summer of 1990, we finally succeeded in making the office a center of energy and creativity and work. The office was buzzing with people, ideas, and emotions.

We reached out to other programs in the prison: We did presentations and seminars in the Family Violence Program, the West Wing, and the Nursery, where women had been voicing fears and questions. We developed a puppet show for the children visiting their mothers for a week during the summer.

Suzanne Kessler wrote about that transitional period:

Probably more women got AIDS education and counseling at Bedford during those months than in any other community at that time. From my records I calculated that ACE had direct contact with over a thousand women through prison orientations, workshops, seminars, or counseling. This was the kind of data the AIDS Institute (the funding source) was interested in. Reflections from my journal suggested a different kind of evidence of ACE's impact on the prison population:

"Every time we do a seminar, the women come up to us afterward and say, 'So when are you coming back here next week to do another one?'

When ACE members walk through the tunnels, it's not unusual for someone they pass to say, 'Hey when are you calling me down to the ACE office?' or 'How can I join ACE?' . . . Sometimes I think ACE is a magnet for all the generalized anxiety and discontent in prison. . . . AIDS is the issue that brings them to us, but we hear a lot more."

COPING WITH DEATH
AND OVERCOMING GRIEF

By the fall of 1990, we had begun to feel comfortable using the office. Our new coordinator, Jacqueline McDonald, community liaison Yolanda Rosado, and civilian counselor Dee Holmes came to work with ACE and stayed for almost two years. During that period, our work focused on education, counseling, and caring for women in the infirmary. We worked throughout the facility, but it was the office that was a center of energy, creativity, and work. It buzzed with people, ideas, and life. Yet, as the deaths increased, so did the grieving. The office became a center for that as well.

Often, when a woman died, word spread throughout population, and the ACE office was the place where people gathered. We sat around the long table. Sometimes there was silence. Sometimes there was just the sound of crying. We have a tradition of telling stories about the person who had died. We try to remember the things that made us laugh as well.

* * *

I remember when Carmen died. We all got together. It was raining that day; it rained for days after that. Everybody was crying, and I remembered something Carmen had always said when she was sick: "When I die, it's going to be raining, and when that rain hits you, you're going to think it's water, but it's really going to be me pissing on you." And sure enough, for about a week it rained, and I was soaking wet with water, but I knew it was Carmen's piss.

* * *

Each time a woman from the prison died of HIV-related illness, we made a quilt for her. In that period, it became such a regular event that we began to store paints and material for the next quilt, which we knew would be needed all too quickly.

* * *

I remember several times when we had three tables at a time covered with white material and groups of people painting quilts, because the deaths had come so rapidly. "She told me she wanted a purple car on her quilt." "I'm going to put a pack of Newports because that was always on her mind." "I'm putting the sun because she loved sitting out in the yard." On and on as the blues and purples and reds and green paints filled the white material, trying to capture the spirit of the sister who had passed.

* * *

We held most of the memorials for our sisters at the office. At Sonia's we played salsa music. Sonia had overcome PCP pneumonia again and again, committing herself to make it out of Bedford to get to her daughter and grandchild's house in Boston before she died. Against all the odds, she made it out on parole and lived with her daughter and granddaughter for a few months before she died. At her memorial we recalled her strength, her humor and example.

The memorials were also filled with grief, with the goodbyes that people needed to say. In our long room, we would hang the quilts with yarn and paper clips through the little holes in the ceiling boards. We lined the chairs up facing the quilt or quilts. Someone would bring down a tape player and the favorite tapes of the person who had died, and at 3:30, women would come to the office for the memorial.

One thing about the memorials: In the street the funerals were so plastic, but here people knew that it could be them.

At Carmen's memorial, which was held in the chapel before we had the office, Romeo opened by saying,

Farewell. Goodbye. Those are all the pat phrases people used to say. I won't be seeing you anymore. Somehow none of the phrases seem to apply to me and you, because I'll be seeing you and hearing your laughter and feeling you in the spirit I call memories.

Feeling as I do about you, the loss of your nearness to me is as profound as the loss of a child from a parent. For seven years I've seen through the mask you wore to keep others away from you. Fear of getting too close, when all along your façade was transparent. In it I saw only your loneliness and desire to be loved. I'm glad I saw through that mask, because the gift I got from you in return is priceless to me, Carmen.

When we held a memorial for another Carmen and Rosa, who were in the founding group of ACE, we felt the loss of our first generation of leaders. Kathy played a song on her guitar that she wrote to honor those that we have lost:

A TOAST TO THOSE WHO ARE GONE

(adapted from the Phil Ochs song)

Many's the hour I lay by my window
And thought of the people who carried the burden
Who were locked up in prison and searched out an answer
And ended their journey unwilling heroes.
Many are the women who have been part of ACE,
Women who have brought all their fears and their courage.
They've spoken in whispers, they've spoken out loud;
Finding strength in themselves,
They gave strength to their sisters.
So here's a toast to those who are gone,
Sisters with whom we laughed and cried,
And a toast to the ones at the end of the line,
A toll of the bells for all who have died.

Sometimes the deaths were just too many, and we felt overwhelmed and exhausted.

When word arrived that a sister had died, the coordinator of ACE used to make a phone call to the living units and ask for the ACE members to come to the ACE office. In the spring of 1992 there were so many deaths one after the other that when I would get a phone call to come to ACE, I would lose my breath, my heart would start beating fast, and I wouldn't want to go, I just didn't want to hear about one more death.

We faced death not only among our sisters who were here or who had been paroled, but in ever-increasing numbers among our family members and friends. Most of the women in this prison have at least one person who is close to them who has died. In some cases entire families have been devastated.

MY FAMILY

My only three brothers and my sister have been infected with the virus. I guess my biggest fear is knowing that if something happens to them, I'm not going to be able to see them. Two of my brothers live in Puerto Rico with my mother, while my other brother lives in Detroit. My sister is doing time upstate. The one that I'm closest to is the oldest one. He's gay. We can talk about everything—there are no secrets between us. He didn't want to tell me when he found out, because he knew how I would feel. Because he didn't want to tell me, my mother told me. So then I told my mother to come and visit me with him, so he could tell me himself. He was scared, he thought I was going to change toward him, like his friends did.

When he came to see me, I acted like I didn't know anything. I let him tell me. And when he told me, he saw it didn't change the way I felt about him. He didn't let me drink from his soda can, and I got mad.

My family knows what type of work I do here. The next-to-oldest, he's the one that's real sick. We didn't get along that well on the street. He told me himself. I had called my mother, and she was crying. My mother couldn't tell me, so he got on the phone and told me. That's when he told me about my sister-in-law, his wife—she's sick too. My nieces so far have tested negative.

My youngest brother, he's just twenty-two years old. He's not open about his status. He's got a lot of anger. He got it from sex, from the first girl he ever had. He turned gay after that. I'm waiting for him to tell me about his status, so I can give him more information. He says he got it from this girl, because she had thrush in her mouth. I told my mother that I wanted to talk to him, but she said not to talk to him now, because nobody else in the house knows about it. But yesterday my mother told me in front of him and his lover.

My sister, she's HIV-positive, she's doing good. She says she's tired of jailing, she doesn't want to die in jail. She writes to me.

I probably escaped AIDS by being locked up. God knows what would have happened to me if I'd been out in the street running. I'm angry doing so much time for something I didn't do, but God knows I'm thankful for being locked up, because I would have been dead.

I got involved in ACE before I even knew any of my family had AIDS. One of my lovers had it—it's all crazy like a nightmare.

How does my mother deal with it? It's very hard for her. She stays by herself, and she doesn't talk about it, unless I call.

I don't know what the future holds, but I plan to do work around AIDS when I get out. I think it helps to be able to talk to all my family. I help them look for information, and maybe that helps. With my second brother, when I found out, I tried to get him to go to support groups with his wife, but he's not ready for it. His wife is in denial; she thinks my brother is going to get well. He might get well, but he might not.

In Puerto Rico it isn't the same as it is here. Support groups don't exist except in one town. They got hot lines, but that isn't as good as a support group. I barely sleep because I know that one day I'm going to get a call telling me that one of them died. I pray to God to at least let me out to spend a couple of days with them, if they are going to die.

My mother gives me strength, she talks to me, she tells me to be strong. If I'm not strong, she's going to get weak, she doesn't need one more in the family to go down. She needs all the support she can get.

After I wrote this piece, I received the news that my brother in Puerto Rico died. My fears of losing him came true.

* * *

Remember Us

In memory of my loving sister Yvette

I think of you often and remember us,
    I miss you dearly, "Yvette."
I remember you as a little baby, so beautiful
    and so soft, "My little white girl."
I remember the happy moments we shared your
    beautiful smile every time you smiled.
I remember the times we had in Kaiser Park,
    where we shared a beer or two and talked
    of things we felt most deeply.
I remember those happy moments hanging out at
    Corn Queen and the Polar Express at Coney Island,
    where to watch you dance was a pride that only I enjoyed.
I remember those special days we shared
    with the family on the beach and
    fishing with Pops on the pier.
I remember our pain, our tears, and the sadness,
    we felt when you told me you were positive.
I remember your phone calls, and your letters where
    we expressed our loneliness and our love for each other.
Yvette, I often sit alone and think of how you
    died and still I find it hard to understand
    why did I lose you?

Yvette no one but you could ever understand
just how much my heart aches for you.
I love you little SISTER and ALWAYS WILL.

Remembering you with love always.
Your sister, Aida

* * *

AIDS activists outside talk about the problem of survivors' guilt in the gay community. We, too, experience this. Many women express guilt, wondering why they are alive when so many of their friends and families have died.

* * *

One person I'll always remember is Jeannie. When we were teenagers we married into the same family. We were best friends, but we called ourselves sisters. I remember going to the doctor with her when she found out that she was pregnant. I have so many memories of her; singing in the park, going dancing, having fights, taking our children Jasmine and Lil Albert to the park, the memories go on and on. Our lives were good together, we were just kids. . . .

I was a year older than Jeannie; she always looked up to me. Unfortunately, there came a time when I wasn't much to look up to. I was getting myself involved deeper and deeper in the drug scene. I remember one day we were in the kitchen of my apartment. I was shooting heroin. Jeannie said that she wanted to try it too. I said no, but she persisted and eventually I gave in.

A couple of years later, I moved from Brooklyn to Queens. Distance and time separated us . . . life went on. Eventually, I wound up in Bedford. One day I was in the hospital building and someone called me. It was Jeannie. I was so happy and yet so sad to see her here. Who would have thought back when we were kids that someday we would wind up in prison doing time away from our children?

Jeannie tested positive for AIDS. I was devastated. I had been tested twice but I tested negative. While Jeannie was here, she informed me that many of our friends we had shared needles with had died. This was all both painful and very scary for me. In addition two of our brothers-in-law also died of AIDS-related causes. What a nightmare! Jeannie was so scared. She quickly began to get sick. I spent lots of time with her in IPC. I remember the day when Jeannie was to go home. She looked beautiful. I walked with her as far as I was allowed and we said our goodbyes. We hugged and cried, and for my own sense of sanity I made her promise that she would wait, but her eyes told me something different.

One day while I was in the school building one of Jeannie's friends told me that Jeannie died. I couldn't believe it. AIDS had struck again. The guilt that I felt was overwhelming. Why did I ever let her shoot drugs? Why didn't I fight harder to stop her? And why have so many of the same people that I shot drugs with died and I was still alive? I'll always wonder if I hadn't allowed Jeannie to shoot drugs, would she still be alive today?

* * *

Coping with death from a distance is part of the prison reality.

* * *

Dealing with death in prison can leave you confused and in disbelief. Receiving a message from someone that a loved one is gone gives you a lot of room for denial. You can easily refuse to believe, because it doesn't seem real. Even if you can accept that they passed while you were still in prison, how do you cope? How do you deal with the need to touch their things, to go to all the "familiar" places that are filled with that person's memories? You really never know for sure if you have begun to deal with their loss until you've had the opportunity to face these things.

* * *

And then, if you are able to go to the funeral, you face another set of experiences. Some women are confronted with an awful choice.

* * *

When my little brother died several years ago, I was angry and lost. Angry that I was here and not with him when he needed me. Angry that my mother was alone to deal with this. She didn't deserve that . . . I let her down. But I was also lost in the prison process that controls our ability to participate in the death and dying process. When a member of our immediate family is dying, we can request either a deathbed visit or to wait until they die and go to their funeral service. That's a hell of a choice! My little brother was in a coma, so the choice was unbearable. I chose to see him alive one last time. My family contacted my counselor here and gave her the verifications she needed . . . doctor confirmation that he wasn't expected to live long, that my family believed he would want me there. . . . Paperwork was done and approval sought for my trip to his hospital room. It took two and a half days before everything was worked out. On the third day, I would have seen him, had he lived that long. I found out about his death four hours before I was scheduled to go to his bedside. I no longer had an option; I was going to his funeral.

* * *

Provisions for funeral trips and deathbed visits are by nature "security-focused" rather than focused on our emotional needs and our families. The worst part for many women is being "chained to their pain," being prevented from running into their family's arms or reaching out and touching the hand of their loved one in the coffin.

* * *

I had already been told before we arrived, "The handcuffs stay on while you're at the funeral service." As we walked into the room where everyone was, I could see everyone turn to look at me. All of them had already been crying, it was a terrible thing to see. But the look on their faces when I shuffled in the door was worse—it is not describable. I had on shackles on my feet and you could hear the chain drag in the quiet funeral parlor. My hands were cuffed and a metal chain was wrapped around my waist and hooked through my cuffs. If I had ever had any illusions of wanting to be there to comfort my mother, they were shattered when I saw her looking at me standing there. At that moment, I wished it were me who had died. I'm twenty-three years old and in prison for drugs. That's bad enough, but at that moment I felt like I was a serial killer or some hideous creature all chained and cuffed. That's how I felt, because that's the way it seemed I must have looked to them. And no one wants to be cuffed when their family is hugging you and your hands are tied together, hurting, and you can't hug your family back, standing there . . . almost in reach. One thing that's a blessing is that some of the officers are considerate and have compassion. I wanted to hold on to my father's hand in the coffin, but with the cuffs it was hard and awkward. It upset my family when I struggled trying to, so I just whispered to my dad, "I'm sorry. Please look past these things and see me, please see that I love you and I'm sorry. Forgive me." I never want to go on another funeral trip again while in prison, but if I lose more of my family, I know I'll go anyway, regardless. It's just so shameful, so degrading, and it leaves you without the very things you went there for—to say goodbye in your own way, to hold someone who is crying, and to be held when your heart is coming undone.

* * *

ACE became a lightning rod for people's feelings of loss. We knew we had to find a way to help people express their grief, to help them survive it, and to help all of us survive it. We began a quilt project for women to make small quilt squares for their family members and friends. When we put up the sign-up sheet, more than a hundred people signed up on the first round to make quilt squares.

In the beginning of the epidemic, we were full of hope for a quick cure and were energized by our own mobilization. But the death toll rose, and a cure is not in sight. We have confronted many of the same feelings that people doing AIDS work outside of prison are facing: powerlessness, passivity, and cynicism. We look for strength by connecting to people outside the prison who are also involved in AIDS work, by addressing issues beyond the prison, by reaching past our own sorrow to help others, and by expanding our ability to meet people's needs.

THE ACE CONFERENCE

At an ACE meeting, the superintendent said, "Why don't you have a conference?" It was a perfect idea, a way to reach people we had no other access to, a way to share our struggles, our story, and our work. The themes would be the difficulties of fighting AIDS from inside prison walls and our need to link up with other people who were also fighting this virus on the outside.

It took over four months of solid work to put the conference together.

* * *

It was so stressful putting the conference together. I just kept thinking of how important it was, and kept working. I really couldn't get excited about it at that point. I just wanted it to happen. We needed help from the outside, but we also had a lot to offer them. Not that many people were reaching out to us, so we knew it was time for us to reach out to the rest of the world.

* * *

The guest list included inmates, prison civilians, administration, representatives from the other prisons in New York State, hospital workers, parole representatives, and community agencies. Many of the people who had made ACE possible in the very beginning, whom we had not seen for a long time, were also invited. It was scary, stressful, and exciting.

* * *

I waited years for it to happen. We burned out the copy machine twice and the computer once trying to put it all together. It was a lot of work, but I had a lot of hopes that went with it. I wanted people to understand what we were doing and why. AIDS work in prisons depends on peer education, and it was a chance to show them it truly works. We also wanted people outside prison to know that even though we are prisoners, many of us care about the fact that people are dying from AIDS. Not everyone who makes a mistake stops caring or being human.

* * *

Each of us was responsible for a part of the conference. This was the first time many of us spoke publicly. There were panels, a play, and four different workshops. The workshops included Parole Process and Community Linkage, ACE Guidelines (creating a peer counseling and education program in other prisons), Women's Issues Surrounding HIV/AIDS, and PWAs Empowerment in Prison.

* * *

It was during the planning of the conference that our big banner was created. It's a large quilt with the names of all the women we've lost embroidered on it in different colors. I was really pleased with it as I worked on it. When we finally hung it that day in the gym, however, it suddenly looked different. The impact on me was just tremendous. I just looked at it and realized just how many women there were who would only be with us in spirit on that day. I cried. My eyes were full of tears all day. It was overwhelming, just the fact that we had come that far to reach that day.

* * *

There were numerous positive outcomes from this conference: Representatives from other prisons, such as Albion and Mid-Orange, exchanged ideas for building programs about AIDS. In addition, we began to build a network of communication for the women who were transferred to Albion. Parole representatives agreed to explore the possibility of women on parole, normally not permitted to associate with one another, to meet when dealing with AIDS-related issues; women from ACE educated people from the outside about AIDS in prison and about women and AIDS and demonstrated the strength of open PWAs. For the women in ACE, we saw the social impact and felt our own personal accomplishment. We had become organizers, inspiring others beyond the prison, encouraging AIDS work in other prisons, the Division of Parole, and women's communities.

ACE WALKATHONS

We have held two walkathons. When we first thought about doing a walkathon around the issue of AIDS, the question that came up was what did we want to do with the money we raised. We knew that we wanted to give some of the money to a children's organization or hospital, but we had no idea where to find one. We sent letters to different places, but received no answer. Then we heard about Incarnation Children's Center through a civilian from the Women's Prison Association.

* * *

Sister Bridget came to meet with us. She shared a presentation about the babies with us, and from that moment on we knew that our hearts would be open to the Incarnation Children's Center. We are able to place a face to the many children who are suffering with HIV/AIDS as we are here in the prison.

* * *

In our Second Annual ACE Walkathon, in 1994, women in Bedford Hills walked around the small prison yard to raise money. Most of the 250 women were connected to AIDS through the death of at least one close friend or family member or by being HIV-positive themselves. But they were walking to raise money for the babies who are HIV-infected and reside at the Incarnation Children's Center, and for the women who are sick in the IPC infirmary and for ACE projects.

The yard was decorated with multicolored cardboard balloons, each painted with the name of a baby from Incarnation Children's Center who had died; two life-sized cardboard figures of long-distance runners, representing women surviving and thriving with AIDS; a rainbow of hands with the names of past and present ACE members; and our large quilt with names of each of the women from Bedford who had died, all hung up along the fence. Each woman wearing a red ribbon, we walked for several hours along with some community AIDS workers. The sun shone down on us, and the atmosphere was upbeat. A loudspeaker filled the yard with music from salsa to Motown to Queen's "We Are the Champions," silenced only when the music paused to allow the reading of names of those who had died—at Bedford, among friends and family, and the babies.

The Walkathon allowed women to feel that they could help others, not just be the one needing help. And it was not just a feeling: the women of Bedford raised $8,000 in pledges from correctional officers and civilian employees at Bedford and from friends and family, money that will concretely make a difference in people's lives.

GOING HOME ON PAROLE

For many women, leaving prison raises both hopes for a new life and fears of whether or not we can make it. PWAs face added issues and need a lot of preparation.

* * *

I started working on my discharge planning for six months before I went out on parole. I needed to make arrangements for my medical care and housing and for an outside support system, and I decided to get myself involved in AIDS activism on the outside so I could prevent myself from going back to using drugs. I wrote job applications to outside AIDS agencies to work as an educator. Once the board granted me parole, I wrote to residential programs for ex-offenders and told them my approximate release date. I got an acceptance from Providence House. In September 1990, four days before I left to go, Providence House called me to say that there were no beds available, there was an emergency situation. Instead I was to be released to the Parole Resource Center, an emergency shelter that I desperately wanted to avoid. Then Providence House called me, they had a bed for me, but my parole officer was dragging his heels about letting me go. I called Terri Wurmser, the client services specialist at the Division of Parole, to advocate for me. I got into Providence House, and a civilian ACE staff member took me clothes shopping and then drove me to Providence House.

* * *

For Katrina, going to Providence House instead of an emergency shelter meant that she had a chance to make it. At Providence House she was surrounded by people who cared, who supported her dream of becoming an

AIDS activist, and who were there for her each day when she came home after looking for a job. It helped to have familiar faces, including the director of Providence House, Sister Elaine, who directs The Children's Center at Bedford Hills and works with women and their children while in prison.

Another woman, Jay, was not so fortunate, even though she had a civilian community counselor helping her. Although a good discharge planner can make a big difference to a person's survival on the outside, there is no guarantee that the woman will get the support and resources that she needs.

* * *

Jay wanted to go home to her kids, but she was afraid of telling her family her HIV status. In addition, she didn't like the neighborhood she was going back to because of pressures to use drugs, which would get her rearrested. Yolanda, our civilian discharge counselor, started working with her. I remember hearing an argument Yolanda was having with somebody over the phone. Apparently, Jay was going to be sent to a shelter upon release, and Yolanda wanted her to go to a halfway house, which would have been easier for her because there was more supervision to help her with her status and addiction. They released her to a shelter anyway. Jay kept in touch with Yolanda by phone once or twice and then she went to her brother's house. We found out later that Jay had gone back to using drugs and that her brother didn't know where she was. A few weeks later her body was found in the railroad yards where all the old trains are parked.

It hit me that no matter how much we try to help some of the women in here, if we don't have a better support system out there, then they will go back to using drugs. When you're working with your buddy and they tell you that they don't want to leave and then you find out that they have died, you doubt yourself as a person and as a buddy. You wonder if you really want another buddy, and that probably when they go home you'll lose them too—the failure of the system and of their own problems.

* * *

For PWAs, having an emotionally supportive environment is critical. They are dealing with powerful emotions, as well as the concrete problems of survival.

* * *

Now having the opportunity of comparing the difference between the sense of community inside the walls of Bedford Hills Correctional Facility to the "outside," I can say there is no comparison. Regardless of the loss of so-called freedom by being behind bars, I have said many times that I wish I was back inside with my supportive community of ACE. Maybe it isn't fair to compare, because it is a unique environment—we not only met together as a group of women sharing, discussing, and exploring new ideas around AIDS issues, we also lived together.

* * *

ACE HOME

Many women leaving prison have said that they needed a buddy, someone to show them how to deal with setting themselves up for medical and addiction treatment, and someone who would be there to support their choices—a buddy who's been there herself. Often a woman returns to an abusive relationship or to an environment where it is difficult to refrain from using drugs because she cannot afford to live independently somewhere else.

ACE always had a dream of having ACE in the outside community for women who leave on parole. We knew as soon as we created ACE that there was a great need for a supportive community for women who are PWAs when they leave prison. It required having enough ACE members who had already been released from prison and who were able to create a sister organization on the outside. By 1992, that condition existed. We were ready to create ACE HOME. It was made up of women who were touched by ACE when they were in prison—either as a member or as someone who had been helped by it.

* * *

I came to Bedford in 1989. I had my HIV test here. In the back of my mind I knew that I had the virus. I met Katrina when she came into the back units to do AIDS education, and I told her that I had the virus. I didn't make any plans for when I was coming out. I went back to the same life I knew, and I was back in Bedford in 1990. I saw Katrina again. So many of my friends had died from HIV and drug addiction that I wanted to know more about ACE. I never joined ACE as a member, but I came and stuffed envelopes in the ACE office and I read every piece of information that I was stuffing into those envelopes. I left Bedford again, went back to my three kids, and immediately started working on my drug addiction. I went to Narcotics Anonymous, and their advice was to keep busy. They could only help me with my addiction, they couldn't help me with my HIV. And none of the AIDS groups gave priority to my needs because I was asymptomatic. That's when I started seeking out support groups, that's when I started helping to build ACE Home.

* * *

ACE Home set the following goals:

Provide a Mentor/Buddy Program
. . . Meet the woman prior to her release date from prison to assess the needs she will have upon release;
. . . Meet her, if at all possible, at the Facility when she is released, escorting her to the Department of Social Services and other agencies for health care, social services, housing etc.
. . . Bring her to ACE Home support groups, twelve-steps meetings, and other programs of recovery.

Sponsor Regular Support Groups
Provide a nutritional meal, a safe environment in which women can talk about the issues that they are confronting, and transportation assistance, if needed, to be able to attend the meeting.

Sponsor Empowerment Workshops
Teach women to access agencies, fill out forms, and advocate on their own behalf; present HIV/AIDS-related issues; discuss how to go on a job interview, family violence, parenting issues, stress management, etc.

Making Referrals
To agencies that can help with the problems that women who are HIV-positive are facing.

How ACE Home Came About

Just as the creation of ACE broke new ground within the criminal justice system, so did the creation of ACE Home. In 1992, after a number of preliminary meetings about the idea of ACE Home, Jacqueline McDonald, ACE coordinator, arranged a meeting in the prison between ACE members; Ann Jacobs, executive director of the Women's Prison Association; Terry Wurmser, client service specialist of the Division of Parole; and two ACE members who were released and on parole—Katrina and T.J. The key problem presented by the idea of ACE Home was how to get permission for ex-offenders to meet with other ex-offenders on the outside. Any socialization between ex-inmates on parole is usually considered a parole violation.

Terri suggested that ACE on the outside might be able to meet in the Parole office building. This location wasn't ideal: we knew that women would be afraid to meet there. Some women kept their HIV status secret the entire time they were in prison and would not jeopardize their privacy by showing up to an ACE Home meeting in the Parole office. ACE asked Ann Jacobs if WPA would consider taking on this project; Ann said that she would propose it to the board. Terri subsequently obtained support from Parole for women to meet on the outside.

The founding meeting of ACE Home occurred inside the prison and involved current ACE members in prison and those women who were now home on parole and who would take responsibility for building ACE Home. The superintendent agreed to let the women on parole into the facility whenever necessary for the development of ACE Home. This decision also meant breaking new ground. Once a woman leaves prison, she needs permission from both parole and the superintendent to come back into the prison. It is not unusual for permission to be granted after six months for a personal visit. It *is* unusual, however, for permission to be granted to come back and participate in a program. Soon after our reunion meeting, we got a letter from Ann Jacobs offering the WPA as a meeting space for ACE Home. She also said that ACE Home could use the kitchen for group meals. We were thrilled.

In helping other women, ACE Home members have also helped themselves. Being a member of ACE Home gave some of the women a purpose and identity, a sense of confidence and self-respect that helped them overcome the tragedy of AIDS.

* * *

I get such inspiration when I go into the prison to do outreach, I can't even sleep the night before. I know the ladies have heard it all before, but it's different when they heard it from their own kind. I went to speak at Riker's Island, and there were inmates against the wall, women inmates. The commissioner of corrections was there that day also. And when the ladies saw me walking down the hall they said, "Yeah, they don't never clean up the place until people from the commissioner's office come in."

And I happened to turn around and said to one of them, "I'm you, you're me. I stood in these walls and said the same thing you said." One of the ladies hollered, "I know her, that's Linda! She's been in here." They can understand where I'm coming from instead of hearing someone reading books and then telling them stuff. It doesn't work like that. When they heard it from me, they kind of felt it.

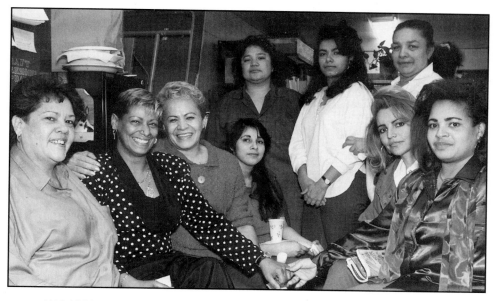

WOMEN FROM THE HISPANIC SECTOR OF ACE, 1992-93
Left to right: Violeta Acevedo; Doris Moices; Carmen Olivera;
Migdalia Martinez; Ana Maria Rodriguez; Sandra Ospina; Marleny Agero;
Gladys Franco; Awilda Gonzalez.

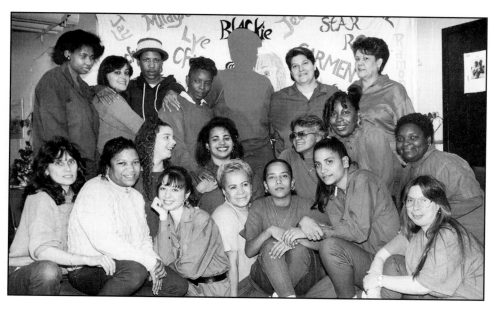

A GROUP OF ACE INMATE STAFF AND ORGANIZATION MEMBERS (1992)
Top, standing, left to right: Gloria Edwards; Ruth Rodriguez; Donna Harvey; Joanne Brown;
Cathy Salce; Violeta Acevedo.
Middle: Bonnie Forant; Awilda Gonzalez; Aida Rivera; Doris Romeo; Lisa Osborne
Bottom: Kathy Boudin; Viniece Walker; Lisa Finkle; Carmen Olivera; Betsy Gonzalez;
Rachel Luna; Christine Forsythe.

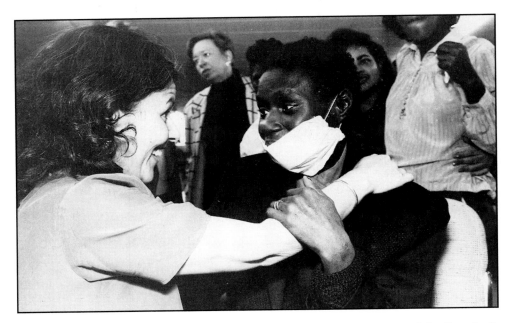

In October, 1991, ACE held a book party to celebrate the completion of the first draft of *Breaking the Walls of Silence.* Katrina Haslip, who had been out on parole for a year, an AIDS activist during that time, had asked the Superintendent to have such a party, perhaps knowing that it might be the last time that we would see her. Katrina died six weeks later

Below: Carmen Royster, a PWA and founding member of ACE, (center) with Judith Clark at the ACE book party. Carmen died twelve weeks later.

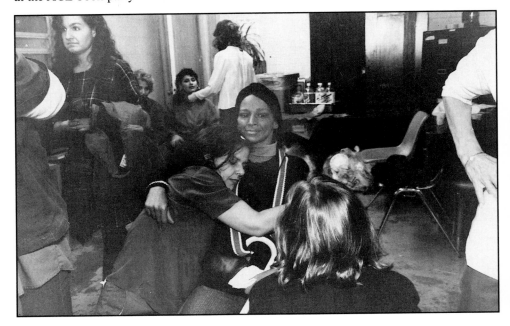

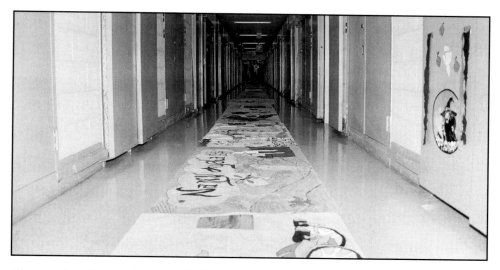

The corridor of a housing unit. Quilts are laying on the corridor floor, by the women for their sisters from Bedford Hills who had died. After a memorial is held for the women, the quilts are sent to the Names Project and become part of the national quilt.

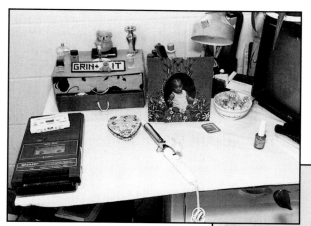

INSIDE A CELL:
A cardboard makeshift shelf resting on two cabinets.

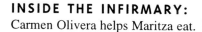

INSIDE THE INFIRMARY:
Carmen Olivera helps Maritza eat.

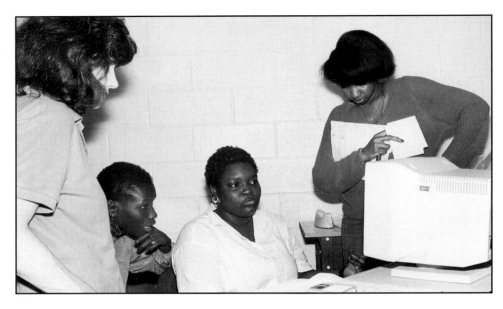

AT WORK IN THE ACE OFFICE
Left to right: Kathy Boudin; Katrina Haslip; Lisa Osborne; Gloria Edwards.

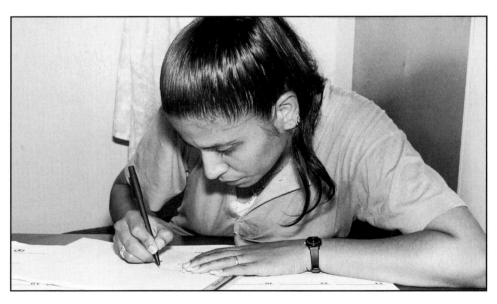

Rachel Luna goes over a list of names after doing orientation for the new women who just arrived at Bedford Hills Correctional Facility. She will ask the civillian counselor to call the women who signed up to come to the ACE office for support and education.

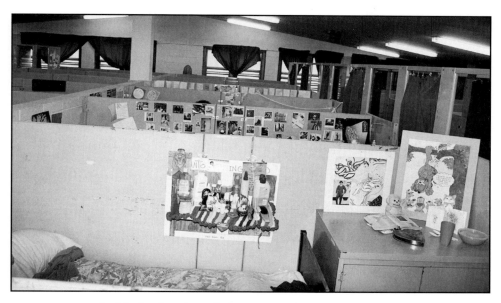

Inside the dormitory living area of the "backbuildings,"
where ACE first did educational outreach.

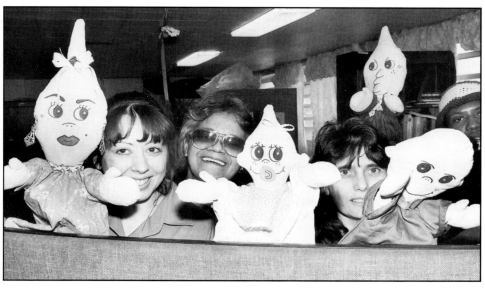

The puppet show "Once Upon A Virus." ACE members put on the puppet show
for children visiting their mothers in The Children's Center.
Left to right: Lisa Finkle; Aida Rivera; Kathy Boudin; Donna Harvey.

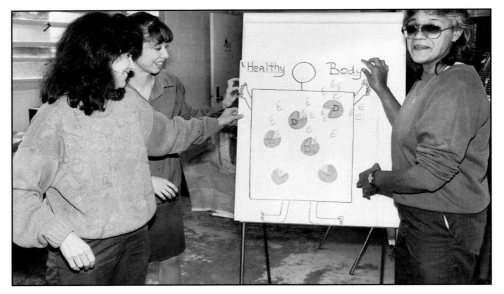

TEACHING THE WORKSHOP "What is HIV/AIDS?"
Left to right: Kathy Boudin; Lisa Finkle; Aida Rivera.

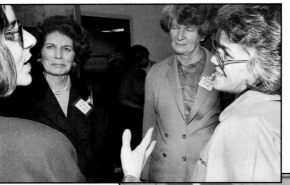

Debra Levine and Aida Rivera speak with two women from the Women's Prison Association.

Left to right: Aida Rivera, Katrina Haslip who is visiting from parole to help write *Breaking the Walls of Silence*, and Doris Romeo in the yard outside the ACE office.

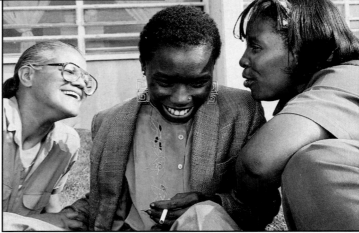

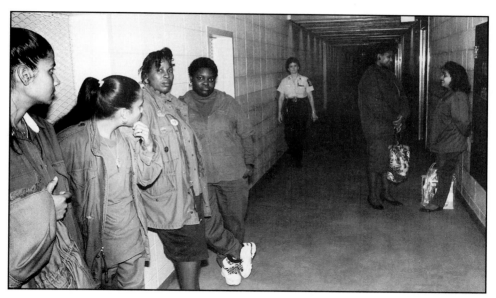

ACE members standing in corridor waiting for an officer to open the gate.
Left to right: Rachel Luna; Betsy Gonzalez; Doris Romeo; Lisa Osborne; Awilda Gonzalez.

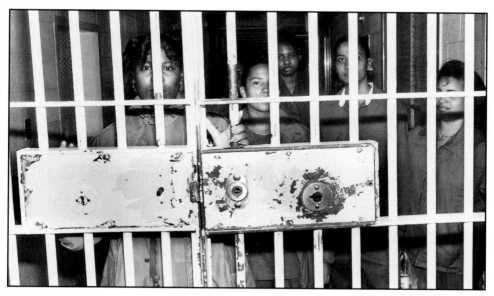

Women waiting for an officer to open the gate.

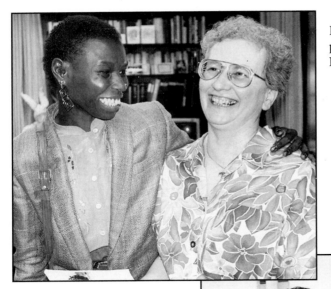

Katrina Haslip, after she was
paroled, and Superintendent
Elaine A. Lord. (1991)

**PEER COUNSELING
IN THE MAIN YARD**
Left to right: Joanne
Brown talks with Awilda
Gonzalez

ACE members walk
toward the yard.

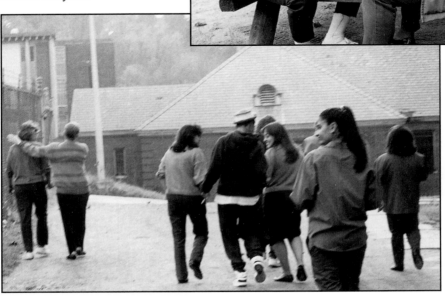

6
The Day-to-Day Work of ACE

PEER SUPPORT AND COUNSELING

Peer counseling—I'm just impressed that we can do it. I didn't know what kind of potential we'd have as peers. We speak the language that each of us understands. Even if it's silent, even if it's with our eyes, it's something that each of us seems to understand. I know I wouldn't want someone from the Department of Health trying to educate me about IV drug use when they haven't even taken a Valium. How could they give me helpful hints? I would feel that they are so out of tune with reality that I wouldn't be able to hear them.

ACE counsels women who are facing painful, frightening, traumatic times: a woman experiencing the death of a husband, brother, or sister; a woman who discovers that she herself is HIV-positive; a woman who was feeling healthy and now is breaking out into sweats and fevers and fears she will die any day; a woman who is going home to a family that she fears will reject her because she is HIV-positive.

Fear and stigma encircle our counseling. A woman may not want to come to the ACE office because she is fearful that it will reveal her secret that she is HIV-positive. Yet she needs to talk. We can meet in the yard, exchange words while waiting for Commissary, or give a hug while passing by the mess hall.

As *peer* counselors, we sometimes need to contact a professional within the prison to offer counseling services we are not equipped to provide. But we are able to meet essential needs: to care enough to listen as women express their feelings, to help them to define their choices and to make their own decisions, to provide the information that necessarily accompanies HIV/AIDS counseling. We are here seven days a week, at all hours. ACE members live on every unit and work in every workplace. As peer counselors we do a job that could not be done any other way. There would never be enough money to hire enough people to meet the emotional crises that HIV/AIDS has created for our community. In our work, some of us use the word "sister," some use "client," but however we say it, as peer counselors we are here for the women.

We deal with several counseling issues: the experience of taking the HIV-antibody test; preparing to go home and the issues that HIV/AIDS raises; living with AIDS; grief and loss.

Taking the HIV-Antibody Test

More and more women are taking the HIV-antibody test. We have learned the importance of counseling before a test. Often an ACE member goes with a woman when the blood is drawn. The waiting period of weeks is one filled with enormous anxiety, and we try to be there for her during that time.

If a woman finds out that she is HIV-positive, she is then faced with a profoundly new reality and needs a lot of support. She also needs as much knowledge about the virus as possible. We explore with her what is happening to her body, what her options are in terms of medication and diet, and who might be of support to her in and out of prison.

* * *

June 28, 1990, is a day I'll never forget. It was on that day that I found out I was positive for the HIV virus. At the time I had been an ACE member and an HIV/AIDS educator for about a year and a half. I had also worked with many HIV-positive women, encouraging them to go on and not to give up. But on June 28, all the positive, empowering things I had said to others went right out the window. My first thought was, "Oh, God, I'm going to die." I've never been so afraid in my life. I felt like: Why me? Why now? I mean, I was no longer doing anything to put me at risk. I was no longer promiscuous. I wasn't using drugs anymore. I was getting my life together. I was in a drug program, going to school, and doing what I enjoy doing—helping others. It's strange though, that once I found out my status, I didn't want to do anything. What for? I was dying. I finally understood how all the women I spoke to felt, and how nothing anyone said to me and nothing I knew about the virus meant anything. It took lots of tears and support from my ACE sisters for me to finally tap into my knowledge of HIV/AIDS and begin to accept my diagnosis and the fact that I was not different from the women I had viewed as clients.

* * *

If a woman tests negative, we want to do the best we can to help her stay that way. We educate her and explain to her that she has choices regarding sexual and/or drug practices. Being educated and learning about making the right choices can help stop the spread of AIDS.

Women Going Home

We work with women who are HIV-positive in the months before they go home on parole. They may need to make a clinic appointment, get their medical summary from the hospital here, apply for their ADAP card (AIDS Drug Assistance Program), or get housing. Housing is a central yet difficult issue, because often the most accessible housing for a woman may be a place that is not a positive environment for her:

I had one lady that had a drug problem and she wanted to get paroled to her sister's house. She had talked to me on several occasions about her sister, who got high. I put a few ideas out there for her but in a form of a question such as: "If you go and live with your sister, would you be able to keep from getting high?" "Are you strong enough to walk away from that temptation?" "Can you be in the same room with your sister and watch her get high and not want any?" I then let her know that if this was the only housing she had, that I would help her find a place to stay, such as a drug-rehabilitation program. I just couldn't come out and say, "Look you can't go there," so I gave her a few ideas and encouraged her to make her own choices. I also told her that her parole officer would have the last say on her place of residence. He would have to be the one to investigate and see if he approves of the environment. If he feels that the environment isn't good, then we would have to start all over again. That's one of the reasons why we start this process early.

* * *

Housing is one area for which we need a civilian community liaison in order to do the work. They can pick up the telephone, develop options they are familiar with, and build a network of contacts in the housing and social service world.

Our prerelease counseling also addresses hard emotional issues that a woman will face when she goes home:

"My kids don't know about me. I didn't want to tell them while I was here. But now I can't put it off anymore. I wonder if they will accept me."

"I know if I start to get sick, I'm going back to drugs. I won't be able to take it. But I don't want to hurt my children any more than I have."

"I'm going back to my husband. He's HIV-positive. I think he infected me. I have a lot of anger, but I also love him and I want to be there for him."

Whether it's children, a mother, a husband, or how to have safe sex, it is always also a question of how to face the world, how to come out of prison already bearing the weight of that experience and label, and how now to live with being HIV-positive "positively." It is about building up self-esteem and courage.

Living with AIDS

Women who are HIV-positive come to ACE to talk about many issues. They talk about their fears of dying, of suffering, of telling their families, of whether they can have a child, or of what to tell their children. For women in ACE who are PWAs, peer counseling raises special challenges.

* * *

I've been a counselor now for two years in ACE. Mainly I work with other women who are HIV-positive. Oh, yeah, I forgot, I too am HIV-positive. Sometimes I have to admit it gets really hard for me to remain a counselor and not speak from my own experience, identifying the similarities between me and the client, instead of helping them see their options. On the one hand, it feels good to be able to relate to and understand who you're talking to, but that same understanding can sometimes not be so good. Sometimes I sit and listen to women talking about all the medical problems they're having, or mental problems, and I say to myself, "Is this what I have to look forward to?" Sometimes I just want to run away from ACE, away from HIV/AIDS, and just pretend neither of them exists, but then I remember the women I work with and how their just seeing me sometimes gives them hope, so I go back to work. After I meet with my ACE counselor and get rid of all my negative feelings, I'm then ready to counsel. You see, I'm not just an ACE counselor, I'm also a client.

* * *

In addition to one-to-one support, ACE also has had PWA support groups and support groups for women whose loved ones are HIV-positive. These we call a significant-other group.

* * *

To me, a support group is good because it helps you adjust to your illness. You can see other people who have the disease living a long time. When I was in a support group, it helped me overcome my denial and fear that other people wouldn't accept me. They've been through what I've been through. Some are doing better, some worse, but we know we're in the same boat and we can help one another.

* * *

As women and as prisoners, we have many issues that may or may not be AIDS-related. We refer women to programs that can meet other needs of theirs: Children's Center, Family Violence, ASAT (Alcohol Substance Abuse Treatment). We don't always sit around and discuss AIDS. We talk about our children, our families, drugs, or just different experiences in our life, in and out of prison. A lot of the time we laugh. In this work—let alone in this life!—you have to have a sense of humor.

> It's difficult getting out
> of Bed. These Days.
> Yet I know what lies ahead
> will require me to force
> the muscles to me
> standing on these painful leg bones.
> I'm remembering when I was
> the best on my feet.
> I could dance
> on the tip of my toes!
> I grasp on to those moments

I'm on stage with the lead
part, of *Grease*.
Wow!! Whee!!
There I go, I'm without
limits, without the pain.
The dance of the 50's,
Do you love me? Do you love me?
Now that I can dance
Watch me now. I do the
mashed potatoes, I'll do the twist.
I could shake, shake. Do you like
it like this?
It's difficult getting out of bed
These days.
But not in my head.
— Doris Moices

We are prisoners first, counselors second. We are subject to rules and regulations that often interfere with our counseling. We might be in the middle of a session, when everyone is suddenly ordered back to their housing unit. Or a plan for a counseling session may be affected by an unexpected outside hospital trip, a dental appointment, or a visit. Prison is on the one hand regimented but on the other hand filled with appointments over which we have no control. Frequently, a person whom we have been counseling is transferred—"drafted"—to another facility. This means we cannot put closure between ourselves and the woman. We can only hope that when she reaches her destination, someone will be there to pick up where we left off.

Not every woman wants to be counseled by an inmate. Some feel that we don't know enough, while others feel that it gives us too much power as inmates or they fear that we'll break confidentiality. In these situations, it is helpful to have a civilian staff person available as a counselor.

Our Training

We have had formal training through the New York State Department of Health HIV/AIDS Pre- and Post-Test Counseling Certification Program. We also rely on our own experiences. We analyze them, formalize them and then teach counseling to new ACE members. We pose questions that we continually reexamine: What is counseling? What are the qualities of a good counselor and of a bad counselor? What is the difference in being a peer counselor versus a counselor who is a professional? What are some of the problems peer counselors may run into? What is the difference between a friend and a counselor?

It is this last question that best captures our experience as peer counselors. We counsel the same people with whom we share our lives and sometimes friendships. As a friend, we may be much more passionate in imposing our concerns, hopes, fears, and ultimately judgments, whereas counseling involves helping a person define her choices and allows her to make her own decisions. We often find ourselves wearing two different hats, and sometimes we have to choose which one to wear.

* * *

I had been doing counseling work for some time and thought I was very effective at it. I had even begun to perfect certain aspects of my counseling. Several months and hundreds of clients later, my best friend revealed to me she was HIV-positive. Suddenly, my counseling techniques went out the door and I immediately responded to her as a friend. This was to become the beginning of numerous nights of personal conflict with little sleep and one hell of a dilemma.

I told my friend what her HIV diagnosis actually meant—that there was this big difference between HIV infection and AIDS; that it did not necessarily mean that she would immediately progress on to AIDS; this new information did not have to mean instant death.

We talked about several topics: Risk-Reduction, Significant Others, and Treatment. Yes, treatment . . . treatment that she did not want to receive and that she believed she did not need. That's when I'm certain that I lost my counseling ability and fell into my friend role. I could not understand how she could share her diagnosis with me as a counselor and then expect me (as her friend) to accept the reality that she did not wish to be treated!

I was frantic! As a friend, I thought of making an appointment with the doctors for her and then just taking her there. As her counselor/adviser, however, I knew she was entitled to make her own choices, regardless of how I might be affected. I could not think in terms of "empowerment" for her. My idea of that was my advocacy for her and my holding her hand. It meant being there for her, because she was my friend. Yet I knew that it was becoming overwhelming and I had to detach myself somehow. I knew that I could not detach myself from our friendship and do only counseling. I knew that she needed both a counselor and a friend and that counseling alone was simply not applicable to us. I could not counsel her about treatment options and have her take in none of these choices. Nor could I convince myself that in time she would come around. In fact, I was not willing to wait and see. If I failed as a counselor, it was okay, I could live with that. But I could not accept my ability to fail as a friend.

IPC – OUR INFIRMARY *

IPC was a place where nobody wanted to stay. One woman told me that she was going to die, because this was where they put people who were going to die. Just looking at the place made people feel this way. Because of this overwhelming feeling, we knew that ACE had to make a difference in IPC. A group of the women from ACE started going to IPC. We started cleaning, painting, and at the same time taking care of the women who were sick. Comforting them and making them feel alive again. We let them know that they don't have to feel alone, that they have friends in ACE. They also understand that they are not there to die but to live life to the fullest.

If you look through the crisscross metal grating of the locked gate that separates the infirmary from the medical-clinic waiting area, you see a short corridor lined with doors that open into rooms. The infirmary is small, holding at the most twelve people, but it is vital to us because it is where people are struggling for their health, and often for their lives.

The infirmary houses women who are too sick to be on their regular housing unit but not sick enough to be in one of the outside hospitals that take Bedford's women. Some women are in IPC for a short time, recovering from a leg injury, a burn, an operation, or perhaps their first opportunistic infection of AIDS. Others may live there for as long as six months or a year, if they are chronically weak and need constant care.

IPC is at the heart of our work because it is about life and death. Everywhere in the AIDS movement, people have struggled to make it less about dying and more about living. And ACE, in this tradition, grew out of the early attempts to transform IPC from a place of isolation and death into a place of healing and life.

---

*The next two sections are "IPC-Our Infirmary" and "Medical Advocacy. While our experience has taught us that inmates can play a critical role in caring for sick inmates in the infirmary and as medical advocates working in cooperation with medical personnel, the utilization of inmates by the prison medical department has expanded and contracted at different points in ACE's history.

As ACE members, we work in IPC along with other women—porters, aides, nurses. Job assignments fade into one another: we may help the porters to buff and clean, we help the nurse's aide change sheets and bathe women; we accompany wheelchair-bound women to church or to their visits; we pick up their packages in the package room if they need our help. We serve as medical advocates to the women housed in the IPC unit so that they can better understand what is being said to them by their doctors. Underlying any particular task is the human connection between the women housed in the IPC unit and our ACE members. What makes the difference is the friendships that grow. That alone is life-sustaining.

When we look at the rising numbers of people who have HIV/AIDS, we see that there are not enough funds to pay civilians to meet the daily needs of those who are sick. The role of ACE members and the other women who work in IPC is critical. A stark illustration of this is in the twenty-four-hour medical watch. The administration and the medical director have numerous times asked the ACE organization to provide twenty-four-hour care for a woman. A dozen or more ACE members sign up for six-hour blocks of time to cover as many days or weeks as are necessary.

We know that some of the women do not have long to live. A woman may be just twenty, twenty-five, or thirty years old and the HIV virus is already getting her. She no longer wants to fight this illness. Reluctantly, we have to face the fact that we cannot change this. But we attempt to change how these last months are spent. We share laughter, we share warmth, and we share our dignity.

Some of the women who are sick may not have close family members, and their friendship with an ACE member may become the most important relationship in their lives.

* * *

I met Sheryl H. during one of my regular visits to IPC. Sheryl was in need of help, but when I asked her if she needed it, she said no. Sheryl had gangrene on all ten fingers and toes. One day I heard someone crying in the ladies' room. It was Sheryl. I asked if something was wrong. She answered, "no." So I left, only to come back again and attempt to talk to Sheryl again. One day I just sat on her bed and I told her I wasn't leaving until she would tell me what was wrong. That broke the ice between us, and a bond was formed. Sheryl expressed her fears and her pain to me. She allowed me to braid her hair and change the bandages on her fingers and her toes.

Sheryl was granted parole, but two months before her release her gangrene began to get worse. She was moved to the outside hospital so they could operate. They planned to cut off all her fingers and toes. This was hard for Sheryl to accept, but she understood that this had to be done. I felt really sad, because I wanted to be with her but we knew this was impossible. But I was glad it would be done.

Then I heard that she sat there for a whole month alone and they didn't even operate. I thought I'd never see her again, she would be released from there. But when she realized she wasn't getting the operation, she demanded to come back so she could say goodbye. She had only a week until she would go home. But she had gotten much sicker, and when she came back I looked at her and I knew that she wasn't going to live long. I've been around enough to feel that death look. The day she was supposed to be paroled, she died. As much as I tried to prepare, I could not stop the pain of her loss. But I feel good because she's one person I got to say goodbye to—because she came back to say goodbye to me.

* * *

For others, who may be suffering from their first opportunistic infection, IPC may be a safe haven, a space in which they can absorb the reality that they have HIV/AIDS, to say it out loud to others and gather the strength to face the outside. Emma talks about this:

The next big thing I had to face was the fear I had of being rejected by my loved ones and my friends—of being alone with this. That's when I began to educate myself about the HIV virus. The biggest step for me, however, happened when I was hospitalized in 1991. I was in IPC. I was scared to go there, I was feeling isolated already, and I was afraid that being there would make it worse. While I was there, I made the decision to let people know that I was infected with the HIV virus. In fact, I wanted *everyone* to know. I couldn't stand feeling bad about my status and keeping it a secret. I was tired of fearing rejection. I told an ACE worker named Gloria. She listened and asked me questions, but she didn't turn her back and reject me. Soon, I had begun telling others and begun finding that I had family and friends in the facility. The women who were patients with me in IPC became my family. The doctors and nurses and the ACE women became a part of it and added to the caring. While I was there, ACE came and gave us Christmas parties and did activities with us. They did nurse's aide work for the women who couldn't bathe themselves or change their sheets. They helped keep the place clean and were always there to talk with us as counselors.

When it came time for me to go, I was scared to leave, because I had their support there and encouragement. I didn't know how population would accept me. It was while I was still a patient that I decided that I wanted to be an ACE member and that I wanted to work in IPC. The other patients were my friends and family—now that I'm out and working there, that hasn't changed. The women in IPC are my friends, and we are family.

* * *

As caregivers, we want to be women who can be relied on. But we don't want to foster passivity and dependency. We ask one another, how do we help women to be independent? When do we do too much? And when is it right for us to cut back on what we do because the woman is ready to do more for herself?

I remember when there were fifteen of us working around the clock, day after day with Nay Nay. Some people said, "Hey, she really can feed herself now and she can move herself from the wheelchair onto the bed." Other women said, "But when I'm with her, she can't do any of those things." I was one of those people. Then one day when Nay Nay was really hungry and she couldn't get anyone's attention, I saw her wheel herself in the wheelchair, get the bread, wheel herself to the microwave and make her sandwich. I just shook my head. I knew I had been had for many days now.

* * *

When a woman goes out to the outside hospital, we cannot go with her. We have to depend on the doctors, nurses, and civilian staff for information on how she is feeling and if and when she is coming back to the prison. It is difficult to just sit and wait for news of someone whom you have cared about for a long time. The most difficult time is when you fear that it is the last time you will see someone.

* * *

I knew Carmen from the outside, from when she was seven. So when she got sick here, I was like her big sister. I spent months by her side in IPC. We talked about her son who had died, about my sister who had AIDS, and about herself and death. When she said she wanted to die, I said, "Stop talking like that." But after a couple of months I came to the realization that she was going to die, she was getting sicker, and she talked about going to be with her son and my sister. She helped me deal with death.

I had this fear that one day I would come to IPC and she wouldn't be there, so I spent as much time as I could with her. One day I went upstairs for the 6:00 count; Kathy stayed with her, massaging her legs. It seemed like the longest count. I was in my room, I kept waiting. As soon as the doors opened I hurried down the hill with Maria. It was raining, and as we hit the turn before the hospital Maria said, "Look, there's an ambulance." I saw it and immediately thought of Carmen, and I ran toward it. The medics were carrying Carmen out on a stretcher. I said to her, "Carmen, where are you going?" She turned to me and said, "Where the fuck do you think I'm going?" She was coming in and out of reality, pointing to the rainy sky and talking about the stars.

When I went into the hospital, I wanted to curse everybody out. When I went into IPC, I saw Kathy sitting on a couch and I started yelling at her, "Why the fuck didn't you call me? You knew she was leaving," and I started to cry. Kathy started to cry and said, "I told them to call you but it was count—you couldn't come during count." We held on to each other and cried. It took a moment to realize that the superintendent was standing there. She told me she had to send her out, she was too sick to stay. That was the last time I saw Carmen. She died about a month later.

All of us who have worked in IPC have gotten exhausted from it. Perhaps someone we were close to died, and simply being there meant feeling too much pain. Sometimes we have left for good, sometimes for a break.

I've been visiting IPC since sometime in 1988. You get burned out. You watch people suffer and die and wonder, Could it be you, and when it's your time, will somebody be there for you? It scares you and it hurts. I stopped for a while in 1989, for six months, because a very close friend of mine died.

* * *

Despite the problems, our work in IPC makes a tremendous difference. Sometimes we meet a woman who seems so sick that she won't live more than a few days. Then, over time, with care and love, we watch her move back into life. One of these women, Sheryl T., tells about herself:

In 1990, I took the test, because I had been using drugs all my life. I was feeling good, but I started breaking out with herpes. I had a rash—I guess it was shingles. I was going for surgery for a skin graft, and they tested my blood. I didn't know anything about AIDS at the time. I really didn't believe when the test came out positive—I took a positive test result as a sure sign of death. I got paroled and started using again. I stayed out for a year. I told my kids while I was out—they were ten and nineteen.

I went back to selling and using drugs and violated my parole. I came back to prison and got sick. I kept losing weight, I couldn't walk by myself. I went to IPC, and the doctor put me in isolation while waiting to see if I had TB. After I came out of isolation, I got sicker. During this time, I really didn't have any feelings, I really didn't care. I felt alone. I had no one I wanted to share my feelings with. I was in the outside hospital for a month and a week. I was real sick. I had visits from my brother, my sister, they even sent for my son, brought him down from Attica because they thought I was that sick.

When I came back to Bedford, I only weighed ninety-seven pounds; now I weigh one hundred and twenty. I remember, I had to be in the bed twenty-four hours a day. I got up only when Gloria showered me. I was very weak, I couldn't feed myself, I couldn't drink or swallow, my speech was very impaired. I had to have Pampers on twenty-four hours, I couldn't go to the bathroom, I couldn't sit up, I felt bad. And all I wanted to do was smoke cigarettes, at the time I didn't care what kind I smoked. I didn't care about eating, and Lisa and Aida used to bring me food all the time. Aida had a lot to do with me eating. I didn't want to do anything, and she used to come and talk to me. She made me start caring; she and Gloria were my backbone. Then so many people started coming down. Indio worked with me all the time, Lisa O., Lisa F., Kathy, Doris.

Now I'm able to do a lot for myself. I can hold my own juice, I can stand up, I can go to the bathroom, I go to church every week. I'm very thankful that I stayed around to see my first grandchild, because it looked like I wasn't going to be here. My hope is to live a longer life, that they will find a real cure for HIV. I go to the parole board in November 1993.

I'm a fighter. I've been sick a lot. I fought it all. I'm surprised I'm saying this much—I'm a very shy person. In a way, I haven't really dealt with being HIV-positive. I don't really accept it. I feel like I'm just the same as I was before.

* * *

In 1993, Sheryl was granted medical parole under the new early-release program for prisoners with terminal illnesses. She spent six months in a nursing home and is now being cared for by her family, after being released on her regular parole date.

MEDICAL ADVOCACY

It is crucial for anyone who is HIV-infected to get good medical care and to have a good relationship with her health providers. ACE has been able to create a medical-advocacy process, in cooperation with the medical department, that contributes to this effort.

Medical advocacy is in part a formalized system: we have permission to accompany a woman into her doctor's appointment when a woman is dealing with HIV-related issues. We use a permission form to accompany this process. HIV, like other serious illnesses, gives rise to fear. Fear can freeze a person: she can forget to ask questions, she may not hear what is being said; the technical language itself can be hard to understand; perhaps she does not want to know what is happening because it is too frightening. It helps to have a friend along, one who is also educated about HIV, who can help ask the questions, remember what was said, and be there for support. Other times, we may not go in to an appointment, but we can help a woman define her questions and we can urge her to write them down and then to come back after the appointment to talk about what happened.

Even women in ACE who are HIV-positive, who teach others about AIDS and who may be medical advocates for other women, may want a person to go with them to their own medical appointment.

* * *

I didn't want AZT. I didn't like how it made me feel. I wanted an alternative. I needed an advocate to go with me, even though I, Katrina, was able to help other women. I needed an advocate to help me get through those medical appointments, to be able to talk without crying, without yelling. In order to get something accomplished, to help me make a list like I helped other people do. When I went in and asked for DDI, which hadn't been approved yet, the doctor would cut me off. I was persistent, I cried, I told him he would allow me to die without an opportunity to try other drugs. I told him just because I refused AZT doesn't mean I don't care about myself, I just didn't agree with them. It was good Kathy was there. She would intervene when I couldn't respond. She presented questions when I couldn't.

* * *

Medical advocacy is also informal—a network of communication that stretches between population, ACE members, and medical personnel, be it nurses, lab technicians, doctors, or the medical director. A woman may be sick on a living unit. She continues to have fevers, and she can't get the doctor's appointment that she needs. If we pass a doctor whom we know, we can say, "Anna has been sick for too long. Can you please make sure she gets an appointment?" or we can ask Liz, the ACE coordinator, to call the medical director, Dr. Griffith, to bring the problem to her attention. It takes a constant effort on everyone's part to make this informal network work, but it is a necessary "net" to catch people who need help.

The AIDS epidemic left us feeling frustrated, helpless, and frequently angry at doctors who didn't have the answers: not the cure we needed, nor clear predictions of what would happen to our bodies, because HIV affects each person differently, nor certainty about medications. We learned from the recent traditions set by the women's self-help movement, the PWAs who support each other in the effort to get good medical care throughout the country, and the medical advocates who are now on staff in many hospitals. Active involvement in our own medical care, support for one another, and dialogue with doctors and medical staff has helped us overcome our feelings of helplessness and has improved our medical care.

Nereida Ferran,
Medical Director, Bedford Hills Correctional Facility, 1988–1992. Presently medical doctor at St. Clare's Hospital, Spellman Center:

> The concept of ACE is sorely needed at many correctional institutions: AIDS counseling and education provided by a group of well-informed, caring, and dedicated peers, who through a well-planned training program acquire the knowledge for counseling others on AIDS prevention and living with AIDS issues. Having peers providing this service facilitates the process of communicating key information in a culturally, ethnically, and gender-sensitive manner and in a language that can be understood. The recipient also gets the comforting support of people who can relate to (and understand) their life experiences.
> And it works!
> The women would listen and ask questions and learn about AIDS in a much more relaxed and freer disposition than one could find in a traditional educational environment. I was delighted to hear them asking very intelligent, informed, and pertinent questions during the multiple times we met.
> Their role as a peer support group complemented our work in the medical area. They were in many ways an important part of our outreach effort by maintaining an alert eye among the population to identify women in need of medical care who were not accessing available services because of fear, distrust, misinformation, language barriers, or pure hopelessness. They would bring the problems to our attention or at times personally bring the patient. They would empower other women to begin

taking control of their lives by making informed decisions about their health and lives. They were able to reach an extensive number of women that educators and health professionals could not approach because of a shortage of resources, communication problems, lack of cultural awareness, indifference, etc. . . .

I, not so secretly, admired such dedication to their vision and to one another. It was for me an eye-opening experience to witness the degree of sharing, love, and compassion expressed to the women hospitalized at the facility infirmary during the periods of illness and vulnerability. They would cook, groom, pamper, listen, celebrate, support, laugh, and cry with the very frail or dying as well as with those going through less trying moments. They would practically erase the words of isolation, rejection, loneliness, and stigma from the daily vocabulary of those patients, to replace them with love, friendship, acceptance, and hope.

Some of the problems encountered in correctional facilities affecting delivery of care have to do with lack of timely accessibility to services, due to security-related restrictions and language barriers, as well as a shortage of out-of-facility specialized services. This fact made it imperative that patients not miss scheduled outside appointments. The ACE women assisted in the process by alerting us anytime they found such mishaps, as well as by acting as interpreters and "buddies" for the women in order for us to attend to the specific problems presented. In a system like corrections, where the population has such a high incidence of HIV disease, as well as multiple other medical conditions, and with such an active movement of inmates in and out of facilities on a regular basis, it is relatively easy to inadvertently overlook patients with problems. In view of the shortage of staff that is prevalent in government institutions, as well as the unnecessary abuse of services by some patients, to have a group like ACE as an "inside observer" of the population helping to discern the real need from the superfluous was a welcomed favor. We were glad (and lucky) to have them, and I firmly believe that their program and curricula should be expanded to similar institutions. This type of organization is also a valuable and untapped training ground for effective peer counselors who, when released to the community, will find these skills are also needed. Their special work gave meaning to many lives and certainly could be a solid step toward rehabilitation by getting inmates involved in helping others and empowering one another in the process.

I finally want to express my respect and regard for the dedicated work of the ACE leaders and founders, because their resilience and commitment to the project has made it the success it is and has touched the lives of many . . . including me. It was a privilege to have met and worked with such a special group of women, and I certainly hope that their excellent work and contribution get the attention and support they deserve.

Best wishes, sisters!

EDUCATION

The underlying motivation for our educational work is the recognition that "knowledge is power." We do educational work for many purposes. One is to help prevent the spread of HIV infection. Another is to allay fears and challenge stigma. A third is to give people tools for attaining better medical care and taking more responsibility for their health.

How and where we do our educational work changes, and is determined by the particular circumstances and needs at any given time. Sometimes we hear of arguments due to fears about AIDS in the back-building dormitories. We'll do a rap group there. Or when TB emerged as a major health problem in the prison system, we educated ourselves with the help of the medical department and brought in outside speakers for population. With the growing awareness of STDs (sexually transmitted diseases), ACE developed a series of workshops on women and our bodies, presenting them to women in the Facility drug program—ASAT—and then in Spanish to ACE Latina members.

The following are three examples of our education work:

Orientation

Every woman entering the New York State prison system must first come to Bedford Hills reception. Once here, she spends a short period of time going to doctor's appointments, getting paperwork in order, getting prison clothes, and being tested, processed, and classified. Once out of reception, some women stay here, but most are taken to one of several other female prisons in New York. Although this time period is generally an overwhelming one for women, it is also an opportunity for ACE to reach each of the women entering the prison system.

The level of anxiety among these women is enormous: anxiety about casual contact and about the possibility or actuality of their own infection. In the short time they are here, just having someone to talk to makes a tremendous difference. Those women who will stay on are able to make their first contact with ACE.

Once a week, several of our members go to the units where the new women stay and present a mandatory HIV/AIDS orientation. During a two-hour question-and-answer period, women also have a chance to hear the concerns of others and to talk one-on-one if they choose to.

Rap Groups, Videos, and Discussions

Reaching out to large groups in orientation or workshops has many advantages, but the pain and stigma around HIV often create other needs for those dealing with it. We've found that confidentiality and feelings of acceptance and support are often more easily achieved in small groups focused on particular issues. Many PWAs who are working out whether to be open about their status choose to first "go public" in a small rap group.

* * *

I had never talked about my husband's death, unless it was privately to a close friend or two. Then I went to a group on Testing at ACE. There were only five of us, so we got to know one another pretty good and to feel comfortable. Once a few other women began talking about why they were there, I realized my pain and fears weren't too different. I finally said what I had kept thinking for a year: "I'm scared to test, because I'm afraid he made me positive like him. I loved him . . . but I don't want to die like he did." The group made a real difference in my life.

* * *

The ACE Puppet Show

In a female prison, children and motherhood are integrated into everyone's life and thoughts. Here at Bedford Hills, we have the Summer Program, in which mothers have their children visit for five days each year. Many of us who were learning about the HIV virus also wanted to be able to talk to our children and to other mothers about HIV. It took time to figure out the needs of the mothers and children, create consent forms, and develop a program that allowed mothers to be able to participate in the educational process, but it was worth it.

After each show, we handed out coloring books to the children that had the same story in them that the puppets told.

As it was going on, some of the kids started talking to the puppets, giving them information, asking questions, or yelling at them for stigmatizing another puppet. . . . Overall, the show was a success. . . . Having the support and input from the Children's Center director, Sister Elaine, made a big difference. . . . For me, the nicest thing about doing the puppet show is knowing that we are reaching a new generation; children who will one day, we hope, deal with this virus better than we have.

Our education is not solely about a presentation of facts. We try to identify the feelings and attitudes that impact on how people deal with facts. Why would a person who knows that you cannot get HIV/AIDS from hugging a woman who has the HIV infection still be tense and even reluctant to hug a woman with the virus? Why would a person who knows that having sex without a condom could be inviting death not use a condom? Why would a woman who is HIV-positive not want to become informed about HIV or medications? Education, to be meaningful, must involve the whole person, and when we present information we explore these kinds of issues.

Our presentations take into account that our population is made up of Afro-Americans, Caribbeans, Puerto Ricans and women from all over the rest of Latin America, white women, gay and straight women, older women and adolescents. We have to have different voices to reach different ears. We usually work in diverse groups, often three, four, or five of us working together in a presentation.

The very process of teaching changes our own understanding of what we need to be focusing on. For example, our experience of talking with women about HIV/AIDS prevention and the rising problem of STDs necessitated empowering them with the knowledge of their bodies that women are often denied. Thus, we developed a new curriculum, called "Women and Our Bodies," which includes sessions entitled Understanding Our Bodies, The Menstrual Cycle, STDs, and Reproductive Choices. This curriculum, already a core part of our work, is still in its early stages of development. We have used this curriculum with women in the drug treatment program, the community preparation program, and the nursery, and it has been carried out in Spanish and in English.

We have adopted the saying "Each one, teach one," knowing that only by continually inspiring and generating new teachers from our peers will we be able to meet the challenge of AIDS: there is no cure, so the heart of hope in AIDS work is education, both in prevention and "surviving and thriving." Thus, Part Two of our book describes our educational philosophy and methods and the educational curriculum that we use.

7
Our Stories

For this chapter, some of the women who are presently active in ACE have written their own story. For some of us, this represents our first attempt to articulate our lives; others of us have written our stories before. The voices are as distinctive and diverse as we are.

Lisa Osborne

The first thing I think about is that I'm spoiled. My mother was willing to put herself aside to make sure I had something I needed or that I was fed and clothed. There were times when my mother would go without to make sure that I had. I remember her wearing the same pair of shoes for three or four years, but every year I would get different shoes and different outfits and be dressed like other children in the neighborhood. I grew up in Brooklyn. I've lived in apartment houses, I've lived in projects. I have an older sister, she's fourteen years older than me, so it was like I had two mothers and they both were incredible. My sister was more the disciplinarian, but she always explained why. She would say, "You have to go to bed and stay there, but I'm making you do it because . . ." It made us very close.

My mother's from the church. She was raised religiously. Her idea of a party is four people sitting there with a cup of tea. I used to think she was square. My mother is like my pillar of strength. Even when things are hard, or it seems like, "Ahhh, I can't win," she still keeps going. She's like the Energizer Bunny—she keeps going and going and going.

When I was in high school, I went from wanting to be a nurse, to wanting to be a vet, then a physical therapist. I got something from my sister. She's always pushed me. "All Lisa has to do is to get it in her mind that Lisa *can* do it, and Lisa can do it." She puts me up on a pedestal. We were estranged when I first got arrested, because she couldn't deal with coming back and forth to prison. But I got real angry and frustrated and wrote her a letter, and things are better now.

When I turned sixteen, it seemed like everything went cuckoo. I knew everything, Mommy didn't know anything. Halfway through my sixteenth year, it was, "You can't tell me anything." I was the typical adolescent, worried about my friends, looking good, being popular. My mother didn't drink or swear, she was very protective. Most of my friends would have an eleven o'clock curfew. She would want me in at ten, and I would rebel and say "So-and-so's mother doesn't make her come back that early."

I started using drugs, experimenting when I was thirteen, but doing it more seriously when I was sixteen getting ready to turn seventeen. I notice that I go by extremes. My mother would say, "I want you home by eleven," and I would sit there and get defiant and not come back for two or three days. She would have a fit. I was on self-destruct. I can't think of why. I worried more about what my friends would think about me, because I'm a big people pleaser. I wanted to be liked. I think part of it came from the fact that my family doted on me. I was like a little princess—well, maybe not princess, but to my mother and sister I was as close to perfect as a child could be. I was so used to everyone liking me that I needed that from everybody.

I dropped out of school at seventeen, May 1985. I had one more year, but school bored me. So I just stayed home, and by October I was going crazy, plus I felt bad that I didn't have a diploma, so I signed up for the GED, and by the end of November I took the prescreening and they told me I would take the next test in January. I started studying on my own a week before in order to take the test—my mother thought I had been going to school. When I got my diploma, I passed it with a 270. It was so high that I am down as a Martin Luther King High School graduate, not just a GED. I had signed up for a business class before I was arrested. I had applied to Medgar Evers and LaGuardia Colleges because they had physical therapy classes. I got arrested in March. I was supposed to go in that April to talk to the colleges about financial aid, classes.

During this time I was hanging out with friends and using drugs. I knew an individual who used to sit there and say, "I need you to babysit, come over and let's have a few beers." I would think of her as a friend, and she was encouraging me in my rebellion. I got arrested.

I got to Bedford when I was twenty-one, because I spent eighteen months on Rikers when I was fighting my case. I had to take a plea, since the judge told me he would give me fifty to life if I lost at trial. So at twenty years old, I said to myself, Whether I'm innocent or not, I'll take it. When I got to Bedford, after I saw that I wasn't going home, I said, Okay, I'm not going home for a while, with a sentence of 8 ⅓ to 25 years. I said, What am I going to do? When I got here, an individual who I had met at Rikers told me to meet her in the yard, and she came with a rundown for me about all the programs that exist. We both were adolescents, and at Rikers Island, adolescents can't go to college, and she said to me, "We can go to college here." Actually, she discouraged me from ACE. She said that all they do is talk about AIDS, and it's depressing enough. It's funny that the one thing she told me to adamantly avoid is the one thing I enjoy the most.

I have really grown up in prison. It's within the last three years only that I've now become more me-oriented. I'm more concerned about what I think of me, whereas in the past I would almost beg, borrow, or steal to be liked, to fit in. I wanted everyone to like me, but I'm okay with me now, and I know not everyone will like me. It took me years and years to come to that. I have my bachelor's degree, and I have been a teacher's aide in business education class. Now I'm twenty-five. When I was arrested, I was eighteen getting ready to turn nineteen.

My sister has always instilled in me a pride in being black, but an "Oh, yeah, I'm black and society's going to try to keep me down" kind of pity song. My sister always said although society might close a lot of doors, if you struggle and do the best you can do, you'd be surprised at what you can do. She taught me about role models, Malcolm X, Martin Luther King. When I sit there and think about the virus, I want to be like Rosa Parks. I'm not going to the back of the bus on this one.

I would like to be able to help others the way I do in ACE on a larger scale when I am released. That's why I'm hoping to be a health advocate, to advocate for those who need medical care and to advocate for a cure.

* * *

Anonymous

I was brought up on a farm down South. To me, I was poor, because my parents left us down there with my grandmother, so that they could earn money in the North, but my grandmother had her own farm, a garden, animals, and I was always the favorite of everybody and I got my way. I was a spoiled kid growing up. I was so spoiled that my father used to tell us that if we stepped in dog mess, we should just leave our shoes there and he would buy us a new pair of shoes. I used to constantly come back barefoot. That's how spoiled I was. And I still have some of those ways with me; if I can't get my way I still act spoiled. And I did it to my son. It was all about me. If you weren't in my family, I didn't care about you. My family was my world for me.

When I was twelve I moved up North with my parents and my sisters and brothers: I have two sisters and two brothers. I went to school. I wanted to be a teacher, and my mother wanted me to be a teacher also. While I was in school it seemed possible, because when I was in school I was a good student. I also wanted to be a stewardess, because I loved to travel. But then I started playing hooky from school, when I was about sixteen or seventeen, and when you start playing hooky, you begin to hang out in the street, and I started drinking a little, a little wine. I guess I left school because of peer pressure, because all my friends were cutting out and I wanted to be down with them. So I cut out, and we just had fun, had a good time.

I was getting ready to graduate. We had a field trip. I forget where we went. I had stolen a fifth of liquor from my mother, and I turned the whole boat over, and a few of us could have drowned, and somebody told on me, and I got suspended and that was it. I didn't graduate. I could have gone to another school, but I didn't go—that was the end of my school days. Ever since then I went downhill—being in the streets, getting high, drinking, smoking reefer, which I never cared for, doing it because everyone else was. And then I got farther into drugs. I started going to Manhattan a lot. I always had money because I was selling drugs.

I saw this girl who I had been going to school with. She had been the cutest girl in the whole school, but she looked so bad. I asked her why she had changed. She told me she was using drugs. I couldn't believe it. I started sniffing to see what would happen to me. But she told me she was shooting. I told her to hit me, I wanted to try it myself, and I got hooked. And then I wasn't making the same kind of money, and I started doing bad, doing illegal things, and the drugs controlled me. I got arrested before this arrest, for possession of a weapon. I got bailed right out. I had copped out to come to Bedford, but the judge recessed the case and I didn't go to court. I wonder if I had had to do some time whether I would have ended back here for this new case, homicide and robbery. Twenty-five to life.

I believe that if I was still in the street, I would be dead. But being in here, I went back to school, GED, now I have my bachelor's degree. ACE was my first jailhouse family, and the sharing and concern that we gave to one another means that I now reach out to other people. And the virus made me look at myself and where I come from. I was in the streets and the streets are very mean—it takes a strong person to survive them. I was able to survive them. I didn't catch the virus by shooting drugs. I used other people's works, I can't say I had a clean pair of works. It's by the grace of God that I didn't catch the virus. That's one reason that I dedicate myself to the work I do, because it could have been me. I have walked down the same paths, and when they get sick, I take it personally, because I know it could be me. Being involved in ACE changed me. It helped me grow.

I'm a mother. It has been hard, because I left my son when he was so young, when he was five; now he's nineteen. I can never recapture those years, but at least within those first five years that I was with him, we created such a bond that no prison, no bars can break it. He still looks to me for advice, and we have been tested over the years and we passed that test. At one point I used to say he and my father were the only things that kept me strong in here, but since my father died, it's my son. We've had our bouts with him getting into trouble. Even though my mother's there, and aunts, he still feels alone, because I was his mother and father and now I'm here. But we've been able to talk, and he told me that he's very angry at me because I'm not there to punish him when he does something wrong. But we've cried about this and it helped. When he was young, he wanted to be a police officer, but when I got arrested that changed. Just like it affected my life being here, it affected him. I look at him, and he's grown up to be a fine man now—he can cook, he can dress—and I feel good, but I feel sad because he learned those things without me. I wasn't part of that. He's still my baby, but in all reality he's not that five-year-old. Now I have to talk to him about safe sex. It's hard. At one time he used to visit a lot, and now it's not enough, and I question his love, I ask him, "Don't you love me?" and he says, "Yeah, mom, I love you, but I have my girlfriends." And I know I want him to enjoy his life. By my early twenties I was incarcerated. In my late teens I was on drugs. I feel that the best things that happened to me besides my son's birth are I got involved with ACE and God came into my life.

* * *

Ruthie Rodriguez

I was born and raised in Brooklyn by my parents. I have a sister and a brother. When my father first came here from Puerto Rico, he sold apples and oranges from a red truck. That's how he got started. He worked very hard, seven days a week. Now he owns several stores. I admire him for his strength and determination. My mother was a paraprofessional and went to college while trying to raise three kids. My love for books and education in general comes from her. We were a typical family. My greatest love as a kid was animals. I remember always feeling sorry for stray dogs, and bringing them home and putting them in the basement. My largest collection was twelve. I used to steal food from my mother and give it to the dogs to eat, until one day my mother got hip and made me get rid of them.

I was a very bright student, an A student. I was also very over-protected by my parents. When I went into the sixth grade, I rebelled. I guess I wanted to be a boy, because in my family my brother got everything. He was the one who was allowed to go outside while I was only allowed to go out for half an hour a day. I never had friends over, and I never played games. I was always told that my brother was allowed to stay out and play baseball because he was a boy, but I wanted that too. When we misbehaved, it was always, "Wait till your father comes home," it was always "the man." I didn't understand why being a man meant that you had the power, you had control, whereas it was the mother who did everything. She had the babies, did the housework, and had a job. So why did the man have control? I always had a need to prove that I could do what a man could do, and not only do it but do it better.

When I went to the sixth grade, I joined a gang. I fought a lot. I wanted to wear boys' clothing. I wanted to be a boy. I wanted to have control. I started playing hooky, and on my fourteenth birthday I shot drugs for the first time with a thirty-two-year-old man. And I loved it. And it was downhill from then on. At that point I lost control, or so I thought. I know now that you can't lose what you never had. Once again, the men in my life had the control. From the leaders of the gangs, to the drug dealers, to the boyfriends. I went from one abusive relationship to another, and I saw no way out. A lot of people till this day ask, "Well, why did you stay?" What was I supposed to do? I was young, a teenager, hooked on drugs, no education, female, and Hispanic, living in the ghetto. There was no way out. I had a lot of anger in me. My life was led in a self-destructive, negative way. I ran away from home at the age of fourteen, and I've been running ever since. I can't blame anyone for it, for I made my own choices.

Even though I wasn't going to school, I read a lot. I used to read love stories, and the newspaper. It was a habit for me to read before going to sleep, if I didn't nod out first.

The best thing that's happened to me is that I have a daughter who is now fifteen years old. I've tried to build a relationship with her that gives her pride in herself as a woman. I want her to believe in herself and not to put limitations on what she can do. She wants to be a singer, and I encourage her. What I've tried to build with us is mutual respect. I'm always telling her she's great and that she's the most important thing in my life. We talk a lot about her and what's important to her in her life. I feel lucky that we are as close as we are, because we've been away from each other for over eight years now. When I feel down, I call her and we talk. She motivates me and she gives me strength. She's really proud of me. I think she likes the combination of a hip mom with book knowledge. There's times when people try to put me down. I have an aunt that told my daughter in a negative way, "You're gonna be just like your mother." My daughter turned around and told her, "I hope so. What's wrong with my mother, anyway?" It's hard being a mother from prison. That's been the hardest thing for me, being away from my daughter. But we've both learned acceptance. I could never make up the time that we've lost to her, but I try to do the very best I can from in here.

When I first came to Bedford I was still rebelling. I used to get in trouble a lot. I basically grew up during my eight years in prison. I was twenty-four when I came here. I've had a lot of pain, but I've also had a lot of good times here. The people I've met have made the difference. I was taught how to do my time constructively. You try to live your life to the fullest, in whatever way you can. When I first got here, I made a calendar that had three thousand six hundred and fifty days on it, the length of my sentence; it was hanging on my wall. Every day I'd get up and cross out a day. I was punishing myself, until one day a friend of mine came in my cell and tore it off the wall. Every holiday I'd lock myself into my cell. I felt that I didn't deserve to be happy. I'd caused too many people too much pain. I was finally taking a look at myself. And I didn't like what I saw. I knew it was time to make a change. I had to make decisions. Although it seemed like an eternity, I knew I was getting out someday. I'm still trying to prepare for that day. I feel that I've done pretty good for myself. I finally went to school, and I have my four-year bachelor's degree from Mercy College, which made my daughter very proud. And I discovered that I have artistic talents that I hope to use someday. I'm happiest when I draw. My loves in life are children, animals, and art.

When I look back at it all from a distance, being in the street and getting high gave me an education that college just can't give you. And now, coming to Bedford, I have both—I have street knowledge and book knowledge, and if I use them right, they will take me a long way.

Without the people whom I've met here, none of this would have been possible. Before I came here I heard some weird stories about the women. But none of them proved to be true. I learned the true meaning of friendship here. That's not to say that everyone's my friend, but those who are, will be forever. I have one particular friend who after being here went home and has stuck by me ever since. Here in Bedford with my friends, I don't have to be ashamed of what I've done, because all of us here have made mistakes. We look at life differently; we have an appreciation for life that people in the free world take for granted.

In terms of ACE, I guess it's a need to help someone who could have been me. I've shot drugs, I've been promiscuous, yet I'm still alive, and I'm HIV-negative. Maybe there's a purpose in my life after all—who knows?

* * *

Windy (Awilda) Gonzalez

When I came to jail nine years ago, I was twenty-four years old. I didn't have any sense about it. I was very naive. I thought everything was about me—I was very spoiled. When I got to Bedford Hills, I found myself very lonely and very scared. I had a sentence of fifteen years to life for sale and possession of drugs. I knew I had two choices. I could keep going the way I was before my arrest, or I had the choice to do my time constructively and try to improve myself. I could choose to help myself and help others.

I grew up in Puerto Rico. I have a big family—fifteen uncles, four brothers from a different father. I never lived with my mother. I think she was trying to save me from sexual abuse. At first I lived with my grandmother. Then I thought I was going to go with my mother, but she sent me with my aunt. My grandmother loved me. She thought I was an angel. But my aunt was very military, a good provider of material things and a good woman, but I didn't get the love I needed. I was raped as a child, sexually abused, and when I was seventeen years old I left home.

I came to the United States when I was eighteen. I had a lot of dreams, and I had a grant, and I wanted to go to college and be a lawyer. I went to live with my friend and her father. After a while you feel like you have to move on and not bother people. I was making $75 a week. Sometimes I would be hungry in the classroom. Sometimes the teacher would have to give me tokens. Then I moved into a little studio, and I had a sewing machine and a small table. When I first came here, as part of the college I was in—Boricua College—they gave us internships to earn a little money. My first job was in the Commonwealth of Puerto Rico office as a counselor. It's as if I always had the skills to be a counselor. I dealt with people who had immigrated like me, and I would help them with forms, or help them locate people, immigration issues. Then I went to work for Reality House Youth Assistance Program. They offered me a job in the summertime, since they liked my work. That's when I found out that I really loved to work with kids. Then I went to work for Family Court, Juvenile Delinquent Section. I did field work for the lawyers who were defending the kids. I made a little more money then, but things were a little tighter, since I was finishing my two years, graduating. I wanted a ring and I wanted more. I looked for jobs. I had a job with the CETA program, but it was terminated, but I had already moved, rebuilt my life around that job, in a law department for worker's compensation, and it fell through and I was left out there. Then my little sister came to live with me—more money. Every time I went to apply for a job, they said I was overqualified. I didn't understand that. I was in this country two years later struggling to make a living. I was proud. I wasn't going to take welfare.

I trusted someone who was supposed to be part of the law. I chose to believe somebody who asked me to do something and got in this mess. I was young, I was ignorant, very naïve. The DA stressed that because I was so well educated and had work experience that I should have known better, but sometimes you end up doing things for survival, and you don't see options.

When I first arrived at Bedford I wanted to hold on to being young, to catch that moment and never let it go. I didn't want to walk out of here bitter. And it made me such a silly girl, and I did things like throw snowballs, things that I didn't do as a kid because I had so many responsibilities. I felt free. I paid a price for that. I wanted to trust eveybody. Everybody was good. I trusted everybody, and I learned that that wasn't true. And now I don't need to buy friends, I don't need to buy material stuff, I can stay alone, just lay there, write poetry, knit.

When I came to jail, I didn't know anything about AIDS. In 1989 I went and found out that I had cervical cancer, and they said to me that I had to take an HIV test. I said, "I don't have a problem with that." I don't use drugs; I had been a lesbian for many years, so I didn't have a problem with that. And I was not scared at that point. So I went and I gave the blood, they did the blood work, and when they finally called me to give me the results . . .

By then I knew of ACE, since ACE had started, but my mind was into other things. I was concentrating on improving myself, and at that time I wasn't ready to get involved with ACE. I was very involved with the Hispanic women here and getting some therapy for my problems, before I got involved with something that big, and I knew that ACE was going to be big. I knew from the beginning, from the enthusiasm that the women showed, it made me realize how big and positive this was, but I wasn't ready at that point.

The nurse came out. She gave me the impression that something was wrong, and I panicked. I sat there on the bench, and I said, "Damn, I have to do some inventory here; wait a minute. I don't use drugs but I have slept with people, you know. I have had sexual relatonships with people." I got real scared. Then I finally got in, and then again the nurse gave me this reaction that made me feel "Damn, I got . . . this virus!" and my heart was pumping and I was terrified. And then she told me I was negative, and at that point I had been incarcerated for four years, so it was a relief, but I realized that I didn't know anything about AIDS. I have tried to better myself so much, yet I don't know what's going on, what's happening around me. And I said to Aida, "Well, look, I have to take these workshops. I want to learn," so she invited me to come to the workshops. At that time they didn't have anything set up in Spanish, for the Spanish women, and I said, "You know what? I'm really good in Spanish, in translating. Why don't you let me translate the workshops?"

Working in ACE has been good. It has also been painful. I have worked side by side with a lot of PWAs, and working with these people, it's like, "Why am I complaining?" I have no right to complain. These people are living, and they're doing so good, and they are there for me. A lot of times they have given me support. So I want to be here. To me ACE is a source of strength. It's like a reminder that "Hey, you're a fortunate person, and you have so much to give. There's somebody out there that needs you. I have gained a lot out of knowing that I can comfort somebody.

Even though this has been such a bad experience, spending so many years in prison, in a way I'm also grateful to have come here.

You know, I have a lot of dreams. I want to go to ACE Out as a volunteer. I have a lot things I want to do, and I know I'll do all of them. I have a good base—a good, good base—and it's sad to say, but this place gave it to me. And I guess also the little things that my mother, my grandmother, and my aunt taught me, values—all this has made me realize that I have another chance.

* * *

Anonymous

I was a young child growing up in a house with domestic violence. It was one of those houses in which no one talked about it. Nothing ever left the house, so you would go to school with a big smile on your face that meant nothing. Everyone lied about everything. In our home was a world of pain, but outside of the house everyone acted as if the painful things didn't happen. It didn't stop the terrible things from happening, it only made you learn to minimize them to yourself and others. But the things that happened were terrible. The things I remember most about childhood are confusion and fear.

I grew up in the suburbs until my young teens, and then I lived in the country. There was no place to go socially when I needed to connect with others. I liked it there, but it was lonely. My life was frightening and yet also boring and middle-class. I was born in this place where middle-class people kept everything clean. They didn't share their dirty laundry, they held a job, smiled at everyone they met. But at home some of these people were beating each other up. To me, middle-class meant you went through everything everybody else went through but the rules of social behavior said that you don't talk about it to others—or even to yourself.

At thirteen I met my first and only boyfriend. He showed me what I thought was love and affection. I believed I needed him in my life and fell very hard for him and our relationship. Within a short period of time, it became abusive. Compared with what was going on in my home, it did not seem like true abuse. Slowly, it became more and more violent, but by then I'd left behind my family, had no friends, and didn't have the strength left to keep fighting pain and fear. I didn't see it at the time, but he slowly gained more control of my life than I had. It probably wasn't hard, since I'd lost most of who I was in the long years of violence with my family. Somewhere in me I wanted to leave, but I only knew a few sure things about life: (1) I didn't matter, and (2) my life didn't matter because I didn't. I felt trapped in a nightmare and didn't even know I was allowed to wake up, that I deserved to. Once you get to the point where you are more afraid of the unknown than the consequences of staying, it's hard to leave. I stayed with him for eight years. One day I guess it hit him how bad it had really become. He told me to leave, and if I didn't get out at that moment while he was letting me, he knew he would kill me later. I was scared to death. I'd tried to leave before and he had come after me. I thought it was a trick, but I was tired of being that afraid within my family and with him. If I didn't leave then, I knew I never would. While I had that one chance, I took it.

I came to prison less than a year after I left him. One part of me wants to avoid thinking about my life before as much as I can. I didn't like my life, but I didn't know how to change it. It wasn't the life I wanted to lead, and I wasn't the person on the outside that I was on the inside. I settled for things because I didn't know how to make them any different. When it got unbearable, I went the whole cycle from being lost in it, to fighting it— then at a certain point I just gave in and stopped caring, just got up every morning and went through the motions. As a child you can't change very many bad things in your life, and by the time you grow up, sometimes you no longer realize you're allowed to want change, you never even learned how to try. Prison is a sad way to stop that cycle.

Being in prison has been kind of two-sided. In one way, it's been a chance to be away from all the things that were controlling me and all the things that were frightening. A place to be safe, where I am somewhat in control of my own life, making my own decisions without someone intimidating me, threatening me. I've learned to trust God, and see how beautiful life can be as He intended. I first found out who I was in here also. It was a surprise that I am someone I can like. Now that I'm the one living my life, I have begun to be able to have my first dreams and visions for myself. But that's also frustrating, because now I'm doing twenty-five years to life just at the point where I could imagine having a good and happy life for the first time. I've spent time here working on many of the things that weren't right about my family. A lot has changed. We want to be a family for the first time, and we're beginning to know now what a family means, yet I can't be with them. I guess just finally knowing that it could be will have to be enough.

ACE was the first place that I had interaction with women. My mom wasn't really in my life, even though we lived in the same house. It was strange for me to see so many adult women who were nurturing, who interacted with one another. Women who allowed one another to talk openly about abuse, drug problems, sexual issues . . . and they didn't feel disgusted, ashamed, or frightened about it. I couldn't even deal with that at first. ACE has been a safe place to work where no one has judged me, and where they have let me grow. I've sort of allowed ACE to be a substitute for the family I've always wanted and still don't have.

Knowing now how much hurt is in this world of ours, I could never live a life that ignored it. One day, when I'm out, I want to offer services in the community. We need a lot of people to get out in society and help. Our world suffers from drug addiction, homelessness, illiteracy, abuse, neglect . . . and not enough of us are offering any help to those who need it. ACE is wonderful for me because I am able to really help people. Our clients are women who are HIV-positive, HIV-negative, with children, without. They come from all paths of life, but they all were on paths that ended up in prison. The important thing now is that they all have the possibility of a future that is healthy, happy, dignified, and productive. That's one reason this book is important, because sometimes we all need to hear that, to believe. I sure wish I had *before* coming to prison.

* * *

Judith Clark

I grew up in Brooklyn, in the fifties and sixties in a Jewish intellectual family. In many ways, my life, if not exactly the model I saw on *Father Knows Best,* was typical for that time and place: walking to public school every morning, riding my bike around the neighborhood or hanging out with my friends after school until my parents, who both worked, came home. Every Friday, my father took my brother and me to Coney Island to play Skee-Ball and eat at Nathan's, and he drove me to music school every Sunday. But I always had the feeling that events "in the world" were more important than family relations or day-to-day life.

I was a "red diaper" baby, which is to say that my parents were communists when they were young, active in social and labor movements of the 1930s through the 1950s. For me, that meant growing up in an atmosphere of social concern and political activism, but also feeling the fear and tension of McCarthyism. I was a quiet kid, for years inhibited by a speech defect. So it came as a surprise to my parents and others when I grew into an outspoken, rebellious teenager.

In 1963, when I was in junior high school, black parents throughout the city, supported by teachers and others, called for a school boycott to demand quality, integrated education. I was one of the few students in my school to join the boycott, and thus began a lifetime of involvement in civil rights and human rights movements. In college, I joined Students for a Democratic Society (SDS) and helped found one of the first women's-liberation groups. After a year, I was expelled for organizing a sit-in. Instead of going back to school, I became a full-time organizer. Full of righteousness and fury, I was always at the more militant, confrontational end of the movement (that's putting it mildly). I didn't go back to school until twenty years later, when I came to prison.

In 1971, I spent nine months in jail in Chicago, for charges arising from demonstrations. When I got out, I was haunted by the fact that I did a relatively short sentence for all my charges, while people I knew in the black and Puerto Rican movements were getting killed or imprisoned for years. During the seventies, many of the people in the antiwar movement were settling down, getting jobs, having families. The mood of the country was changing. The war in Vietnam was ended, and people felt like what they had been struggling for had been won. Yet I knew so many people who were in jail—Native Americans from AIM [American Indian Movement], Black Panthers. I saw what was happening in Africa and Latin America, and I looked around at the conditions here, and said, "How can they say things are better?" I felt crazy with guilt and anger, driven to do something to make people notice. I worked to support people in prison and on trial.

So many people from various movements were lost during those years. I spent a lot of time going to courts, prisons, and funerals. Years later, when I was in prison, I remember calling my friends in San Francisco when the AIDS epidemic had struck, and their saying, "There's a holocaust and no one is paying attention." I flashed back to those earlier times, in the seventies. I remember, at one funeral, a father saying, in anguish, that it goes against the natural order for parents to have to bury their children. That's happening now with AIDS.

One thing that I find ironic is that during the seventies, I helped organize support for class-action lawsuits by women at Bedford Hills. Little did I know! The day I arrived here at Bedford, the officer who photographed and fingerprinted me handed me a copy of the *Powell v. Ward* settlement and said, "Read this carefully. Women fought very hard for the rights that you now have." I realized that insofar as we have rights and important programs here, it is because people inside started with nothing and worked to create them. Sometimes when you're handed something on a platter, you don't understand what it took to get it. Perhaps that is part of what led me to realize, when AIDS became a crisis, that we had to do something ourselves.

I've been openly gay since my early twenties, and I lived in large households of women and children. I was always a bit of a bossy mother hen and loved talking with people, sitting around a kitchen table, or standing on a street corner. When there's a problem, you organize and do something about it! There was always a whirlwind of people and happenings, stress and chaos. Good training for living with sixty women on a floor in here!

When I think about my life before prison, I'm glad to have been active in international and domestic movements, to have known people who were part of changing the world. But I'm not proud of how I went about it—the violence and recklessness. I always wanted to have children. Finally, I took the plunge and had a baby girl. What a joy! But it also created a crisis, because I needed to reorganize my life and priorities. I knew it and wanted it but couldn't face changing my life. Instead, I felt driven toward escalating recklessness that culminated in actions in which three people were killed and many lives and families torn asunder.

I've been in prison for twelve years. That's half my adult life. I have a life sentence. Many people come to prison as teens and grow up in prison. I was an adult when I came into prison, but it was here that I began to deal with my personal self, with realizing that I needed and wanted to change. The hardest thing for me has been my separation from my daughter, and building a meaningful relationship with her has been central to my life inside. It pushed me to rebuild my relationships with my family; to confront painful issues of loss, guilt, and remorse; and to reassess my sense of commitment and identity. I'm lucky to have family and friends who have helped me all along the way.

I've spent five of the twelve years in prison in one form of isolation or another. So it's a good thing I like solitude and self-reflection and do yoga every day. I write and I paint. I went back to school and received my bachelor's, and I recently completed my master's degree in psychology, writing about the experience of long-termer mothers in prison. In part my interest in psychology grew out of my own internal explorations and in part grew in response to the mental-health crisis in the prison. Prisons are the dumping ground for poor and homeless mentally ill people today. And, of course, working with ACE has been a major part of my life.

ACE provided me, as it did others, with an opportunity to be productive. It is one thing to look at one's past and feel remorse. But we need opportunities to take what we've learned and transform our feelings into positive action. To be part of the solution.

Aida Rivera

In 1983, I was arrested in Brooklyn and charged with the sale and possession of drugs. I was sent to Rikers Island, and a year later I was sentenced to fifteen years to life. On December 10, 1984, I was sent to Bedford Hills to serve my time.

I grew up in Brooklyn, in Coney Island, and with eight brothers and four sisters, life wasn't easy. We were on public assistance. My mother, in a way, was the one who kept order in the house. She was the one who disciplined us. My dad was the easygoing one. I love both my parents very much, but my dad was my teacher and my soulmate. He taught me to see things through his eyes.

There were two things I enjoyed doing with my dad, and those were fishing and going to the junkyard. I remember going fishing with my dad. He always woke up at five in the morning, started the coffee, and got the gear together, and by six-thirty we were on our way. My dad considered himself a real live fisherman. The man would fish anything out of the water.

My father wasn't just a fisherman, he was also a junkyard man. The junkyard was his paradise. Everything and anything he found was good. Our first blender came from the junkyard, but it burned out after a week. One of the things we never ran out of were combs, because it didn't matter where my father found a comb, he always picked it up and brought it home. He used to go fishing and come back with a couple of fish and a pocket full of combs. He would say, "Why bother to buy them, when I can find them? Why pay for them? He would put the combs in hot water and soap and say, "See? Now we have combs." So we never ran out of combs.

My parents are both from Puerto Rico. My dad spoke a little English. My mother didn't speak it at all. We grew up talking English to them. In turn, they answered us in Spanish.

When I was in high school, things were hard, times were hard. We didn't have enough money for so many people. And at sixteen, I decided one day, instead of going to school, to drop out and find a job. And I found a job where my father used to work, in a yarn factory. I got hired, and every day I'd start out for school but I really went to work. They knew my father. And finally I had to tell my mother, and she was upset, but I was sixteen so there was nothing she could do. After there I worked in a doll factory in Bay Ridge, and it was then that I found a way to make better money—drugs. As for me and drugs, I was a casual user—I wasn't into shooting and sniffing. I had a habit, although I didn't see it as that at the time. It took me till I got here to figure out that that was true. When I was arrested, I had five kids. I was selling drugs for the easy money.

When I first arrived at Bedford Hills, my attitude was to take care of myself and the hell with everyone else. The bottom line was that I just wanted to do my time and not concern myself with anyone else. I had my own problems, which were my sentence and the fact that I wanted to see my five children that I left behind. Anyone with a problem was on their own. Whatever problem they had was their own, not mine.

When I was in the street, it was different. If anybody needed my help, I was there for them. I was dealing drugs, so it was easy for me to do whatever I had to do for whomever. I had the money. I remember one time my mother called me about some lady. Her infant baby had just died and they didn't have money to bury her, to lay her out in the funeral, and I just went and gave the lady her money. And I didn't know her. It was like I cared enough to do that. But once I came into the prison, I didn't want to be bothered with anybody's feelings.

Then, in 1987, I found out that my sister was HIV-positive. I had no understanding nor any knowledge of what HIV/AIDS was. I decided that it was time to get off the merry-go-round completely, step back and take a real good look at myself. I had to figure out what I really wanted to do with myself. Did I want to continue living the life I was leading or make a change for the better? I realized that instead of my sister being HIV-positive, it could have been me. In prison, arts and crafts was the first place I went to when I came here. I remember making this ugly cup—to me it looked so beautiful. Then I made a vase. And I realized that I could do things. I was amazed that I could do all these things, it was a whole different experience for me. And I guess every time I had a problem or crisis, ceramics became a way of expressing what I felt. I actually won first prize with a vase that was called *A Sandwich*. It wasn't even supposed to be in the competition. I had made it for a friend, and when I went in to pick it up, I found out it had been sent to an art show, a Department of Corrections art show. I was amazed that not only had it won first prize but someone had bought it.

In 1988, I joined ACE. I wanted to learn more about the virus that my sister had. To do so I knew that I had to get an education, so I went back to school. After nine years as a high school drop-out, I found that going back was not easy. Getting involved in ACE changed my life. I began to look at things differently. I started caring about other people, even people I did not know and might never see again in life. In 1989, I received my GED.

Today, in 1992, I'm about ready to get my associate's degree and I'm working on my bachelor's degree. Today I know who I am and what I want to do with my life as well as where I'm going in life.

* * *

Kathy Boudin

I was born in Manhattan—Greenwich Village—during World War II—in 1943, to be exact. To most of my friends here, that seems like ancient times. I am obsessed with concerns of aging. I've recently turned fifty. Yet, so many people I have known in prison have died in their twenties and thirties from AIDS that I feel very lucky to have lived so long.

I grew up with my father and mother and brother. My grandparents were Jewish immigrants from Europe, and although we were not rich, we lived in relative comfort. There was a lot of emphasis on education and learning. My father was a civil liberties lawyer, and he gave me a love for sports and chess. My mother was a wonderful poet. From both of them I inherited a concern for social problems. In my childhood I was aware of the unjust persecution of people for their political ideas during the Mc-Carthy witch hunts. I used to go to folksong concerts sponsored by trade unions that my father represented. My first demonstrations were to protest the testing of the atom bomb and the release of radiation into the air. At nine years old I decided I wanted to be a doctor, and I held onto that dream until I was halfway through college. I worked toward that dream by working most summers in medical-related jobs: as a counselor for a Fresh Air Fund camp for handicapped children; as a counselor at a camp for blind children; volunteering in a hospital.

My other love was sports, and I used to fantasize about being the first girl to be allowed to play in the Little League, or the first batgirl for a major-league team (about thirty years later my son was a batboy for a day for the Chicago Cubs).

In the summer before my third year of college, in the sweltering heat and humidity of New York City, I was studying calculus as preparation for medical school. I remember hearing about students like myself who were dedicating their summer to struggling against segregation in the South. I was frustrated just being in a classroom studying math; medical training seemed so long, and being a doctor offered the possibility of helping only one person at a time, while the movement offered the chance to completely change society. I felt an urgency to become part of the struggle, and I put my plans to be a doctor forever behind me.

When I graduated from college, I joined a group of students in Cleveland, Ohio. We moved into poor neighborhoods to help organize against poverty and racism. I became close to a group of Afro-American women on welfare and some Appalachian families who had left West Virginia when the mines closed. I began to see America through the eyes of those who didn't have an equal share in the wealth of this country, who were denied equal housing, health care, education, because of their race and class.

I loved the work in that community, learning from people whose background was very different, being able to teach and use some skills from my background. Together we felt ourselves part of a movement: We organized to make immediate concrete changes: to get a streetlight for a street where a child was killed; to get a late welfare check; to have a rent strike to get rid of rats in a building. We also felt part of a much larger movement for what we thought of as "real change" in the United States.

When the war in Vietnam began to accelerate, when throughout the country black communities were in rebellion, I wrestled with the idea of being a lawyer, and even briefly attended law school. But I was drawn into the day-to-day work of an organizer, and I continued that work. As more and more black people were killed—Malcolm X, Martin Luther King, and the hundreds of people whose names are not well known—I became especially preoccupied with the responsibility of being white in a society divided by race and class. I wanted to totally throw my lot in with the struggle for freedom.

It is difficult now to recreate the sense of possibility, of the hope, urgency, and desperation of those years. The horror of the war in Vietnam, and my awareness of the different ways blacks and whites were treated and the ways in which my own birth opened up possibilities that another person's birth would not, created in me a moral crisis and constant questioning as to how to live in a society and world so divided by racism and privilege. That crisis drove me to act in extreme ways, that commitment led me to feel that I should be willing to sacrifice totally for my beliefs.

I spent twelve years underground. I thought about my life almost entirely around determining what was the most important thing I could do to make a difference in our society, trying to take my cues from history, from what was happening in other parts of the world. There were things I enjoyed—spending time in nature, sports, learning Spanish, seeing a good movie, friendships. I found myself tied into youth culture: becoming a vegetarian, hitchhiking as a way to move around. I worked in many of the unskilled jobs that women often have: cleaning houses, waitressing, being a saleswoman. But my guiding goal was changing society.

There were many changes during those twelve years, however, including the end of the war in Vietnam and the disappearance of those strong movements. In my mid-thirties, I was no longer sure what to do, and I also felt the clock ticking as a woman in terms of having children. I was living with woman friends and their children, and I knew that if I wanted a child I would have to have one soon. I had always been worried about how as a woman I could both raise a child and also continue work. But the women's movement made me feel I was not alone in trying to figure this out, and most important, I was moved to do something that *I* wanted to do, for *me,* not a social goal, but fulfilling a personal desire. I gave birth to a wonderful son, with David Gilbert, his father.

Tragically, I didn't understand how to put the different parts of myself together. I was arrested fourteen months after my son was born. While I don't want to talk in detail in this context about the activities surrounding my arrest, I want to say they were wrong. The violence produced a tragedy for those who were killed and injured and for their families, devastating my own family and others as well.

After my arrest I started on a path toward earlier important threads of myself in my earlier life. In prison I've spent time teaching, counseling, and developing programs about foster care and parenting, adult literacy, and AIDS. I went back to school and got a graduate degree in education. In prison I have grown to love writing. It has been a way for me to work on understanding my own experiences.

ACE has been a community for me inside prison, a place where I have developed important friends, and it has been one place for me to do work that makes me know I am not just spending my time in prison waiting to get out, but I am doing something meaningful with my life now. It is paradoxical that out of this tragedy of AIDS, ACE has given me and many others both a chance to do something about the AIDS epidemic and a chance to grow as teachers, counselors, and organizers.

An important source of strength for me in prison has been friends. Friendships have always been important to me. I've had very good friends in prison and have been very lucky to be close to family and friends outside.

Along with many other women here, I work on being a mother from prison, helped by the existence of the Children's Center. My relationship with my son has been both the source of greatest sorrow of being in prison and also the source of greatest joy and energy. In my most difficult times, my focus on him has given me strength: making Christmas presents each year for him and his brothers; reading books that he is reading; having water fights during the summer program. This winter my son was visiting me and it was snowing hard. For the first time in our lives, we were able to actually play in the snow together—we got permission to play on a patio next to the visiting room. We built a snowlady, which in the lives of most mothers would have been part of a normal winter. To us it felt as though a small miracle had occurred. And now I am just waiting and watching for that moment, not too far off, when he will stand tall enough to look me in the eyes.

* * *

Gloria Edwards

I was born in Curaçao. Curaçao is an island—24 square miles—off the coast of Venezuela. You can walk around the whole island in one day. One of the main things when I was growing up was gambling. In a small town, that is mainly how we supported ourselves—cockfights, dogfights—sports that Americans might consider barbaric, we do. Drinking also started at an early age, even as young as eight years old. My grandmother still lives there. She is 107. I grew up with a lot of people around me—twenty-four cousins, another brother and sister—but my brother Desmond really raised me from two months old. He is fifteen years older than me. My mother died in childbirth, and my father killed himself two months later. I guess I always was afraid of abandonment, especially from Desmond.

I came to the United States when I was fifteen for the first time. My brother was in the Vietnam War then. I got a visa because he had been in the war and could become an American citizen, and he sponsored me. And I had an aunt living in Brooklyn, and I stayed with her for about two months. And we heard from Desmond. He came. It was 1970. And he reenlisted again for another twenty-four months. He was in charge of a platoon, and they were in a dugout, and it was Thanksgiving Day. He went to get some more dinner, and when he came back to the dugout, the dugout had been bombed and all his friends and platoon were killed. That's why he reenlisted, to go back, and he later told me, to die with them. But he came back out in 1972.

At first life in the United States was strange; in my country you could leave the door open, not worry about your jewelry. Also, the racism was reversed. My country is ruled by black people. The first time I remember

I was hit by this was in a bar on Lexington Avenue, and the man behind the bar told me, "We don't serve your kind." I didn't understand at first what he meant, since in my country, black people have the power and probably there is discrimination against whites. I said to the man, "What do you mean, you don't serve my kind?" He said, "I don't serve black people." I ordered a beer, and one of the guys who was sitting there went back and got the beer for me. I found out later that he was the owner. But by then the other guy had already called the police. Later, I used to go back to that bar, since the owner was all right, just not that bartender.

Once my brother got out of Vietnam, we moved to another place in Brooklyn. Then about six or eight months later, I met the man who I would marry. We got married pretty quickly.

When I came here, I didn't speak English, since they don't speak it in my country. But now they are teaching English in the schools in Curaçao because there is a developing tourist industry.

My husband was born and raised in Harlem. We had two daughters. It was hard for him. When we got married, we had about three hundred people at the wedding; two hundred were my family. His mother lived in Harlem, and after the reception we rented a hall in Brooklyn. When the hall closed, we wanted to go some place, and we finally divided up—the black West Indians went to Brooklyn, and the black Americans went to Harlem.

In my country, you don't cut the wedding cake until the second Sunday. You get married on a Saturday. Then on the second Sunday everyone comes back to the bride's house to cut the cake. So for my wedding, I had two second Sundays. We make black cake, and we cut a hole in the top and keep pouring wine in it, and by the second Sunday it is nice and strong.

You should have seen the look on my husband's mother's face, she kept asking, "When are you going to cut the cake?" We said we can't— nobody gets cake until the second Sunday. In between, you go away on your honeymoon.

I've been in Bedford Hills for a little more than two years. I have at least six more to do. It's been easier than I thought it would be. I thought it would be a place where people beat you up all the time, people attack you. I think when you're out in the community and you hear about prison, it scares you to death, like someone is going to beat you in your sleep.

Here, for the first time in my life I'm able to relate to women and trust them. This is the first time for me. Even though I'm a woman, I was never able to relate to women. I've always looked at women the way men look at them: backstabbers, gossipers, not to be trusted. I grew up only around boys. But boys were more respected and had the power. It was as if I was always competing with them and trying to be like them. Even now, I hear in my head "Boys don't cry. If you're strong, you don't cry." And even though my head tells me that's not true, I feel like it is, in a way. And so even though I was a woman, I was always ashamed of being a woman. I always wanted to be a man. I felt best when I got dressed up, made up, flirted. But that was it. I think I thought the only way to be a woman was sexually. In here, I have run into women who have been confident in themselves, who have turned out to be good friends and have supported me. And even though I was scared at first about trusting women, I have no regrets. I've been fortunate.

Being in ACE has affected me a lot. It helped me to talk my feelings out more, rather than just keeping everything bottled up. It's helped me to keep my temper, because I really like working with the ladies in IPC, and so I try to reason things out. My job is important to me. I would feel guilty being in lock if something happened to Sheryl and I wasn't there. I'm able to laugh at myself a lot more. I hope to go to college while I'm in prison.

Getting arrested and being in prison has wrecked my life, it has wrecked my family. This started with what happened to my brother. Desmond told me that if I were indicted, he wouldn't be able to live through it, and the day of my indictment, he had a heart attack and died. The destruction and losses have continued. When I get out of prison, I think I want to go back to my country and continue working in health and AIDS. My country is a small country. There's only one hospital, and there are clinics. When I get out of prison, I will be in my forties, if I'm lucky.

* * *

Katrina Haslip

Last Will and Testament, written upon leaving Bedford Hills on parole in September 1990.

I, Katrina Haslip, being of sound mind, except when suffering from dementia, or half-himers, do swear that the following are my wishes, to be duly executed upon my departure from Bedford Hills. That I leave my worldly possessions to the following:

To KATHY BOUDIN AND JUDY CLARK: For all the times that you asked me questions about myself, my personal life, and my own growth.

To you I leave my condensed version of the story of my life, which should answer all your questions, to be divided equally between the two of you.

To Aida Rivera: I bequest to you my treasured Vaseline case, so that you will never forget how it looks, and for all the times that you hid it from me. Now grease your lips!

To Dee (Debra Irving): I leave to you my medium-size replicate doll, Dreads, as a reminder to you that I am your dreaded sister.

To Maria Hernandez: ACE has acknowledged your worrying ability. In honor of that recognition, I leave you with my official pendant, my pink worry stone. Worry much!

To Pearl Ward: I leave you with my name, Katrina Haslip, in exchange for yours, which I will be using on job applications, since you hold a bachelor's degree. Thank you kindly.

To Romeo (Doris Romeo): I leave you with a gift certificate of unlimited value for your use to use only at Bricetti's for gum on a regular basis. Send Elaine for it—it's only right down the street.

To Agnes Alvarez: For your assistance with any/all of my problems, in regards to this office, my personal affairs, and your attentive ear, I leave to you a set of earphones, so that you will not have to listen to the others when I'm gone. Block them out, honey!

To Barbara Ford: To you I leave a manual on how to run ACE. Please use it.

To Linda Malmberg: To you, I leave population, for which you will be doing a lot of counseling. Good luck!

To all the pwas: I leave you with hope, that you, too, are capable of becoming empowered and strong. Lean on ACE, they are the key to your empowerment and strength. Thanks to them, I can now go anywhere and stand openly alone as a PWA and feel wonderful about myself. Know that the same experience lies ahead of you. Be well!

To all the other ACE members that I have not listed by name, I have not forgotten you. Continue your commitment, and know that I will go away torn but strong.

AFTERWORD: REFLECTIONS

1992

Change is inevitable. ACE is not the same now as it was in the beginning.

Before, ACE was a mission, a dream, a *voluntary* effort that mobilized the energies of our community. We were self-defined and self-determined to an incredible level, given that we were functioning in a prison. As prisoners, we are so powerless that the process of helping ourselves, with no civilian structure directly affecting us, unleashed in us energy, self-reliance, and a sense of ownership. We always knew the superintendent held the ultimate power, but when things were running smoothly, she gave us the space, and we felt footloose and on our own, squeezing time in between our institutional jobs to do AIDS work, making it up as we went along, drawing on our own personalities and imagination where we lacked resources and structure.

Then ACE became a funded project and an institutional program. We got an office, and some of us became paid staff, able to devote a lot of the day to AIDS work, while others were voluntary members of the larger organization. We had policies and procedures to follow. Civilian staff were hired, which helped because they could do what we couldn't. They had access to outside agencies, were able to use the phone to call inmates to the office, and could keep our office open on a regular basis. All this enabled us to be more accessible and reliable, more professional. Now, when we went out to living units and classes, or to orientation of new inmates, we could follow through, because the civilian staff could call individuals and groups to the office. For a while we had a civilian counselor who facilitated grief groups, and a community liaison counselor who helped women prepare for going home. We got official training and certification as pre- and post-test counselors. The ACE office became a true haven for PWAs and for others who needed a place where someone cares, a place where they could be themselves and find the support they needed.

But there was a price for all that. Before ACE had an office we were everywhere, moving throughout population. Now we tend to spend more time in the office, with the women coming to meet with us there, and so our presence in population is much less.

Even if we were still a voluntary program and didn't have an office with civilian staff, there probably would have been a change: by now that early period of energy would have ebbed. Today the situation around AIDS is different in Bedford, just as it is in society as a whole. When we first started, the silence and fear around AIDS created a desperate need to talk, to find support and to learn about the epidemic. ACE was about breaking the silence. That was a moment in time, and we played a role inside Bedford that such a moment called for, just as others were doing outside. That sense that we were doing something very important for ourselves, for our sisters, gave us a mission, a unity, a commitment. When we went to speak, it was explosive. As people committed to make a change, when we got that kind of a reaction, it gave us the energy.

Now, talking about AIDS isn't new; it's even become boring to many people. In part, this reflects the positive changes that the struggle has brought with it: a much greater general knowledge about AIDS, less fear of getting it from casual contact, more support for women who are HIV-positive. But in part it reflects the acceptance of something that seemed unacceptable before — the deaths of so many young people.

There is a continuing need for ACE, as the numbers of women who are HIV-positive increase and the need for support and prevention grows. Stigma toward women who are HIV-positive still exists.

* * *

It was a day before my birthday, autumn 1992, and everything was just completely out of control. Someone very special to me was told her father died. I was extremely depressed and scared, because I know I'm a candidate for developing full-blown AIDS. I had finished work for the day, so I went back to my unit and got into the shower. Another inmate walks into the shower room. She opens my curtain and looks in, keeps insisting I tell her who's next to shower. I didn't answer, because I wasn't the only one there. Yet she begins to holler at me, so I say, "Miss, please just don't open my curtain again." She starts cursing now, telling me I'm a miserable bitch, and "What, do you think I want to come in there and catch AIDS?" Those words hurt me to my heart, so bad I just lost complete control. It made me feel as though I was shot down and killed. My reaction was only to respond by defending what little pride I still had. All of a sudden I found myself in a violent rage. I just didn't care what came behind it. So before I knew it, we were both physically going at it.

* * *

It's 1992 and it feels to me like we are losing ground, in terms of a rise in stigma and a sense of passivity among women in population. Maybe it's similar to what's happening on the streets these days. The epidemic has been with us for so long that people take it for granted and it's harder to mobilize to fight to change things, or to promote safe behavior. Many women I know do not want their HIV status to be known because of fears of stigma, so they don't reach out to the needed resources in ACE. And there is little discussion or consciousness-raising or solid information about new developments outside the ACE office. Then, too, the TB epidemic has people scared, yet most are ignorant about the facts.

One day, I walked onto my floor and saw about fifteen women sitting around the rec room with hospital masks on. I thought it was some kind of early Halloween joke! Did I walk onto the set of *General Hospital?* I asked several of them what was going on, and all they said was "You have to be careful; can't tell what's going around these days." Finally, someone explained that the women heard a rumor that one of the women on our unit had active TB and had refused to stay in IPC. Of course, it wasn't true. But I realized we had hit a new low.

* * *

1995

It has been seven years since the beginning of ACE. The epidemic is worse, and we are fortunate to still have an organization in prison committed to struggling with AIDS. As we read back over our early history and the more recent years in ACE, we can say that we've made it through the storm. We've confronted low times, yet we've been able to adapt to new conditions, to create new ways to cope with an epidemic that is entrenched in the prison system as well as throughout society. We have lost the first generation of PWAs, but new voices are speaking out, self-assured, discovering their own strengths and going on to inspire others. Some of the people who created ACE have died; many have gone home, yet new women are coming forward. ACE has a renewed sense of optimism, of confidence, in being able to make a difference. We're reaching out to the women in the Nursery, to the reception women coming into Bedford, to the substance-abuse program, to the unit for women with special emotional problems. The care for women in the infirmary is as loving and consistent as it has ever been. The office no longer feels like a trap; it is both a springboard from which we reach out to others and also a place where people can be sure that they can find support and a sense of unity. Many activities take place in the office: individual counseling and medical advocacy; memorials; prerelease planning; Sharing the Sunshine (women knit slippers for the women in the infirmary and booties for the babies at Incarnation Children's Center); a T-shirt project; the memorial quilt and wall hanging; making a banner to go to Washington to bring ACE into the Mothers Against AIDS march; a PWA support group; outside speakers; a journal workshop; a two-week program for all new inmates; quilt making; planning our walkathons; and ongoing education for population, including a focus on women's health issues. We know that the past cannot be repeated, and the present has urgent tasks. We believe that as prisoners, we owe a debt to society, and ACE offers a way to give something back, as we combine work that mobilizes and empowers with necessary services. And, like everyone else, we fervently hope for a cure.

This book is primarily about life in prison. Our lives inside can feel very insulated. The "free" world seems very far away. We crave energy from people and events on the outside.

Occasionally, events occur that remind us that our energy inside can also reach outward. One such event occurred in the winter of 1992–93. After years of demonstrations, meetings, and lobbying by AIDS activists, particularly women, the Federal Centers for Disease Control (CDC) agreed to change its definition of AIDS to include several symptomatic illnesses that HIV-positive women in particular get. Thousands of women who were previously excluded from adequate medical diagnosis and treatment and financial entitlements, despite their illness, were finally now acknowledged.

Our own sister, Katrina Haslip, made an important contribution toward this hard-won advance. According to an article in *The New York Times,*

> . . . Since her [Katrina's] release in 1990, she has talked about her infection at conferences, protests and in one-on-one outreach work. She has met with CDC officials in private, and berated them in public, as she doggedly pushed for the new definition that she says will help get women tested and the disease diagnosed early, when treatment is more effective.[1]

Tributes to Katrina in the media when she died described her as a black woman, a Muslim, an ex-prisoner, and a member of ACE who left prison and went on to play a powerful role as a spokeswoman for women with AIDS. Reading these articles gave us a sense of pride and power. What we were doing inside mattered on the outside.

Katrina was a part of us who went everywhere. We felt we were with her in Atlanta, Washington, Rikers Island and Sing Sing, the International AIDS Conference in Italy, and everywhere else she spoke.

---

1. Mireya Navarro, "An AIDS Activist Who Helped Women Get Help Earlier," *The New York Times*, November 15, 1992.

Katrina had a dream and a commitment while in prison. She wanted to take her own experiences as a PWA and an organizer to become a voice for the voiceless when she got out. And she did.

Before she died, Katrina said, "We emerged from the nothingness, with a need to build consciousness and to save lives. We made a difference in our community behind the wall, and that difference has allowed me to survive and thrive as a person with AIDS. To my peers in Bedford Hills Correctional Facility: you have truly made a difference. I can now go anywhere, and stand openly, alone without the silence. . . .

PART II
THE ACE CURRICULUM

8
Empowerment Through Education

ACE'S EDUCATIONAL PHILOSOPHY

Our approach to education embodies *peer* education in its essence, and we believe it is best suited for the task of enabling our community to mobilize itself to deal with HIV/AIDS. Our peer education takes a problem-posing approach. We present issues as problems to be examined, problems facing all of us, drawing on the knowledge and experience of the women being trained. This approach assures dialogue and encourages both the sharing of ideas and respect for differences. It also is the beginning of empowerment when our participants see that their ideas and experiences are important and respected.

There is a particular role open PWAs have played in our educational work. The participation of PWAs lets us talk about not "them," or "those people," but "us." PWAs speaking about the medical issues communicate a sense of hope because those of us who are PWAs are coping and surviving. PWAs can bring humor to the situation in ways that outsiders cannot. Finally, PWAs introduce a personal element to educational work—those of us who are HIV-positive are real people *living* with HIV/AIDS.

Most of our educational groups include people who are HIV-positive and who are not HIV-positive. This reality creates a need for special sensitivity. For example, one woman who is HIV-positive may be working through fears about having a sexual relationship; another woman who is not HIV-positive will say, "I would never have a relationship with someone who is HIV-positive." How do we have a group discussion about sexual relationships that can draw out everyone's feelings and doesn't leave people who are HIV-positive feeling worse? Although there is no simple answer to this kind of question, it means that educational workshops require creativity and awareness about the personal situations of people we are teaching.

TEACHING TECHNIQUES

The teaching techniques we have used are directly related to our educational philosophy.

Traditional Presentation of Knowledge

Trainers must be prepared to systematically present information in as clear a manner as possible. Visual aids are extremely important in the presentations. Much of the information will be new and will focus on medical and scientific data. It is crucial to reinforce what is discussed orally with both written and graphic representations. Handouts that allow people to deepen their understanding after the session is over are important, because they give participants something to take back to their housing units. Finally, newsprint or easel pads are useful for recording brainstorming sessions.

Brainstorming

This technique involves asking participants to share their ideas or feelings about a particular question, and a list is developed from the responses. It can be used for a number of goals:

a. It encourages everyone's participation and helps diminish fear of criticism. Everyone, after all, is just bouncing around some ideas.
b. It draws on the participants' knowledge, and it creates a bridge from what they know to what they are going to learn. It also helps the teacher find out what the participants already know, what level they're at.
c. It facilitates problem solving.

Role-Plays

A role-play simulates an actual situation in which a dilemma is being worked out, with the participants taking the roles of the people in the situation. A role-play allows both participants and observers to express feelings and creates a safe environment in which many of the complex issues related to HIV/AIDS can be expressed. It allows people to see things from new or different perspectives. A role-play can have different endings; how it plays out will vary depending on the personalities of the participants, their relationship in the role-play, and many other variables. The same dilemma can be worked on with as many variations as there are people.

Small-Group Discussions

Whereas large-group format is useful for passing on information, smaller groups, where everyone can talk on a more personal level, create an atmosphere of trust where real feelings and attitudes can emerge and be shared. Small groups may range anywhere from five to ten people. These groups have proved to be critical forums for discussions of stigma, sexual issues, HIV testing, and cultural issues. Small groups also provide a forum where women who are uncomfortable about speaking publicly—as many women are—can participate.

THE ACE CURRICULUM: EDUCATING OURSELVES

The ACE curriculum is embodied in nine workshops, each one lasting approximately one and a half hours. The entire series provides an extensive process for learning the information presented and exploring issues related to HIV/AIDS. The workshops are organized into the following topics:

1. HIV/AIDS: A Shared Concern
2. HIV/AIDS: A Social Disease of Stigma, Blame, and Prejudice
3. What Is HIV/AIDS?
4. HIV/AIDS: Treatment Strategies and the Role of the Nonexpert in Getting Medical Care
5. HIV/AIDS: Transmission—How HIV/AIDS Is Not Transmitted (Casual Contact), the Role of Drugs, Transmission from Mother to Child, and Blood Transfusions

6. HIV/AIDS: Sexual Transmission
7. HIV/AIDS: Testing
8. Women and HIV/AIDS
9. Living with HIV/AIDS.
   The workshop series meets three objectives of ACE's program:
   a. To provide an in-depth education for those who want to learn and talk about HIV/AIDS-related issues for their own personal reasons.
   b. To provide a process for encouraging women to become ACE members, so that ACE can continually involve new people. This is particularly important in a prison because people are constantly leaving the prison either for home or for other prisons.
   c. To provide training for ACE members to develop their abilities as peer educators. Usually, the different workshops are taught by teams of two to five women who work together to prepare and to carry out the workshop.

The nine workshops were developed as a series to educate individuals who want to have a deeper understanding of the HIV/AIDS epidemic than it is possible to get in a single-session presentation. Nevertheless, each workshop can be used alone. The curriculum is the basic material used by ACE not only in the nine-week workshop series but in the many situations in which we do educational work—orientation, video and discussion groups, classroom presentations. The groups presenting the material are constantly adapting it and developing it to meet the particular context in which it is to be used. We encourage you to do the same.

No matter how original, factual, and thorough a curriculum is, it is just a matter of words on paper. It takes *people* to give life and meaning to the information and teaching techniques. The usefulness of the material will be enhanced by what the facilitators and participants do with it. The interaction of the knowledge, ideas, and experiences of everyone in the group will create an education process that helps people change and grow. The background material provides a baseline of information. Read the teaching plans for approaches to teaching this material. Use them, and also develop your own.

Workshop #1
HIV/AIDS: A Shared Concern

UNTITLED

I've become a great
  artist in my mind
As I look up at
  the ceiling
From my hospital bed,
I begin to use my
  eyes as brushes,
    making forms of
      patterns.
Some spaces
  are visual, and
    others only connect.
I'm never alone
As I draw a
  clown.
Other times I focus
  on the side walls
drawing plastered
  creatures
with smiles and frowns.
The plastered canvas
has been revealed.
The exhibition is in my mind.

The infirmary at Bedford Hills, 1995
                   — DORIS MOICES

OVERVIEW

In giving a presentation concerning AIDS issues, there is a need to show and express sensitivity — not only about the information but also about the people who are participating. The goal of the entire workshop series is not just to give information but also to build a supportive community and involve people in the struggle around AIDS. This first workshop tries to create a community that is conducive not only to learning information but also to talking and dealing with feelings around the AIDS issues.

GOALS

1. To get to know each other and share possible concerns about AIDS;
2. To share what the participants hope to get out of the workshop series;
3. To build a sensitivity around one another;
4. To share the history of ACE and how AIDS has affected this prison;
5. To discuss why this workshop series is important;
6. To give an overview of the workshop series;
7. To talk about a common language and about confidentiality;
8. To explain the need for closure throughout the entire workshop series.

TEACHING GUIDE

1. Create small groups of no more than ten participants. Introduce participants. Ask each person what she hopes to get from the workshops and write it on a piece of newsprint. If time permits, ask people why they have joined the workshop series, but be aware that some people may not want to share this with the group.
2. Create a large circle of all participants and then read what is on the newsprint from each group. Comment on the concerns when needed.
3. Introduce ACE members. Talk about the history of ACE, and if there is time, ask some ACE members to share why they joined ACE. Tell participants that there are no certificates or letters to

Parole given. This is purely voluntary and must come from the personal commitment of each participant.

4. Discuss issue of confidentiality.
   a. What does confidentiality mean to participants?
   b. Do a role-play involving embarrassment, shame, and trust. For example, one past situation was that a woman openly stated that she was HIV-positive in the workshops. Later that week, she was waiting to pick up a package and she overheard another participant in the workshop telling someone that she was HIV-positive. She felt very vulnerable and brought this back to ACE. Point out that we cannot guarantee confidentiality, because the people who are participants are not ACE members, yet we hope that there will be a commitment to confidentiality and an atmosphere that is safe.

Discuss the need to let each person speak for herself. For example, a woman may, one week, want to discuss her feelings about being HIV-positive, and the next week she may not want to. It is important not to say, "Well, Ann is HIV-positive, and she said . . . ," because Ann needs to speak about herself when she feels comfortable doing so. Each person needs to empower herself through speaking about herself.

5. HIV-positive or HIV-negative
   Everyone involved in this workshop series has different reasons for being here. For some, there will be very sensitive issues discussed. Ask the group, What does it mean to be considerate of one another? For example, in a discussion, how do we avoid classifying HIV-positive people as "them"? Discuss the terms "victim" and "PWA."

6. Discussion of the Workshop Series.
   a. Importance of the Workshop Series: Through education and understanding, there is a reduction of fear and therefore a reduction in stigma. Through education, a PWA can empower herself: with this medical knowledge, she is able to make personal choices about her treatment and life.
   b. Briefly explain all workshops, time frames, movies, songs, breaks, and the need to be on time.

7. At the end of every workshop, fifteen minutes should be allotted for closure. Ask if everyone is in a good place. Make sure a support system is available. Announce the hours the office is open. End with a closure such as a song.

Workshop #2
HIV/AIDS: The Social Disease of Stigma, Blame, and Prejudice

Introducing the World of Stigma

When I lived in the projects and I got sick, they called the ambulance. They had masks on, rubber boots and gloves, like they were going in for a hurricane or something. The people in the projects told them I had spots on. So I got in the ambulance myself; I didn't want them to touch me the way they were dressed. The ambulance man said to the doctor, "I don't know what's wrong with her, but you better put gloves on because she has spots." They fixed me up and gave me some things for my fever and I went home.

Two days later there was a knock at my door and they said, "It's the Board of Health." I said, "You must have the wrong place." They said, "No, Mrs. K., we have the right place. You have spots and they want you out of the apartment." I said, "Who wants me out of the apartment?" They said, "The tenants all went to the landlord about you, because they have children, and they ain't sure what you got, but they don't want the kids with you." I said, "Well, I ain't moving, because I don't have anything contagious. They'll have to evict me."

All the tenants started talking about me, but I didn't let it bother me. I said to myself, "I'm not moving because I don't have anything contagious."

The next week I took my daughter downstairs to play in the kiddie park, and suddenly all the mothers came down to get their children. When a little girl fell off her bike and I leaned down to pick her up, her mother ran out of the apartment, freaking out on me, saying, "Don't touch my daughter, you have AIDS." It turns out the ambulance driver had told her, and she had told the other women.

All this made me feel awful, because people stared at me, whispered about me, saying, "That's the one. Don't let your kid play with her kid." But I was so stubborn I said I wasn't going to move, I wasn't going to let these people run me out. So they figured they couldn't get nowhere with me. The

Police Department and the Rescue Squad told the people in the projects, at a meeting that I wasn't invited to, that I had AIDS. They tried a lot of things, including calling the child abuse people. Finally, they got me out. They took me to court, saying I had too many people coming in and out and that I had someone living with me. But it took them three months.

When I was in the county jail, they put me in a single room, not on the tier with the rest of the girls. But I said, "You put me back there or I'm calling my lawyer." I heard them in a conference talking about me. Finally, after two days, they put me back on the tier, and as soon as I got back to the tier, a girl whom I had known closely on the street, whom I had let live in my house, she spit on me. I beat her head on the floor, so I never did make it to my tier. I said, "You've got some nerve, eating my food, staying at my house, and now spitting on me." Then they put me back on the tier with two other girls, but everyone had to use the same shower. All I ever heard was, "Don't let that AIDS bitch use that shower, because we have to use it. She's going to get us all sick."

I wrote all this up, and finally I got called before a board of four men to talk about this discrimination.

One of my friends had AIDS. When he got real sick, with lesions, the gas station that he used refused to give him gas. One day my mother was at the gas station after he died. The gas attendant was telling my mother how he refused to give the man gas. My mother said, "Why wouldn't you give him gas? Are you afraid that the AIDS is going to jump off the gas pumps?" The man answered, "Well, I just wouldn't sell him gas no more." So my mother said, "Well, Johnny, my daughter has AIDS, and you better get out from under my hood, because AIDS might jump off of my car onto you." Then my mother called a tow truck and had her car towed to the other gas station across the street.

I try not to let it bother me, what people say. A lot of it doesn't, but sometimes it does. It depends on how I'm feeling that day.

OVERVIEW

The HIV/AIDS epidemic is a medical problem. But along with this comes a social problem, a second epidemic: the epidemic of stigma, prejudice, scapegoating, persecution, discrimination, and blame. The medical problem is affected by racial and national prejudice and discrimination, by sexism and homophobia, combined with fears and stigma about illness and death. This social epidemic has an impact on the medical problem—on money for research and health care, on stress that an individual with HIV infection experiences, and on a community's ability to support people who are sick.

In a period when there is no medical cure for HIV/AIDS, all we have are the human resources—ourselves—to prevent the spread of HIV, to care for the ill, and to move forward on research. Thus, our second workshop looks at the damaging impact that stigma has on the HIV/AIDS epidemic and explores how we can challenge stigma. It is a problem-solving workshop in which we concretely examine examples of stigma in our community and talk about how to respond to them. If we can eliminate stigma, blame, and prejudice, we will actually make a difference in the course of the disease for individuals, communities, and nations in the struggle against HIV/AIDS.

GOALS

1. To understand the diverse roots of stigma and blame associated with the HIV/AIDS crisis;
2. To understand the negative effects of stigma and blame on individuals, communities, and societies facing the HIV/AIDS crisis;
3. To become conscious of one's own reaction to the HIV/AIDS epidemic;
4. To discuss, by looking at real situations, how we can decrease the stigma, blame, and prejudice in the HIV/AIDS crisis.

ISSUES TO EXAMINE

1. Examples of stigma and blame in past epidemics
2. Theories of origin and the problem of blame in the HIV/AIDS epidemic
3. HIV/AIDS stigma: its roots and impact
4. Stigma among us and our community, and what we can do to challenge stigma

BACKGROUND MATERIAL
History: Blame and Stigma in Past Epidemics

HIV/AIDS is not the first epidemic the world has had to deal with. Other epidemics include:

BLACK DEATH (BUBONIC PLAGUE): More than a quarter of the European population—25 million people—died in the 1300s. The social order collapsed: commerce stopped, food production plummeted, courts and police stopped functioning.[1]

SYPHILIS: It appeared in Europe in the 1490s and raged for most of the next century. It was feared until the development of antibiotics in the 1940s.

LEPROSY: It affected millions before the 1940s antibiotics.

INFLUENZA: From 1918 to 1926, it caused 20 million or more deaths throughout the world.[2]

Compare the statistics of HIV/AIDS with the above mentioned epidemics.

The World Health Organization estimates that:

- 18 million people worldwide are HIV-positive, and by the year 2000 there will be 30 to 40 million people with HIV infection.
- 4.5 million people worldwide have AIDS, and by the year 2000 there will be 13.5 million people with AIDS.

The federal Centers for Disease Control estimates that:

- 1 million people in the United States are HIV-positive.
- 401,750 people in the United States have AIDS.
- 53,978 of AIDS cases in the United States are women.

NOTE: Statistics on HIV infection rates are broad estimates, because the incidence of HIV infection is not always reported and is difficult to document.[3]

---

1. Massachusetts Department of Public Health and Massachusetts Department of Education, *Learn and Live: A Teaching Guide on AIDS Prevention,* 1987, p. 49.

2. W. H. McNeill, *Plagues and Peoples* (Garden City, N.Y.: Anchor Books, 1976), p. 255.

3. World Health Organization, United Nations Development Program, *Women and AIDS Agenda for Action* (January 1995); Federal Centers for Disease Control, *HIV/AIDS Surveillance Report* (October 1994).

STIGMA HAS ACCOMPANIED PAST EPIDEMICS

Stigma is a mark of shame, degradation; it makes a person less than human. A past example of stigma involved leprosy. In some European cities, people with leprosy had to wear wide-brimmed hats and ring a bell constantly whenever they went outside in order to identify themselves. This didn't have a medical rationale; it clearly degraded and dehumanized people.[4]

BLAME HAS BEEN ASSOCIATED WITH OTHER EPIDEMICS

People have always looked for someone to blame an epidemic on. Blaming others for a problem is a substitute for dealing with the problem itself. It is, in itself, a kind of contagious psychological process leading to stigmatizing, scapegoating, and persecution, and diverts focus and energy away from the problem. Blame frequently has been based on already existing attitudes and biases:

ANTI-SEMITISM: While the Black Death swept across Europe in the fourteenth century, blame was placed especially on Jews and was followed by the massacre and burning of all the alleged culprits.[5]

NATIONAL PREJUDICE: Syphilis seems first to have appeared in Italy. By 1495, it was in France, Germany, and Switzerland; it reached Holland and Greece in 1496; it was in England and Scotland by 1497 and in Hungary and Russia in 1499.

There was furious debate about whom to blame for the origin of the new disease. Foreigners were usually blamed, especially foreigners who were particularly disliked. The Russians blamed the Poles; the English and the Turks called it the French disease. The French called it the Italian illness, and the Italians called it the Spanish disease. The Spanish called it the sickness of Hispaniola, believing it to have come from what is now Haiti, when Columbus returned from his voyage to the Americas. Scientists still do not know where the fifteenth- and sixteenth-century syphilis epidemic came from.[6]

---

4. Johan Goudsbom, "Public Health and the Civilizing Process," *The Milbank Quarterly* 61 (1986): 166.

5. Massachusetts Department of Public Health and Massachusetts Department of Education, *Learn and Live*.

6. Renee Sabatier, *Blaming Others* (Washington, D.C.: The Panos Institute, 1988).

CLASS PREJUDICE: In 1817, cholera was identified in West Bengal. It spread throughout Asia, East Africa, France, Russia, England, and in the 1830s, the United States. Cholera, linked with lack of clean drinking water and of adequate sewage treatment, is associated with poverty. Stigma against poor people was reflected in the attitude that the cholera epidemic was a just punishment for people who were unwilling to change their lives. "The mass of mankind are, and there is reason to fear, ever will be insensible to the operation of great moral principles."[7]

The Present: Blame and Stigma and the HIV/AIDS Epidemic

Blaming others has characterized the HIV/AIDS epidemic. Haitians, Africans, the United States and germ warfare, and punishment from God have all been blamed for the HIV/AIDS epidemic.

HAITIANS HAVE BEEN BLAMED[8]

In mid-1982, the federal Centers for Disease Control (CDC) defined Haitians—along with homosexual and bisexual men, hemophiliacs, and IV drug users—as a "high-risk" group for HIV/AIDS. This was based on the report that there were 34 Haitians cases and 30 of them denied being homosexuals or drug users. The inference drawn from this data was that perhaps Haitians would provide a new clue to the nature or origins of AIDS.

Haitian physicians criticized this analysis, however, because they said it was not based on adequate data, that cultural biases and ignorance meant risk factors were not picked up. The hospital-based physicians gathering the data spoke no French or Creole, and they had no knowledge of Haitian culture, in which homosexuality is a deeply hidden secret; because the interview was conducted by someone whom they did not trust, those being interviewed were more likely to deny their bisexuality or homosexuality. A Haitian HIV/AIDS researcher asked why 88 percent of the early Haitian HIV/AIDS cases in the United States occurred in males. Then, in 1983,

---

7. Dudley Atkins quoted in Guenter Risse, "Epidemics and History: Ecology Perspectives and Social Response," in Elizabeth Fee and Daniel M. Fox, eds., *AIDS: The Burdens of History* (Berkeley: University of California Press), pp. 197–98.

8. The material about blaming the Haitians for the AIDS epidemic was largely based on the material in Sabatier, *Blaming Others*.

a group of Haitian researchers identified bisexuality as a risk factor in 75 percent of the HIV/AIDS patients, and blood transfusion as a risk factor in 5 percent. The remaining 6 percent had an unknown risk factor.

By July 1983, the New York City Health Commission had removed Haitians from the list of risk groups, and by 1985 CDC removed them as well. But by then the damage was already done, and health officials and the population at large saw Haitians as a risk group.

Stigma against Haitians still has not abated. On April 20, 1990, over 50,000 people demonstrated in New York City to protest a February 1990 Food and Drug Administration memorandum sent to all blood banks, which advised against accepting blood donations from all persons born in, or having emigrated from, Haiti, and from non-Haitians who have ever lived in Haiti or had sexual intercourse with a Haitian. Joseph Etienne, director of the Haitian Centers Council, stated: "This protest is intended to send a clear message to the FDA and the federal, state, and local governments. We wanted them to know that Haitians will no longer allow themselves to be used as the scapegoats in this HIV/AIDS crisis. . . . Today they are targeting Haitians. Tomorrow it will be all Blacks."[9]

The justification for the FDA policy was that HIV was spread predominantly through heterosexual transmission among Haitians, as opposed to other populations in the United States. Statistics on the rising incidence of women infected with HIV through heterosexual transmission throughout U.S. cities make it clear that there is no reason to single out Haitians in terms of heterosexual transmission.

What was the impact of blaming HIV/AIDS on the Haitians?

1. There was an increase in racism against Haitians by combining assumptions about voodoo, sexual practices, and transmission of disease. For example, some people proposed that Haitians may have contracted the virus from monkeys as part of bizarre sexual practices in Haitian brothels, or from voodoo rituals.

2. The United States witnessed a rise of anti-Haitian attitudes directed at Haitians living in this country. By 1980, between 100,000 and 300,000 Haitian refugees had fled the economic stagnation and political repression of the Duvalier dictatorship. Many were here illegally, because the United States supported

---

9. *New York Times*, April 21, 1990, p. 25; *New York Times*, April 22, 1990, p. 34.

that government. By late 1982, these immigrants found themselves categorized as a "risk group" for HIV/AIDS, as "AIDS
carriers." People demanded that they be thrown out.

3. Haitian community workers reported that in some areas the unemployment rate for Haitians was twice that of other black
workers, and that this was attributable to HIV/AIDS.

4. Haiti's tourism industry supported 25,000 jobs in an economy
plagued by unemployment. The HIV/AIDS epidemic literally
killed off the tourist industry. Tourism fell from 70,000 visitors
in the winter of 1981–82 to 10,000 the following year. The political climate bore some responsibility, but authorities feel it was
the HIV/AIDS epidemic that bore the brunt of responsibility.

BLAMING THE AFRICANS

Blood tests that were not very accurate compared with those currently
used suggested that HIV/AIDS had been widespread in Africa for many
decades before it appeared in the rest of the world. This theory was
overturned when newer HIV-antibody tests were used. The African scientists found it both unlikely and insulting that HIV/AIDS would have been
widespread in Africa and unnoticed by them.

Another theory was that the virus might have been introduced to
Africans through green monkeys. This theory was based on speculation
about cultural and sexual practices of Africans. Whatever legitimate scientific inquiry existed around this theory, it was thoroughly distorted by the
racist projections of Western scientists and media. African scientists also
felt that such theories were not rigorously investigated, nor were they
accompanied by equal inquiry about origins in the United States.

The need to discover origins degenerated into the need to blame.
Today, there is a strong current of opinion among scientists that the HIV/
AIDS epidemic is as new to the African continent as it is to the rest of the
world. It probably developed in the mid–1970s in Africa, as it did in the
United States and Europe. Some Africans believe that Western research
into the possibility that HIV/AIDS originated in Africa has been partially
base on slipshod science, motivated by a desire to prove that HIV/AIDS
started somewhere other than in the United States.

What was the impact of blaming HIV/AIDS on the Africans?

1. While the early theories of African origins were often reported
with ghoulish headlines, the evidence of scientific errors was

buried in the back of the newspapers. The racism and national chauvinism that were encouraged by such headlines were left unchallenged.

2. Recoiling from the threat of European racism and stigma, many African governments underreported the prevalence of HIV/AIDS in their countries and were hesitant to allow Western scientists and doctors to work in their countries. Unfortunately, the resources available to African countries and their doctors facing the HIV/AIDS epidemic are much less than what is available in the United States.

3. Throughout the world, wherever African students were studying, they were widely blamed for HIV/AIDS and suffered prejudice and stigma. These countries included Belgium, Great Britain, and India.

4. African reactions can be summed up as follows, in the words of a physician from one of the worst HIV/AIDS-affected Central African countries:

What seems to have happened is that some of the Western press and researchers have used the seropositivity data we supplied, but instead of putting HIV under the microscope they have put our society, our customs, even our love life under the lens. Do you find it surprising that some of us resent this? Whatever goes wrong, whether it is famine, war, politics, or anything else, it is always because we Africans are more incompetent, corrupt, bloodthirsty or immoral than other people. We just got tired of it—we give you information and so often you seem to turn it against us.[10]

THE UNITED STATES AND THE GERM WARFARE THEORY

Many Third World people around the world and in the United States, angered by the United States' blaming other countries or concerned about the genocidal impact of HIV/AIDS on black and Latin peoples, responded by saying that HIV/AIDS was unleashed on the world by germ warfare experimentation in the United States Defense Department laboratory at Fort Detrick, Maryland. Many prisoners have expressed this view.

This theory is difficult to prove one way or the other. Arguments against it include:

---

10. Sabatier, *Blaming Others,* pp. 89–90.

1. Genetic engineering was not sufficiently advanced to develop such a manmade virus at the time HIV first appeared, which was in the 1950s.
2. Why develop a virus unless one's own side can be protected against it? The ideal germ warfare organism would be one that caused disease very quickly, did not spread by itself, and only infected the targeted population, and one for which there was a vaccine to protect one's own side.

On the other hand, others argue that the virus could have been the result of an accident while doing such experimentation.

THE THEORY THAT HIV/AIDS IS GOD'S PUNISHMENT FOR CERTAIN BEHAVIORS

This argument is used to blame homosexuals and IV drug users for bringing HIV/AIDS upon themselves. It has inflamed homophobic attitudes and led to discrimination, assaults, and stigmatization of IV drug users and homosexuals. Women with HIV/AIDS have also suffered from this argument, for they are labeled promiscuous just because they are HIV-infected.

LOOKING FOR THE ORIGINS OF HIV/AIDS

Sometimes people ask about the origins of HIV/AIDS because they are looking for someone to blame for it. But there are legitimate reasons for curiosity about the origins of HIV/AIDS. How did something happen all of a sudden? Where did it come from? Good reasons for asking about the origins:

1. We want some sense of control over our environment;
2. We hope that it might provide answers for a cure;
3. We are curious, and just want to understand.

What are the main theories of origins?

1. HIV/AIDS has been around for a long time. Perhaps it existed in an isolated ethnic group that had acquired immunity to it, so that it rarely caused death. When it spread outside this group and reached people who had no such immunity, it

became a killer.

Diseases familiar in one part of the world when carried to virgin territory have often proved a mortal danger to the newly exposed population. European diseases such as measles and small pox virtually wiped out some North American Indian peoples in the eighteenth and nineteenth centuries.

2. HIV/AIDS came from animals. Some diseases pass from animals to humans—for example, rabies. Blood tests show that forest monkeys in Central and South America and in Africa could act as a reservoir for the yellow fever virus. When carried to urban areas, the yellow fever virus can cause a major epidemic, such as the one that killed thousands of Nigerians in 1987. Trichinosis is spread to humans when they eat uncooked pork. Flea bites spread the bubonic plague. Lassa fever spread from rats.

   Since a virus similar to HIV has been found in monkeys, this theory has gotten attention, but it has not been proved.

3. HIV is a manmade virus, perhaps from a germ warfare laboratory.

4. HIV is the mutation of an already existing virus.

   At this time, it is not known how HIV/AIDS originated; the cause is unknown. It may never be known, just as the origin of syphilis is not known more than five hundred years after it first appeared.

HIV/AIDS: The Roots of Stigma

Stigma toward people with HIV/AIDS comes from other underlying biases:

1. There is stigma against groups already considered outcasts or having second-class status in society. They have already been characterized as inferior or marked or even as disgraceful. HIV/AIDS is simply an added mark.
   a. Negative feelings toward homosexuality/bisexuality and homosexuals/bisexuals;
   b. Racism and ethnic prejudice directed against black and Latin peoples;

   c. Sexism (the view of women as second-class citizens and sexual objects) and anti-woman feelings, especially those associated with women who are prostitutes or who have sexually transmitted diseases—related to the image of "the fallen woman," the woman fallen into sin. Antiwoman feelings often are combined with racism.

2. There is stigma attached to people who engage in certain types of activities, and this also combines with other stigma based on race, class, and sex:
   a. IV drug users
   b. prostitutes
3. There is stigma toward people from other countries; they are considered "less cultured," less civilized. This stigma is apparent in attitudes toward Africa, and it comes from national chauvinism and racism.
4. There is stigma associated with death and serious illness.

What do people gain when they stigmatize others around HIV/AIDS?

1. By seeing others as "bad" or "lesser" and seeing themselves as better, people feel a psychological sense of protection and security from HIV/AIDS, because only "bad people" get such a disease. People believe that because they are not members of the above-mentioned groups and do not indulge in the above-mentioned activities, they will not get HIV/AIDS; they see this disease as directed at the "other," not at themselves.

    I think the stigma will always be there. We, as individuals in this place, stigmatize people in general. I think it comes from how we are brought up. We stigmatize people all the time. The ultimate stigma that people hold on to is toward AIDS. What does stigma do for the stigmatizers? It gives them some power, some type of authoritative feeling.

* * *

2. People also stigmatize those who are ill, out of fear of serious illness and death. People's fear of death and serious illness makes them want to dissociate from people who are sick, as if the mere association could make them more vulnerable. Thus,

they see sick people as "the other," different, and this also gives them a sense of well-being and a false sense of security.
3. People use the negative meaning of AIDS to hurt other people. When two people are angry at each other, even if they are educated, calling someone "an AIDS bitch" is a way to hurt the other person, to insult that person, because AIDS has such a negative meaning.

The Impact of Stigma on Individuals, on Our Communities, and on Society

There is so much stigma associated with AIDS that individuals and communities as well as whole societies are negatively affected. The individual has experienced discrimination: in jobs, housing, medical insurance, schools. An individual is treated with cruelty, and seen as lesser, not worthy of care and attention, even less than human. This creates feelings of shame. Individuals may deny their illness, or choose not to find out if they have it in order not to be associated with it. Stigma robs the HIV-positive individual of the very things she or he needs the most: support, love, medical care, and self-esteem.

The broader society does not give adequate resources for dealing with the HIV/AIDS crisis to individuals and communities who are in stigmatized groups.

The larger society is affected by a loss of its own humanity in its treatment of others, and ultimately, this means the spread of HIV/AIDS is not prevented as soon as it might be. The result is that greater numbers of people become ill.

Stigmatizing and blaming others give people in the "mainstream" the illusion of safety. People believe that because they are not associated with so-called "risk groups"—for example, gays or IV drug users—they run no risk of infection. This undermines the effort to promote safe behavior and to stem the transmission of HIV.

* * *

I feel that the more we learn, the less stigma we have, and if we don't learn about HIV or AIDS, our people will die from being ignorant about the disease. By "our people" I mean black, white, Puerto Rican—I'm talking about saving lives, it doesn't matter what color you are anymore. Stigma is labeling, prejudice.

There was a time when I wouldn't *hear* any information; even though I heard it, it didn't go into me. I knew I was doing risky behavior with sex, but the stigma I had toward IV drug users meant that I didn't pay attention to the information. I just knew it wasn't me, I knew I wasn't like "them." It means a lot when you can say, "I'm in the same boat." I felt that I was better, and all along I wasn't.

* * *

THE HOMOSEXUAL COMMUNITY

Until recently, people thought of HIV/AIDS as a disease essentially afflicting homosexuals and bisexuals. In the early 1980s, when scientists first became aware of the disease, they called it GRID (Gay Related Immune Deficiency).

The larger society denied the seriousness of the disease.

HIV/AIDS took on the character of being a "gay" disease. Because of stigma against gay people, the larger society and the medical establishment did not give it enough attention early in the epidemic when it could have made a difference. This adversely affected gay people and gay communities. It also meant that the larger society was left more vulnerable to the disease, which is not a "gay disease" but one that anyone can get depending on their activities.

The development of HIV/AIDS became a rationalization for an increase in antigay attitudes, discrimination, and attacks against gay people.

The gay community denied HIV/AIDS.

Some gay people feared that acknowledging that HIV/AIDS existed within their community would jeopardize their hard-won status and lifestyle. They felt it would increase repression from homophobic groups, endanger victories against discrimination, and force homosexual men back on the defensive. Also, gay people who found out that they were HIV-positive had to face "coming out," both as PWAs and as homosexuals.

The resulting denial meant a delay in the community mobilization that was necessary to slow down the spread of HIV/AIDS and to fight for the needs of PWAs. Once gay communities overcame the denial of the disease, they became the key force in mobilizing for resources and research to fight HIV/AIDS and stigma. The gay community recognized that its survival was at stake and struggled to change group norms around sexual behavior. This community mobilization significantly slowed down the rate of new HIV infection among gay white middle-class men.

BLACK AND HISPANIC COMMUNITIES

HIV/AIDS is a major problem in black and Hispanic communities. Large black and Hispanic urban communities affected by HIV/AIDS also are facing the desperate problems of drugs, unemployment, illiteracy, crime, racism, and inadequate housing, education, health care, and day care. It is in this larger context that the impact of stigma and the HIV/AIDS crisis must be placed.

Racism affects how society treats the HIV/AIDS epidemic in black and Latin communities.

HIV/AIDS is a sexually transmitted disease. There are many taboos surrounding sexuality, and when people from one ethnic group discuss other people's sexual behavior, frequently racial and ethnic prejudices are involved.

Society does not provide black and Hispanic communities with adequate resources.

The large urban areas that have been so profoundly affected by HIV/AIDS are referred to as "crack-ridden," "violence-ridden," and now "AIDS-ridden" populations. The reality of human beings behind these labels disappears. The broader society does not provide black and Latin communities with the basic human resources that are needed to prevent HIV/AIDS and to care for those who are already sick. Stigma combined with racism, ethnic prejudice, and other social factors means:

- Greater vulnerability of individuals to the disease due to combined conditions of poverty.
- Less of an ability for the individual to deal with the impact of the disease.
- Less of an ability for a community to mobilize to deal with the crisis of HIV/AIDS.

Black and Hispanic communities denied HIV/AIDS.

African-American and Hispanic people are already discriminated against. With the stigma associated with HIV/AIDS, blacks and Hispanics do not want another reason to be singled out. This is one reason why people deny the existence of the disease within their own community. This denial makes it difficult to deal with the existing crisis, because individuals do not get the necessary support and the community does not mobilize to demand help from the government and the society at large. HIV/AIDS is seen as only one more problem among many others. At the same time, HIV/AIDS is a problem so big that it seems impossible to deal with.

Within black and Hispanic communities, there is widespread rejection of homosexuality/bisexuality.

Homosexuality is seen as conflicting with cultural and religious beliefs. Such practices are stigmatized and viewed as a sign of weakness when applied to black and Hispanic men. This isolates and injures black and Latin gay people who now face both antigay attitudes and ostracism as PWAs. It also means that the issue of transmission through homosexual/bisexual practices is not properly addressed. Refusal to share and address these issues in the communities continues to threaten the population of women at risk.

Sexism in black and Hispanic communities, as in the rest of society, affects women around HIV/AIDS.

In the best of circumstances, the secondary status of women means that it is more difficult for women to negotiate safe sex. In addition, unless sexual violence and aggression aimed at minority women is dealt with, the danger of spreading HIV/AIDS through heterosexual contact is great.

PEOPLE WHO USE IV DRUGS AND CRACK

The AIDS epidemic is becoming more and more closely tied to the drug epidemic. Almost half of the new infections are among drug users who shared needles, and increasingly many crack users are also becoming infected. In New York, it is estimated that at least half of the 200,000 people who are addicted and use IV drugs are infected with the HIV virus, but this figure seriously underrepresents the number of cases of HIV/AIDS among IV drug users, because many of them have no health insurance—they have died or will die of AIDS-related infections outside the care of the medical system. Therefore they would not be reported to the CDC. They are considered the second wave of the AIDS epidemic.[11]

Society views IV drug users as primarily "a social problem" and to some degree as people who are expendable. They are often viewed as, and often are, active in criminal activities. The IV drug users' own habits play a role in their inability to get education, treatment, and support systems. On the other hand, politicians and others have argued against funding education and prevention programs for drug users, arguing that they are "uneducatable."

Stigma against drug users, frequently combined with racism and with stigma about illness, has meant poorer health care and support systems. It has meant that they are not accepted into drug trials because they are defined as "unreliable." This means they do not have access to the potentially beneficial new drugs being developed.

WOMEN[12]

Women represent 13 percent of the total AIDS cases in the United States. The proportion of women with AIDS has increased steadily, and it is estimated that women are now contracting the virus at least as fast as men. Women of color have been disproportionately impacted by AIDS: 54 percent of all women with AIDS are black; 21 percent of all women with AIDS are Hispanic; 24 percent are white.[13]

The vast majority of women who have AIDS in New York are black or Hispanic and poor. Frequently, either they or their partners have been drug users. Already such people carry the social stigmas from race, class, or gender prejudices. The result is that the individual woman with AIDS is going to experience less support when she needs it, in terms of psychological, medical, or physical resources.

---

11. Gina Kolata, "New Picture of Who will Get AIDS Is Dominated by Addicts," *The New York Times,* February 28, 1995, Section C, p. 3; editorial, *New York Times,* November 26, 1994.

12. Material for this section was drawn, in part, from Barbara Santee, *Women and AIDS: The Silent Epidemic* (New York: WARN, 1989).

13. Federal Centers for Disease Control, *HIV/AIDS Surveillance Report* (October 1994); World Health Organization, United Nations Development Program, *Women and AIDS Agenda for Action.*

Sexism impacts on women and HIV/AIDS.

Women are viewed as second-class citizens. This is reflected in neglect by the medical establishment. There has been inadequate study of how the disease progresses in women. Women are often excluded from drug trials, which offer some of the only possible treatments for HIV/AIDS. The exclusion of women from drug trials is done in the name of protecting women, because of the danger of harming her fetus. But that approach to the problem means that women are being given drugs that were never tested on women, as well as being excluded from possible existing drug therapies.

Because the majority of women dealing with HIV/AIDS are black and Latin, racism and conditions of poverty combine with sexism to create pressures around women dealing with HIV/AIDS. (See workshop on Women and HIV/AIDS.)

Women are stigmatized for being sexual.

HIV/AIDS is a sexually transmitted disease. When a woman has a sexually transmitted disease, society tends to look upon her with disdain, as if she is amoral, "a fallen woman." One way in which this was seen in the HIV/AIDS epidemic was in the scapegoating of prostitutes. Prostitutes were blamed for being key transmitters of HIV. There has been no real cry of concern for prostitutes' lives, even though female sex workers are at far greater risk of contracting HIV from clients than clients are of contracting HIV from sex workers. In the United States, HIV heterosexual transmission is much more likely to occur from a man to a woman than from a woman to a man. This sexual stigma affects not only prostitutes but all women, since it is often assumed that if a woman is HIV-positive, then she is a prostitute.[14]

HIV-positive women may have difficulty getting an abortion.

Some doctors are prejudiced against prostitutes and IV drug users and will assume that any HIV-positive woman is one or the other or both. They may feel it is not worth the personal risk of infection to perform an operation on an individual against whom they carry prejudice.[15]

---

14. Mary Ide, with Wendy Sanford and Amy Alpern, "AIDS, HIV Infection and Women," in The Boston Women's Health Collective, eds., *The New Our Bodies, Ourselves* (New York: Simon & Schuster, 1992).

15. Commission on Human Rights, Law Enforcement Bureau, AIDS Discrimination Unit, "HIV-Related Discrimination by Reproductive Health Care Providers in New York City," October 22, 1990 (New York: 1990).

Even if a woman can find a doctor, she may not be able to afford one. Because of the stigma around HIV/AIDS, people have lost their jobs, their insurance coverage, and their homes, and in many states abortions are no longer paid for by Medicaid—hence they cannot pay for abortions.

On the other hand, if a poor HIV-infected woman wants to continue her pregnancy, she is more likely to be condemned for that decision than a middle-class woman deciding to take the risk of any other high-risk pregnancy. In part, this is because there is a moral judgment about any disease that is sexually transmitted. Those who contract it are seen as being punished by a righteous God for indulging in certain types of unacceptable behavior.

Stigma gives some women a false sense of security.

Women who are not themselves IV drug users and are not involved with men using IV drugs, especially women of middle-class socio-economic status, see themselves as not vulnerable to HIV/AIDS. They consider themselves "above the other class" that has been greatly affected by HIV infection. Hence, there is a belief that there is no need for safer sex. And while statistically they may be less likely to have a sexual encounter with someone carrying the virus, it is an illusion to feel that they are exempt from danger. This illusion was promoted by media articles and books such as *The Myth of Heterosexual AIDS,* but recent data is pointing out the dangers of heterosexual transmission for women.[16]

DISCRIMINATION AND STIGMA IN PRISON

AIDS is the leading cause of death among inmates in prisons throughout the United States; it is five to ten times more common in prisons than in general society. In New York State, AIDS has been the leading cause of death among inmates since at least 1989, when AIDS-related deaths accounted for 131 of 200 inmate deaths (65 percent). According to a 1992 blind HIV study of New York State incoming inmates, 12 percent tested positive overall, and 20 percent of the women tested positive.[17]

---

16. Michael Fumento, *The Myth of Heterosexual AIDS,* 1989; Kolata, "New Picture of Who Will Get AIDS. . . ."

17. Dennis Cauchon, "AIDS in Prison: Locked Up and Locked Out," *USA TODAY,* March 31, 1995, 6A; New York State Department of Health AIDS Institute, *Focus on AIDS in New York State* (April 1994) ed. Miki Conn, newsletter (Albany, N.Y.: 1984).

The closed prison environment when combined with stigma can create enormous suffering for a prisoner who is HIV-positive. An incident in an Alabama prison, in the early period of the AIDS epidemic, illustrates this: A prisoner who was HIV-positive had to wear a gown, gloves, and mask, and squirt disinfectant over each step each time she left her cell.[18]

Today, some states and counties have laws or official policies that treat prisoners who are HIV-positive differentially; New York States does *not* have any such differential laws or official policies. Some examples of these laws and official policies include:

- Segregation of HIV-positive inmates from other prisoners, and denial of access to the majority of education and work programs that are available to the rest of the prison population. This segregation is explained by prison authorities as necessary to stop the spread of the HIV/AIDS disease inside the prison.[19]
- A ban on prisoners who are HIV-positive from kitchen work, even though the federal Centers for Disease Control says that there is no scientific basis for this policy.
- Denial of access for inmates who are HIV-positive from low-level security classifications, especially those needed to hold jobs outside prison walls, such as picking up litter. These jobs are often necessary for early-release qualification.
- Denial of participation in all early-release programs, such as furloughs and work release, for HIV-positive inmates.
- Denial of conjugal visits to HIV-positive inmates.

The prison authorities' rationale for such differential treatment ranges from the need to maintain management and order among other inmates who have fears of those with HIV/AIDS to the need to respect a public that is hostile toward allowing those prisoners with HIV/AIDS to be let out of prison. Leading HIV/AIDS researchers have said there is no medical reason to discriminate against prisoners with HIV/AIDS. This differential treatment contributes to existing fears and stigma.[20]

Stigma exists among prisoners just as it does in the rest of society. But because prison is such a contained living situation, there is even more

---

18. Conversation with John Hale, spokesman for the Alabama Department of Corrections, Winter 1995.

19. Cauchon, "AIDS in Prison," p. 6A.

20. Ibid.

difficulty in escaping from it. Prisoners have written and talked about having to move from one living unit to another because the pressure against them was so great. Stigma against those who are HIV-positive can combine with racism and/or homophobia to create enormous pressure on a prisoner whose options and openings are already limited.

Stigma can seriously impact on individuals' ability to cope with the AIDS epidemic. For example, homophobia can inhibit frank and honest discussion about safer sex problems; this is particularly a problem in men's prisons. Many prisoners hide the fact that they are HIV-positive in order to escape the stigma and discrimination, and in so doing they deny themselves the medical care that they need and are unable to develop the social support needed to cope with the illness.

RISK GROUP OR RISK ACTIVITIES

Scientists used to speak about "risk groups." They spoke of homosexuals or IV drug users as a risk group for contracting HIV. This was misleading, because people felt that they were safe from getting HIV if they were not a member of a risk group. The risk is not whether you are or feel you are part of a particular group but whether your activity is risky. If you have unsafe sex with someone who is HIV-infected, you are at risk for getting HIV. It doesn't matter how you define yourself sexually. People may not define themselves as IV drug users, but if they use an IV drug once or twice and happen to share a needle with infected blood in it, they can get HIV. Not only is the concept of a "risk group" misleading, not only does it give people a sense of false safety, it also contributes to stigma by focusing on particular groups as dangerous.

TEACHING PLAN

I. How Does Stigma Feel?

a. Give a shocker, a dramatic experience of someone being stigmatized, that all participants can feel. Plan with someone from the audience ahead of time that she will be the target of stigma around HIV/AIDS. Pick a real situation—the more the participants can identify with it the better—or create a situation in which every one of the participants is involved either in being stigmatized or in stigmatizing.

   b. Ask the person (people) being stigmatized about how she felt when it happened.

   c. Ask the entire group, "Have each of you ever felt stigmatized in the way that the person(s) whom you just saw were? Under what circumstances (racial, nationality, gender, illness, financial), and how did it feel?"

II. Brainstorm: Why do people stigmatize? (See background materials for general reasons for stigma and the particular ones associated with HIV/AIDS and illness.) Let facilitator members open up and share their own experiences in stigmatizing people and the process of change that they have gone through. If facilitators are open and honest about their own process, this will encourage an openness among all participants. It is only through an openness about the feelings that cause stigma that we can begin to change.

III. Role-Plays and Discussion: Why are particular groups stigmatized around HIV/AIDS and what is the impact of stigma on a group of people and on society?

Create very short precise role-plays to illustrate the main points in the background materials for discussion of stigma. (This includes homosexuals, black and Latin people, women, prisoners, IV drug users). After each role play, using the newsprint, discuss the main point of what happened.

IV. Presentation on History: Stigma about illness is not new. Stigma toward people with illness is often combined with blame. Present information about the history of epidemics and stigma and the blame toward Haitians and the Africans about HIV/AIDS. This is also a good point in the discussion to explore the theories about the origins of HIV/AIDS.

V. Discussion and Evaluation of Real-Life Situations: How can we eliminate stigma? Discuss real-life situations that people in the group know about, and discuss what people could do in that situation. These situations could be put into role-plays in order to work with them. Two of our own real-life situations, which we put into role-play form, are:

1. Maria sees the coat of Janice, who is HIV-positive, on a chair. She turns to Janice and says, "Take your coat off the chair." She never says anything to her about being HIV-positive, but the underlying tone is that she doesn't want the coat of an HIV-positive person on a chair where she is about to sit. Karen sees this and responds *(various responses and results)*.

2. Joanie is frustrated because she can't find her sweater. She sees that Toni, who is a friend of hers but with whom she frequently argues, is wearing her sweater. Toni is HIV-positive. She starts yelling at her for borrowing the sweater without asking her. Finally, she says, "You're an AIDS-ridden bitch."

A third friend, Denise, intervenes, getting angry at Joanie for her attitude.

In each of the above role-plays, ask:

1. Why do you think one person stigmatized the other person?
2. If you had been observing the scene, what would you have done?

REFERENCE MATERIALS

M. C. Bartnof. "AIDS-HIV 1989 Overview and Update: Overview and Introduction: Why AIDS." From a multidisciplinary survey elective course on AIDS from the UCSF School of Medicine, presented by the AIDS Professional Education Project with support from the National Institute of Mental Health and the Department of Medicine and Psychiatry.

The Boston Women's Health Collective, *The New Our Bodies, Ourselves.* New York: Simon & Schuster, 1992.

Goudsblom, Johan. "Public Health and the Civilizing Process." *The Milbank Quarterly* (1986).

The Harris County Medical Society and the Houston Academy of Medicine. *AIDS: A Guide for Survival.* United States, 1989.

W. H. McNeill. *Plagues and Peoples.* Garden City, N.Y.: Anchor Books, 1976.

Massachusetts Department of Public Health and Massachusetts Department of Education. *Learn and Live: A Teaching Guide on AIDS Prevention.* 1987.

Risse, Guenter. "Epidemics and History: Ecology Perspectives and Social Response." In Elizabeth Fee and Daniel M. Fox, eds., *AIDS: The Burdens of History.* Berkeley: University of California Press.

Sabatier, Renee. *Blaming Others.* Washington, London, Paris: Panos Institute, 1988.

Santee, Barbara. *Women and AIDS: The Silent Epidemic.* New York: WARN, 1989.

Workshop #3
What is HIV/AIDS?

As the disease progresses, it's better to know what's happening to you, but it's also scary, like going to St. Claire's Hospital scared me.

Sometimes the unknown is better than the known. Yet you have to know. Like, if your lips fall off, do I have to use lipstick, what color should I use?

There's always hope, 'cause if you give up on hope, what the hell do you have left? I always tell people, if they don't find a cure, I will. And don't treat me like a pitiful nut, 'cause I felt great until I ran into you—you made me depressed.

Some days I don't feel like smiling, but I manage to crack a joke at least once a day. I want to learn all I can so I can pass it on to others—HIV-positive or not—if it will help them. As for me, as far as being frightened, I mean it's frightening, no matter what. I mean my body is deteriorating all over the place. I never did look like Marilyn Monroe, but now I have all these problems: losing hair, teeth—at least my nails are growing.

I know a lot of things, and there's things you really don't want to know, 'cause it's scary, about the deterioration of the body. There's things you have to know because you're going to have to understand. The thing that gets me through is my sense of humor. If I were teaching this material, I'd do it with a sense of humor.

* * *

I went in search of other long-term survivors, and it seems that I now know more long-term survivors of AIDS than anyone in the world.

I certainly am not sitting on any secrets. I didn't discover the cure for AIDS. There was no single approach that jumped out at me as the obvious way to guarantee long-term survival. When I'm forced to summarize what I found, I say that hope is the necessary precondition to long-term survival. Having hope won't guarantee that you'll survive AIDS, but not having hope seems to guarantee that you'll go pretty quickly.

I have become more convinced, as a result of my own experience with AIDS and from my interviews with about twenty-five other long-term survivors, that there is a bidirectional mind-body connection, which someday we may be able to pin down scientifically. I think the body needs to receive a "live" message. The mind needs to tell the body to fight—that life is precious and worth living. The mind is a great, largely untapped pharmacy, and we've got to find creative ways to mine it. Joy juice is what the body needs to live. And hope is like the air that we breathe; without it, we wither and die.

—MICHAEL CALLEN,
From *Newsline* published by
People With Aids Coalition.

OVERVIEW

HIV is a disease that is new to science. A lot is unknown, but a lot has been learned. This workshop will be a basic science lesson about the body and how it defends itself against disease and the particular struggle it goes through with the HIV virus. We will first look at this process on a biological level and then on the clinical level in terms of how the disease shows itself in symptoms. Learning about these things can begin to give people some way to participate in their own planning and struggle around their health. When people can understand what is happening to themselves or to their loved ones, they become more confident defining and acting on medical and social options.

GOAL

To communicate what the HIV virus is and how it affects the body and causes HIV/AIDS.

ISSUES TO EXAMINE

1. What is HIV/AIDS?
2. What causes HIV/AIDS?
3. How does HIV attack the body?
4. What are the signs and symptoms of HIV/AIDS?
5. What are the cofactors that can affect a person's ability to struggle with the virus?

BACKGROUND MATERIAL

Our Body: Healthy and Sick

During recent decades, doctors and scientists have begun to adopt a biopsychosocial view of health and disease. This means that they see the person in a holistic way: physical, emotional, and social factors all interact, affecting the well-being of an individual. This is particularly evident in medical science dealing with HIV/AIDS.

Illness can be caused by a number of external forces called agents.

- A microorganism, such as the virus that causes the flu or small-pox, or a bacteria.
- Toxic substances, such as poison.
- A force such as electricity.

Illness can be caused by psychological factors.

- Stress is a well-known factor influencing high blood pressure and heart attacks.

Illness can be caused by social factors.

- Malnutrition can cause disease, and it is frequently an indicator of poverty in the lives of children who suffer from it.
- Environmental factors, such as pollution or the noise from airports, contribute to disease.

Individually and in combination, these and other factors cause illness.

Health can be aided by biological factors.

Medicines, often made of microorganisms or chemicals or herbs, can help us get healthy or stay healthy.

Health can be aided by psychological factors.

- Stress reduction.
- Love.
- Activities that are relaxing.

Health can be aided by social factors.

- Living in a nonpolluted environment.
- Stopping smoking.
- Escaping poverty/malnutrition.

WHAT IS AIDS?

A	=	Acquired	Gotten from risk behaviors. Not inherited.
I	=	Immune	Having to do with the system that defends the body from disease.
D	=	Deficiency	A state in which the immune system is not working properly.
S	=	Syndrome	A collection of symptoms or diseases affecting various body parts and systems and together defining a disease (cite HIV-Symptomatic handout).

HIV is caused by a virus that you can get from other people. There is a breakdown of the body's defense system, called the immune system, and this breakdown produces a susceptibility to certain diseases. Often there is a specific cluster of disorders and symptoms associated with HIV, a syndrome. Scientists are also studying the possibility of cofactors, such as other biological, psychological, and social factors, and substances such as drugs or alcohol, which may affect each individual's response to HIV infection and the course of the illness. In this workshop, we will go into detail on how the HIV virus works in the body, but we will also look at the other possible factors that may affect this disease and its treatment. The next workshop will focus more directly on how the biopsychosocial approach relates to treatment of HIV infection.

MICROORGANISMS CAN CAUSE DISEASE

Not all microorganisms are bad; some are good for us. The common term people use for microorganisms that hurt us is "germs." Using microscopes, scientists discovered that there were different kinds of germs. You have heard their names: bacteria, protozoa, fungi, virus. What is special about them is that because they are living, they can reproduce themselves—that is part of what it means to be living—and as they multiply inside our body, they can make us sick. And these microorganisms can be passed—transmitted—from one infected person to another person and she or he can then get sick.

THREE IMPORTANT CONCEPTS ABOUT DISEASE-CAUSING
MICROORGANISMS

1. *Exposure:* This is the actual physical contact with a disease-causing organism. But exposure does not necessarily mean getting sick. For example, you might be in a room where someone coughs and sneezes, and the microorganism in the cough or sneeze may reach you but never enter your body, or it can enter your body in such a small quantity that it doesn't make you sick. Then you are exposed to it.

2. *Infection:* This can follow exposure. The germ or other disease-causing organism can invade the cells in your body. You may never get sick, you may never develop symptoms, because your body's defense system—the immune system—may be able to fight the infection off before you even know you have it. But if you are infected, you are often able to infect other people by passing the microorganism on to them.

3. *Disease:* If, after exposure and infection, the invading organism overpowers the immune system, the disease will be present, in either a mild or severe form.

How do we defend ourselves against harmful microorganisms?

The body's ability to defend itself is called "immunity," resistance to injury from invading organisms. The first line of defense is the outer parts of our body: for example, skin, eye lashes, mucous membrane in our nose, and parts of our throat. Even when harmful microorganisms infect us, we may never know it because there is actually a constant battle being fought against harmful microorganisms in our system. We are not aware of it, because in a healthy person the body is able to protect itself.

THE IMMUNE SYSTEM INSIDE THE BODY

The body's defense—the immune system—is composed of different parts that all work together. It is very complex, but some of the main parts which come into play during HIV infection include the white blood cells (five different groups), antibodies, and certain chemicals.

T4 (T-HELPER) CELLS: These are one type of white blood cell. These cells are very important, because they coordinate the activities of many

Workshop #3 What Is HIV/AIDS? / 213

of the other parts of the immune system and they initially start the immune process.

T8 (T-Suppressor) Cells: These are also white blood cells. They kill other cells that have been invaded by the virus or that have been changed (undergone mutation). They also are responsible for shutting down the whole defense system after the harmful microorganisms have been defeated.

Macrophage: This is another kind of white blood cell. These are larger cells that actually engulf harmful microorganisms.

B Cells: These cells make antibodies. Antibodies are very specific blockers for the microorganism that has invaded the body. B-cells also come in the form of a memory cell. They live in the body a long time and "remember" the harmful microorganism. If the same microorganism attacks the body again, these memory cells rapidly produce antibodies to stop the microorganism.

Antibodies: These are the chemical equivalent of bullets—used to stop the enemies. They are made out of a substance called protein and are very specific for each type of microorganism.

The normal response of the immune system to a viral attack is as follows:

The virus enters the body. First on the scene, the macrophages rush to the defense, digesting the viral cells upon contact. If the macrophages fail to subdue the virus, the T4–cells order the B cells to produce and release custom-designed antibodies and manufacture memory cells to be prepared for future attacks. Finally, the T4-cells tell the T8-cells to get rid of any infected cells and to turn off the attack when the battle is over.

What is a virus?

1. A virus is a very, very small microorganism. Tens of thousands of them fit into the period at the end of this sentence. Viruses are hard to find. An electron microscope, which fills an entire room, must be used to see them.
2. Viruses are parasites. This means they live on or in another organism—called the host—and they use the host's chemicals and nutrients to live and reproduce.

3. Being so small and able to live off their hosts' nutrients, viruses can survive as very simple physical structures. A virus consists of a strand or strands of RNA (ribonucleic acid) surrounded by a layer of protein, and it carries instructions for copying itself but does not have the mechanism for reproduction on its own. Viruses are not cells. They contain no fluid, nor do they perform any life processes on their own.

4. DNA (or sometimes RNA) is like a blueprint for the instructions for building and running every organism—from a tiny virus to a complex human being. A virus uses its host's DNA to write copies of itself. The virus "hijacks" the host cell. Usually, a virus attaches itself to the outside of a host cell and then injects its DNA (or in the case of HIV, its RNA) into the host cell, leaving the protein coat outside. The DNA (RNA) travels to the center of the host cell and attaches to the host's DNA. The hijacked host cell begins to make copies of the viral DNA. Protein for the coat of the virus is also made.

5. Viruses are responsible for many diseases, such as the common cold, the flu, mumps, and chicken pox. Smallpox, yellow fever, and other diseases are also caused by viruses. There is some thought that viruses may cause some cancers, but the evidence is not conclusive.

6. Some viruses, such as the polio virus, live inside a host cell in the body's nervous system; some viruses, such as the flu virus, go into the cells of the respiratory system. But all of them commandeer the blueprint of the host cell to reproduce themselves. They are so integrated into the host cell that it is very difficult to kill a virus once it is inside a cell, because it means killing a lot of cells that the body needs.

What is particular about the HIV virus?

The first important thing to know about the HIV virus is that it picks as its host your immune system, the very defenders of your body against all disease. In particular, it goes into the T4 cells, which coordinate the immune system. This means that the entire defender system is going to be demobilized. So when harmful microorganisms of any kind begin to multiply in your body, there isn't a strong defense system to fight them off, because the HIV virus has weakened the defense system. When HIV is first in your body, you still have a strong defense system. Then, over time, you lose some of your defenders, and you get a little sick because you are more susceptible to infection. With more time and without treatment, you will usually get sicker and sicker, because your defense system can't function.

Technically, no one dies from HIV. They really die from one of the infections that took advantage of a weak immune system—these are called opportunistic infections.

AT WAR

> You should not have revealed yourself,
>   now we must fight
> But you are fighting a losing battle,
>   you won't win.
> You may have your sword,
>   But I have my shield.
> You may be strong,
>   but I'm brave.
> You may try to drive me crazy,
>   but you won't drive me insane.
> You may kill this body,
>   but you can't kill this soul.
> You may come in between me, family and loved ones,
>   but you can't come in between me and my *God*
> Because God created me and not *you!*
> And when the time comes, you shall be
>   sentenced for *Life.*
>
> —CYNTHIA RHODES

Another special characteristic about the HIV virus is that it replicates very fast, twenty times faster than the average flu virus. This means that the number of viruses increases rapidly. Also the virus tends to have a relatively fast rate of binding to its host cell targets compared with the rate of binding between antibodies and the virus.

One of the most significant characteristics of the HIV virus is how great a mutation rate it has. A mutation is a mistake that happens in the blueprint when it is printed. Although mutants are rarely stronger than the original organisms and many of them die, some of them survive, and in time they may become new strains of the virus.

One part of the blueprint for the HIV virus tends to mutate a great deal—namely, the part that designs the protein coat. Since the human

216 / BREAKING THE WALLS OF SILENCE

immune system, including the antibodies, recognizes viral invaders by their protein coats, new mutants may be able to hide from the human immune system, gaining time to replicate and infect more host cells.

Although the T4 cell seems to be the main host cell attacked by the HIV virus, other types of cells also serve as hosts. These include T8 (helper) cells, the macrophage, some brain cells, and possibly cells in the liver. Other possibilities are also being studied.

How exactly does HIV get into the host cell?

The HIV virus, like any virus, has a protein coat. It has particular chemicals that attract it to the protein coat of the particular host cell. It is like a lock and key—a perfect fit. The key fits only that particular host cell, and so the two proteins come together. Then the virus's genetic material penetrates into the host cell, joins with the host cell's blueprint, and is ready to start manufacturing more HIV.

What happens once HIV gets into the host cell?

At a certain point the virus will multiply in the cell, and it may either burst out from it or create buds, which then join with healthy T4 cells, immobilizing them. For reasons that no one understands, sometimes the HIV virus seems to be inactive—dormant—for a long time. People feel good, have no symptoms. During this time, a person can still pass the virus to someone else. What makes the virus begin to replicate and why it takes so long to affect some people and not other people are not understood. Also, people may have a very low T4-cell count and feel perfectly well, have no illnesses. There are still many unknowns about HIV infection.

COFACTORS

Scientists are trying to understand why some people who are exposed to HIV get infected and others do not. They are trying to understand what makes some individuals become sick faster than others and what allows other people to be long-term survivors. They are studying what affects the rate of progression along the continuum of HIV infection. They hypothesize that other factors combine with HIV and influence how the virus develops in an individual. These other factors are called "cofactors." All the possible cofactors listed below are still under study and are being researched by scientists.

EXAMPLES OF COFACTORS:

- *Biological strengths/biological weaknesses* (other microbes or body chemicals).
- *Genetic strengths/genetic weaknesses* (inherited/congenital).
- *Increased stress/reduced stress* (emotional/mental/physical).
- *Substance abuse/staying clean* (alcohol, cocaine, crack, heroin, speed, and all other illicit drugs).
- *Heavy use of over-the-counter or prescription medication/ reducing use* (such as Valium, Librium, Talwin, Darvon, aspirin, cold medicines).
- *Unhealthy living conditions/healthy living conditions.*
- *History of other STDs/safer sex and staying freer of STDs* (herpes, gonorrhea, syphilis, etc.).
- *Frequent viral, bacterial, and/or parasitic infections.*
- *Repeated exposure and/or reinfection.*

UNDERSTANDING THE SYMPTOMS OF HIV INFECTION

The scientific/medical field has tried to chart the development of HIV infection in a person.

EXPOSURE AND INFECTION BY THE HIV VIRUS

When a person first gets infected with HIV, sometimes there are flu-like symptoms. Not everyone experiences symptoms immediately following infection, and even if a person does, she or he may not realize it was because of being infected with HIV. Once a person is infected by the HIV virus, even if she or he experiences no symptoms, the virus can still be transmitted.

Once a person is infected with the HIV virus, the person may feel fine for many years. The person may experience many years free from symptoms of HIV. This is called being asymptomatic. The person may feel fine for as long as ten years or more. This depends on how healthy the person is and on other factors, which are not yet understood.

HIV-Symptomatic (Sometimes Known as PGL— Persistent Generalized Lymphadenopathy, formerly called ARC, or AIDS-Related Complex)

Some of the symptoms a person first develops are listed below. Some of the earliest symptoms often are similar to flu symptoms, but they will last a lot longer (more persistent) or they will come back frequently.

1. For women, vaginal infections
2. Unexplained weight loss of ten pounds or more
3. Oral thrush (a yeast infection of the mouth)
4. Fever of more than a week's duration
5. Persistent diarrhea
6. A dry cough, not caused by smoking
7. Night sweats, of more than a week's duration
8. Shortness of breath
9. Severe headaches and dizziness
10. Fatigue
11. Slow-growing purplish or pink bumps or blotches on the skin anywhere on the body
12. Herpes simplex
13. Herpes zoster, a painful, blistering skin rash usually just on one side of the body (also known as shingles)
14. Swollen gland (enlarged lymph nodes)

AIDS

When a person has certain very serious illnesses and symptoms, the federal Centers for Disease Control (CDC) classifies them as having AIDS. Some of these illnesses are classified as opportunistic infections. They take advantage of a weakened immune system. Others are neurological diseases or cancers. Another is the serious weakening of the body. Some of the more common illnesses that lead to a person being classified as having AIDS include:

Pneumocystis carinii pneumonia (PCP): A common protozoal parasite that multiplies rapidly in the lungs of PWAs and has been the leading cause of death.

Cytomegalovirus (CMV): A virus related to the herpes family. Severe CMV infections can cause hepatitis, pneumonia, retinitis, and colitis, leading in some cases to blindness or chronic diarrhea.

TOXOPLASMOSIS (TOXO): Protozoal infection of the brain, frequently causing brain inflammation and dementia.

CRYPTOCOCCAL MENINGITIS: Infection of the brain lining and spinal cord caused by cryptococcus; can be fatal.

MYCOBACTERIUM AVIUM-INTRACELLULARE (MAI): Deadly pulmonary infection of birds systematically infects the bloodstream late in the course of AIDS. It may also affect bone marrow and cause anemia.

WASTING SYNDROME: Profound involuntary weight loss—more than 10 percent of normal body weight—and/or chronic diarrhea, weakness, and documented fever.

KAPOSI'S SARCOMA (KS): KS is a cancer of the cells that line certain blood vessels. It can be seen on the skin, or it can be inside and not seen. When it is seen on the skin, it looks like bluish-reddish discolorations.

PULMONARY TUBERCULOSIS

ADVANCED CERVICAL CANCER

BACTERIAL PNEUMONIA (SEVERAL BOUTS OF IT)

CANDIDIASIS IN THE ESOPHAGUS

UNDERSTANDING THE DEVELOPMENT OF HIV INFECTION

Scientists are working to understand how HIV infection develops in order to understand it better and in order to know how to treat it. But there is still a lot that remains to be learned, and new understandings are developing over time. The very definition of what is called AIDS is made up by scientists, and it is one that has changed. For example, scientists are continually enlarging the number of diseases that would mean a person can be considered as having AIDS. Originally, when people had dementia, wasting syndrome, or CMV, they were considered to be at HIV-symptomatic stage. Later, so many people died with these symptoms, never reaching what was called AIDS, that these three sets of symptoms and illnesses are now categorized by the CDC as AIDS. On the other hand, PCP, which used to be the cause of death of 60 percent of the people with AIDS, is now a treatable illness, and many people who become sick from PCP get treated and feel fine again, even though simply because they had PCP they would still be categorized as having AIDS.

The very category of having "AIDS" as opposed to being "HIV-symptomatic" is usually very frightening to people, because it makes people feel that they are closer to death. In reality, because of growing treatments for opportunistic infections and the enormous variation in how individuals respond to the virus, the category of "AIDS" does not tell people very much about the overall status of their health or about what their life expectancy is.

There is tremendous variety in how HIV affects people.

- Some people have had an opportunistic infection and thus, according to the CDC, have AIDS, but they feel basically good because the infection has been treated.
- Some people with HIV-symptomatic are fairly healthy; others are quite ill.
- For some people, the illness progresses to death before they are ever diagnosed as having AIDS.
- Some people begin to develop symptoms with high T4-cell counts, and others with very low T4-cell counts may feel completely healthy. At present, scientists do not fully understand how the immune system functions. Therefore, since T4-cell counts are the only thing that they are sure is affected by the virus, there is a focus on T4-cell counts more so than any other part of the immune system. It's very important not to feel, just because you have a low T4-cell count, that you're going to die. Many long-term survivors prove otherwise.

* * *

I listen to people talk about *"full-blown AIDS"* or *"the final stage of AIDS,"* and I'm sitting here and I'm thinking to myself, "Well, I had PCP pneumonia six years ago and I've had this opportunistic infection and that opportunistic infection, and I have twenty-five T4–cells, and I've been in 'the *final* stage' for many years now, but I'm still here, and I wish they would stop using those words, because if I had believed them, I would have died a long time ago, and I'm very much alive.

WOMEN AND THE DEVELOPMENT OF HIV INFECTIONS

For many years, the diseases and symptoms that women who were HIV-positive had were not included in the AIDS definition. In 1982, the Centers for Disease Control definition of AIDS required individuals to have the HIV virus plus one diagnosed illness from a small list of opportunistic infections or cancers. The CDC definition of AIDS was then revised in 1987. The list still did not include gynecological infections such as vaginal thrush (otherwise known as yeast infection or vaginitis), chlamydia, genital herpes, trichomonas vaginitis, gonorrhea, or syphilis, even though these conditions occur differently, commonly, and more severely in HIV-positive women than in HIV-negative women. Even life-threatening diseases such as cervical cancer, multidrug resistant tuberculosis, bacterial pneumonia, and endocarditis were not included.

The implications of this for women have been devastating. If women do not meet the CDC definition of AIDS, they do not qualify for AIDS benefits and disability financial support, including special housing and nutritional allowances. Doctors remain unaware of the relationship between PID (pelvic inflammatory disease), cervical abnormalities, and HIV. The narrow definition meant frequent underdiagnosis and delayed or inadequate treatment of women. It also excluded women with HIV from experimental therapies, since many drug trials continue to require an official diagnosis.

Finally, in January 1993, the CDC put into effect an expanded definition of AIDS. It added three illnesses: pulmonary tuberculosis, invasive cancer of the cervix, and recurrent bacterial pneumonia to the list. In addition, it included those HIV-positive persons who have had less than 200 T cells. These new conditions are commonly experienced by women (and IV drug users). This should lead to earlier diagnosis and treatment of women, because doctors will be alerted to the importance of HIV testing when evaluating such conditions. It will also give women increased financial support, which they need.

The Psychological Impact of Uncertainty

People want to understand what is happening inside them—it helps give them a sense of some control. People want to know: Will I die? Will I be able to continue working? Will I recover my health? What place does my particular T-cell count put me at? But because of the variety of ways that HIV infection affects people, the development of the disease cannot be predicted for any one person based on the general picture. This is very difficult psychologically.

The Social Impact of the AIDS Definition

People who are classified as HIV-symptomatic are often not eligible for the benefits and services people with AIDS receive, even though they may be sicker than any given individual defined as having AIDS and even though they may need assistance. For example, housing allowances and social services support in New York City are greater for people who have been diagnosed as having AIDS. Yet, a person who has not yet been diagnosed as having AIDS may actually feel sicker and need more support than a particular person who has been diagnosed as having AIDS.

Finally, the official CDC surveillance of HIV, in counting only those with AIDS and not those who are HIV-symptomatic, only counts a small percentage of people actually affected. The concerns of people who are HIV-symptomatic are often neglected in health policy and research planning.

TEACHING PLAN HIV/AIDS: GENERAL INFORMATION

* * *

Q: How did you feel when you first started to learn all this technical material?

A: I sat in the workshops but I had no idea I would have to teach. I was just being taught. You try to learn whatever you can. I said, "Help! I have to learn all this?" I used to run to Ethel crying. I knew I could learn bits and pieces, but not in the way I have, in so much depth and able to teach. Sometimes I stop and say, "Lisa, you said all that?" The fact that I can do it makes me feel good—good that I can teach others and that I'm not just a pretty face in the crowd. When I really learned was when I found out I had to teach.

* * *

Introduction

This is the most technical of all the workshops and involves learning about science. It is important to ask questions, because everyone will learn from one another's questions.

In addition to being technical, it also requires a lot of sensitivity. This is because the information that will be given may actually be occurring within some of the participants' own immune systems and mentally it is stressful for them to learn about their illness. One way of dealing with the stress is to make clear throughout the workshop that people can and do struggle with the virus. People struggle using a combination of biological, psychological, and environmental factors. These include medicine, reduction of stress, love, and reduction of risky behavior. This is as important as the destruction occurring in the body, if not more important. Hope should be as much a part of the workshop as the virus hurting the immune system. Even though the workshop is not mainly about treatment, the fact that people can do something about the virus should be part of the workshop.

In our experience, we have found that it is important to have a PWA involved in the presentation, if possible. This helps break fear and stigma in the group by seeing that a PWA is living and surviving with HIV infection. PWAs can also use humor, which helps the group deal with emotionally difficult information. If a PWA is not formally involved in the presentation, it is helpful to involve PWAs who are open and willing to participate in the discussion by talking about their own lives.

We have found that with a large group it is *very* important to break into groups of ten or fewer for discussions, so that people all get a chance to ask questions and retell what they have learned.

A supportive closure is needed to give the group time to absorb the information that was discussed and to feel a sense of togetherness. Possibly an appropriate song, a supportive prayer, and/or a moment of silence will allow this to happen.

In our experience, we have found it useful to have a buddy system or supportive network system. This will allow participants to talk or share their feelings after the workshop.

DISCUSSIONS AND PRESENTATIONS

1. *DISCUSSION:* WHAT MAKES A PERSON HEALTHY AND WHAT MAKES A PERSON SICK?

Ask participants to list things that can make a person healthy and things that can make a person sick. Write these down in two lists on a board or newsprint. Then build from their answers an understanding of how biological, psychological, and social factors are all part of keeping a body healthy or sick and that we have a lot of control over many of these factors. This discussion opens the workshop, because we want to make clear that people can make choices that can affect their health.

2. *Presentation:* Define what HIV means

Tell participants that the goal of this workshop is to explain the immune system and therefore it does not focus on psychological and social factors, even though they are part of what impacts on the development of HIV infection. In the next workshop on treatment, we will examine HIV from a holistic/biopsychosocial viewpoint.

3. *Presentation:* How HIV Attacks the Immune System and Creates HIV Infection and AIDS

This next presentation/discussion is the most technical one in the workshop series. In our experience it has helped to develop a metaphor for the immune system. We have talked about defenders, enemies, the general (T cells), bullets (antibodies), and so forth. This language appears to make a big difference. Equally important is the use of charts as visual aids. It will also help to actually draw the pictures of the process as you are talking, because the motion of drawing helps communicate the process. An additional aid may be to role-play the parts of the defenders, enemies, and HIV, acting out the process of a healthy body defending itself against microorganisms and what happens when HIV attacks the body.

The goal of this section of the presentation is to make certain that participants understand the next three steps (a to c). Using metaphoric language along with the technical language and the visual aids, go through the following steps:

a. How the immune system (defenders) defends the body against harmful microorganisms/germs/enemies.
b. How the HIV virus attacks the immune system (defenders) and how the body starts to lose its ability to defend itself against harmful microorganisms (germs, enemies).
c. How, over time, the opportunistic infections take over, because the immune system (defense system) is so weak.

The above three steps create the broad view of the immune system fighting harmful microorganisms. This is the basis for going into more detail if the group is interested and has followed the explanation thus far. Certain words, such as "T4 cell" and "antibody" will need to be explained, because these are words people hear all the time. There is sometimes confusion about antibodies becoming infected, which they don't. This should be made clear, since it will affect people's understanding both about the HIV-antibody test and the situation of babies having their mothers' antibodies. Also, there will probably be questions about the virus, how it enters the cell, and so on. Depending on the size of the group and the level of knowledge and the time, the presentation can go into more detail, looking at the following information and using visual aids.

Questions may come up here that are more detailed. We suggest waiting until after a discussion of the development of HIV infection and then breaking up into small groups. This is because some of the participants may have questions that deal with the basic information described above and some may understand the basic information but want more details. The small group discussions will best meet the needs of all the participants.

ROLE-PLAY SHOWING THE IMMUNE SYSTEM AT WORK
a. One person is a defender cell and another is a germ or enemy representing the flu or measles. The germ attacks the defender cell, and the defender cell captures the germ.
b. A person representing an HIV virus captures a defender.
c. A third person representing PCP or another opportunistic illness roams around freely as the defender is still held down by the HIV.

4. READ POEM "AT WAR" (SEE BACKGROUND MATERIAL).

5. *PRESENTATION:* COFACTORS

This discussion is important because it will help build a holistic approach to health care as well as give people the tools to understand the complexity of HIV infection. Present the cofactors as factors that can either contribute to a person's ability to fight HIV infection or weaken her or his ability to fight HIV infection. In many cases, a person can make a choice that will affect her or his health.

6. *DISCUSSION AND PRESENTATION ABOUT HOW HIV INFECTION DEVELOPS*

This is a discussion about the way in which HIV affects people clinically—that is, how the disease itself is expressed and experienced. It is a hard discussion emotionally. On the one hand, people want and need to know the information; on the other hand, people with HIV infection or who have loved ones with HIV are personally affected by this discussion. Therefore, the discussion should be frank but sensitive.

From our experience, it is important in the discussion of the development of HIV infection to show the advances that have been made with treatment therapies, that there are many long-term survivors, and the variability in people. Some possible things to present include the following:

1. PCP used to be responsible for more than 60 percent of the deaths from AIDS; now medicines can prevent and treat it.
2. AZT slows down the development of the virus.
3. Several new anti-HIV therapies are being used, including ddi, ddC, d4T and 3tc. These drugs, especially used in combination with AZT or with each other alone, are even more effective than AZT alone.[1]
4. T-cell counts cannot be used as a *sole* measuring rod of a person's present or future health. There are too many variables. Scientists are increasingly using a 'viral load' test as one way to evaluate a person's health and the impact of treatment.[2]
5. People who are long-term survivors might come for the discussion and talk about themselves, and others in the community who have HIV infection might talk about their own struggles, thus reinforcing hope and helping eliminate the hopelessness that surrounds the phrases "last stage" and "full-blown" AIDS.

7. *EXPLANATION*: THE CONCEPTS OF EXPOSURE, INFECTION, AND ILLNESS

Use the visual aids to explain the progression of the HIV in the body and to list the signs and symptoms of each stage. It is important to stress that this is only a general model and that there is enormous variation in how individuals actually experience HIV infection. It's also important to stress that scientists are still learning about HIV infection, so the model will probably change.

---

1. *GMHC Treatment Issues*, Volume 8, Number 9, October 1994
**Positively Aware*, May/June 1995
2. *GMHC Treatment Issues*, Volume 8, Number 9, October 1994

After presenting the broad picture of the development of HIV infection, discuss the particular situation of women and both the psychological and social implications of the way in which the development of HIV infection is defined.

8. SMALL-GROUP DISCUSSIONS

Break into small groups in order to discuss the material. Ask people to retell what they have learned. This is also a time to go into more detail about the HIV virus in the body if people have questions.

    a. Present a chart showing the immune system in greater detail, with the T4 cell coordinating the macrophages, B-cells and antibody production, and T8–cells;

    b. Show a detailed picture of an HIV virus entering a T4 cell, with the CD4 receptor site and the viral protein gp120 attaching to that particular site.

    c. Show the picture of the activity of the HIV inside the T4–cell and how the multiplication of the virus leads either to the bursting of the T4 cell or to the budding of the cell and its attachment to other T4 cells, immobilizing them.

9. *ENDING:* ONE LARGE GROUP

    a. Preview the next workshop by explaining that next week you will be studying the strategies scientists are using to develop treatments and will look at the treatments now being used. You hope to begin the next session with people giving ideas of what might be their strategies for dealing with HIV, given what they just learned about how the virus affects the body.

    b. For closure create a circle of support: Either share a song or hold hands for a prayer, or invite each person who wishes to speak.

    c. After the circle of support, have some time for personal discussions with one another.

       Note to facilitator: Be aware that the most common question is "If I have AIDS, does that mean I'll die?" We answered that question by saying that even though a person is HIV-positive, it should not be assumed that a person will definitely die from it. There are today many long-term survivors; medicines are being worked on, and people are living longer. And the longer one can live, the greater the possibility of a cure.

REFERENCE MATERIALS

AIDS Intervention Management System (AIMS), under the auspices of the AIDS Institute New York State Department of Health. *Criteria Manual for the Treatment of AIDS.* New York: New York Statewide Professional Standards Review Council, 1988.

Burroughs Wellcome Co. *Management of HIV Disease Treatment Team Workshop Handbook.* New York: World Health Communications, 1991.

Feist, Jess, and Linda Brannon. *Health Psychology.* Belmont, CA: Wadsworth, 1988.

Grimes, Deanna E., and Richard M. Grimes. *AIDS and HIV Infection.* St. Louis, MO: Mosby-Year Book, 1994.

Haseltine, William A., and Flossie Wong-Staal. "The Molecular Biology of the AIDS Virus." *Scientific American,* October 1988.

HIV/AIDS and Children: Answers for Caregivers. New York State Department of Social Services. SUNY Research Foundation/Center for Development. Buffalo, NY: 1994.

Massachusetts Department of Public Health and Massachusetts Department of Education. *Learn and Live: A Teaching Guide on AIDS Prevention.* Massachusetts, 1987.

Mass, Lawrence, M.D. *Medical Answers About AIDS.* New York: Gay Men's Health Crisis, 1989.

Mid-Hudson Valley AIDS Task Force, Information Packet. ARCS, 1988.

New York Department of Health. *100 Questions and Answers: AIDS.* New York: April 1994.

"1993 Revised Classification System for HIV Infection and Expanded Surveillance Case Definition for AIDS Among Adolescents and Adults." *MMWR* 41 (December 18, 1992): 1–13.

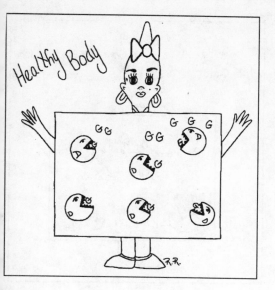

FACTS:
1. Harmful viruses, bacteria, protozoan . . . also known as germs . . . attack our body and can make us sick.
2. Our body fights infection and disease with its defender, the immune system. The immune system fights the viruses, bacteria, and protozoan . . . all the germs that make us sick.

IN THE PICTURE:
In a healthy immune system, when the germs (G) attack the body, the immune system, made up of different types of "defenders" (D), fight back and destroy the germs. Your body is fighting the infection caused by germs.

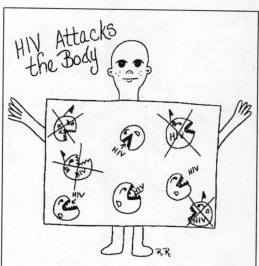

FACTS:
1. HIV, the virus that causes AIDS, attacks the immune system itself.
2. HIV particularly destroys the T-cells, also called CD-4 cells. These cells are defenders which are like generals. They tell the other defenders what to do. Without the T-4 cells (the generals) the whole immune system cannot work.

IN THE PICTURE:
HIV attacks and destroys the defenders (D), the very things that protect us.

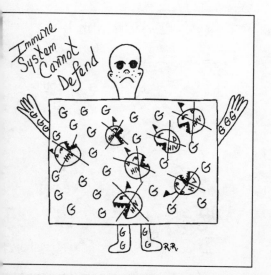

FACTS:
1. As more and more defenders (T-4 cells) are destroyed by HIV, the body's defense system gets weaker and weaker.
2. Then lots of other viruses and bacteria . . . germs . . . can begin to live and multiply in the body, and they can kill us because the defenders are not there to fight back.

IN THE PICTURE:
The person's D's (defenders) are destroyed by HIV. More and more G's (germs) come in and multiply in the body; the person cannot ever get well because there is nothing to fight back with. When a person dies of HIV/AIDS, he or she dies because a bacteria, virus, or other harmful germ made him or her sick and the body's defenders could not fight back and stop the infection because the HIV had destroyed the defenders.

The immune system is very complex. Some of the parts that are important in HIV infection are shown in the picture. "D" stands for "defender," a word for the cells and chemicals that fight infection.

a)T-4 cells: these are white blood cells which help coordinate the other parts of the immune system. The HIV attacks the T-4 cells.

b)Macrophage: these are white blood cells which "eat" or engulf harmful microorganisms. The HIV also gets into the macrophage.

c)B-cells: these are white blood cells which produce antibodies.

d)T-8 cells: these are white blood cells which signal the other immune cells to stop fighting when enough harmful microorganisms have been destroyed.

e)Antibodies: these are chemicals which the B-cells produce; each one is custom-made for the particular germ that it will be attacking.

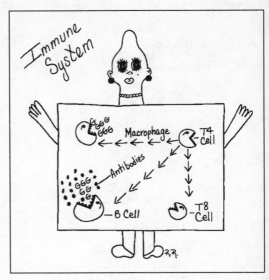

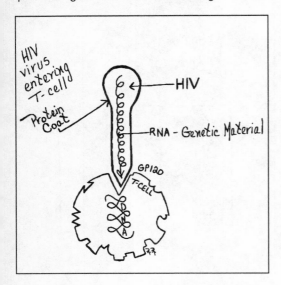

FACTS:
A virus is made up of a core of genetic material called either DNA or RNA. This genetic material is like a blueprint for future viruses. There is a protein envelope surrounding the genetic material.

IN THE PICTURE:
An HIV virus is entering a T-4 cell. It enters in a particular place, fitting like a key into a lock. There is a part of the protein envelope called GP 120 that fits with a part of the outside of the T-4 cell called CD4. Only when these two chemicals connect will the virus enter the T-4 cells.This information is important in scientific research. Scientists are studying whether they can intercept or block the connection between these two chemicals and thereby stop the HIV virus from entering the T-4 cell.

When the HIV virus enters a T-4 cell, different things can happen.
1. Every time the T-4 cell divides (and cell division is a constant process in the body) every new T-4 cell has the HIV virus in it.
2. The virus may multiply in the T-4 cell and create buds with HIV in them. These buds will attach to healthy T-4 cells and paralyze them.
3. The HIV virus may multiply until there are so many that the T-4 cell bursts and is destroyed and the virus floats around in the blood until it infects another T-4 cell.

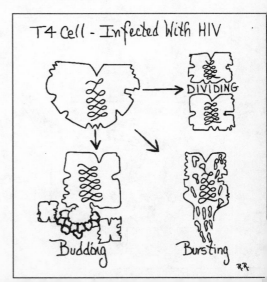

Workshop #4
HIV/AIDS: Social and Medical Issues Regarding Treatment

I never once had to come to terms with being HIV-symptomatic while imprisoned on Rikers Island. I knew that AIDS was in my body, but I didn't give a damn. My only concern was being released while I'm still healthy.

Now I'm constantly reminded of it, its effects physically as well as psychologically. Now I must deal with learning to live with being HIV-symptomatic, being responsible for what I eat, drink, medicines the doctor prescribes or doesn't prescribe, my sleeping habits, having a positive attitude, and many smiling faces.

A part of me craves to know more about this disease, but then at other times I feel as though death will free me from my pain. And then again, I want to know so much more about the AIDS virus, because I want to live. Even though I have come face to face with my illness, I've decided to beat this thing. There is no way that I am going to let some little virus destroy my life. The information I seek helps me to get a better understanding of what I'm up against. The responsibility that I have concerning my health is a big one, but since I want to live I know I will be doing the right thing as I take care of my body. I've always had someone to take care of me, now I have to do it alone. I find myself being discouraged often, because I felt a doctor didn't give me a complete physical or a person treats me as a person with AIDS.

With this education, I've also discovered that I always wanted to know about my body and how to treat it well, but I was unwilling to take the initiative. Now things are clear for me. I can become knowledgeable about this virus, and not be afraid that my learning more will make an abrupt change in my health. I hope to continue on my journey to a happy, healthy, and drug/alcohol free lifestyle just so I can make a difference.

I want to make my family very proud of my accomplishments concerning my work on living with AIDS. I'm still very scared of this illness that can cause death.

OVERVIEW

There are an increasing number of treatment options for people at all stages of HIV infection. They include biological, psychological, and social approaches. This represents a expanding basis of hope. People are living longer, with better-quality lives, through access to treatment and support systems.

Because there are treatment options, people are faced with choices. In order to make choices about treatment, people need to understand what choices exist and be able to make real whatever their decision is. In typical patient-doctor relationships, the decisions are left up to the doctor, but we have found that people can make informed choices if they are enabled to do so through education, medical advocacy, and mutually respectful doctor-patient relationships. They also need to have access to financial support and medical providers.

People ask long-term survivors how they have survived and thrived. Each has made different treatment choices, but the one constant is that all of them have felt that they have taken control in decision making about their treatment and other life choices.

Social factors also impact on the extent and availability of treatment and on the speed and direction of research. Even under the best of circumstances, it takes time for scientists to learn about a new disease and develop treatments. But in the HIV/AIDS epidemic, there have been a number of negative social factors that have hurt the availability of treatment possibilities: the social hierarchy in society and the lack of medical and social services for poor people; government priorities and the lack of adequate resources for medical research on HIV/AIDS; profit being the major interest of companies developing drugs; and stigma.

PWAs and the HIV/AIDS movement have played a major role in struggling to change government policies to expand and speed up treatment research, in pressing for more research funds and treatment options, and in promoting a holistic approach to treatment that emphasizes people's psychosocial as well as medical needs.

HIV infection has not been studied carefully in women. We as a community of women have begun to focus on learning more about women's health in general and talking about how women can mobilize to influence better treatment of women in the HIV/AIDS epidemic. As women in prison, we saw the need to become experts. We sought and received training and read and educated ourselves in order to become educators and medical advocates. We approach this workshop as one means of enabling others to become active participants in their medical treatment and in the broader emotional and spiritual struggles.

GOALS

1. To develop a basic understanding of the treatment strategies based on the information in the "What Is HIV/AIDS?" workshop.
2. To communicate and explore the fact that while there is no cure for HIV/AIDS, there are treatment options that are expanding all the time and are a basis for hope.
3. To recognize the social factors impacting on treatment options.
4. To explore the role of the nonexpert in developing treatment options—the PWA and social movements.
5. To explore the particular treatment issues facing women.

ISSUES TO EXAMINE

1. What are the treatment strategies for HIV infection?
2. What are holistic approaches to treatment?
3. What are some of the questions people need to examine in making choices for their own treatment?
4. Issues of struggle affecting treatment options:
   a. Access to and conduct of drug trials.
   b. Treatment of HIV for women.
   c. Cost of drugs and health care.

BACKGROUND MATERIALS

Goals:

1. To explain the different strategies and give people information about specific treatments.
2. To involve people in thinking about the treatment strategies, challenging the myth that only experts can understand medical issues. To recognize that even the experts disagree and that there is constantly new and often conflicting information about treatment—and that therefore the best hope lies in keeping oneself educated, to be able to make choices.
3. To communicate the enormous progress in the development of treatments for HIV infection that can enable people to live longer and better lives. There is hope!

What are the strategies scientists/doctors are using and what are existing treatments?

ANTIVIRALS/ANTIRETROVIRALS

Substances that slow down the activity of the HIV retrovirus.

AZIDOTHYMIDINE (AZT): The generic name is zidovudine. It was the first anti-HIV agent approved in the United States for treatment of patients with HIV infection. AZT has been shown to inhibit HIV replication in vitro (in the test tube). Studies have shown that AZT slows down progression of HIV disease for some people. Studies continue to try to pinpoint when the optimum time to give AZT is and whether or not it prolongs survival. More recently it has been determined that lower dosages of AZT than were earlier prescribed have the same effect but with less toxicity.

Side effects/toxicity: Bone marrow suppression, including anemia, fatigue, rashes, nausea, myalgia, insomnia, and severe headaches have been experienced in patients receiving AZT. Some people's systems cannot tolerate AZT. Doctors sometimes prescribe erythropoietin to people taking AZT, which replaces bone marrow and thus counteracts the anemia caused by AZT. There is also evidence that the body can build resistance to AZT, so that its effects disappear or significantly lessen over time. Scientists are looking for alternative treatments.

Several other antiretrovirals are now FDA approved for the treatment of HIV infection: ddI, ddc, d4t, and 3tc. These are increasingly being used in combination with AZT or with each other, for greater effectiveness than AZT alone.[note:]

PREVENTION AND TREATMENT OF OPPORTUNISTIC INFECTIONS (OI):

OPPORTUNISTIC INFECTIONS: At least 80 percent of PWAs develop illnesses that would not be serious to anyone whose immune system is

---

Note: A recent development in treatment is a group of drugs called *protease inhibitors*. They work differently than the antiretrovirals described above and are used in combination with them.
GMHC Treatment Issues, Volume 8, Number 9, October 1994

functioning normally but can cause serious illness or death in those with compromised immunity—for example, CMV, MAI, PCP, toxo, and cryptococcal meningitis.

There are many drugs currently used and many more being tested to treat these illnesses or prevent their onset. This is part of a strategy to make HIV infection a chronic, manageable disease, like diabetes or cancer. The development of specific treatments for specific OIs has improved the quality of life for PWAs who have access to them.

One example of an opportunistic infection that has been effectively treated is PCP.

PNEUMOCYSTIS CARINII PNEUMONIA (PCP): PCP has become the most manageable and the most preventable OI.

Drugs that are effective for treating PCP are IV pentamidine, Bactrim, and Septra.

Drugs that are effective for preventing PCP are aerosol pentamidine, Bactrim, and Septra.

It is worth noting that aerosolized pentamidine was first tested and shown to be effective in community-based research trials, rather than trials run by government or private industry. Recent studies have demonstrated that Bactrim is more effective than aerosol pentamidine in PCP prophylaxis and should be used in people who can tolerate sulfa drugs.

The HIV/AIDS advocacy movement argues that there are many potential treatments for OIs that should be tested and are not being tested because of the politics and economics of drug testing. Thus, this has become a major area of social action.

VACCINES

A substance composed of an infectious agent or agents that stimulate immunity by producing an antibody response, protecting the person against future infection by the agent. Smallpox, measles, mumps, rubella, and polio are prevented by vaccines. There are currently approximately thirty ongoing vaccine trials worldwide, according to the National Institute of Allergy and Infectious Diseases (NIAID).

What enables HIV to stay one step ahead of such vaccine strategies?

First, the HIV virus mutates a great deal; thus a vaccine prepared for one form of HIV might not work for a mutated form of HIV. Second, the rate of binding of the HIV to the T cells is very rapid—faster than to antibodies—which means that it is difficult to prevent T cells from becoming infected. Third, since there are no animals that develop the same symptoms of HIV that humans do, the vaccine must be tested on humans, and this raises questions as to how to test it safely and ethically.

IMMUNOMODULATORS

Drugs that alter, suppress, or strengthen the immune system. The goal of using an immunomodulator is to increase the number of functional T4 cells and/or restore the balance of the various components of the immune system. This enables the body to resist opportunistic infections better, to help keep HIV in check. At this time, immunomodulators have not been proved effective or safe—indeed, some immunomodulators have very dangerous side effects and hence are not used to treat AIDS-related conditions (except for Kaposi's sarcoma).

HOLISTIC HEALTH CARE

Holistic health care has a different approach to a person's health than conventional medicine. It sees the body as a system in which the physical, the mental, the spiritual, the emotional all interact with each other. Instead of seeing treatment as consisting of finding the drug, the "magic bullet" to kill the enemy making us sick, holistic medicine works with the different elements of a person to restore the body's natural balances and build up the immune system. The goal is to promote overall health and wellness and build the body's capacity to heal even "terminal" illnesses such as cancer. Holistic health practitioners use alternative means to help build up the immune system. They use nutritional, herbal, and organic compounds that supply minerals and other immune-system boosters.

While one may not appreciate specific techniques, such as acupuncture, there is widespread acceptance of holistic approaches that emphasize living healthfully, exercise, relaxation techniques, visualization, and having a positive mental attitude. All of these approaches can be integrated into any health strategy one chooses. Holistic measures are often used to supplement medical and drug therapies.

Some examples of holistic or alternative health measures are:

ACUPUNCTURE: This is a traditional Chinese therapeutic technique whereby points of energy in the body are stimulated with needles, heat, or massage in order to break up blockages of energy and restore the person's internal balances.

MASSAGE: Therapeutic touching not only is physically beneficial in relieving a variety of physical symptoms, including chronic pain, but can also be psychologically healing and relaxing.

NUTRITION: Paying attention to diet is an extremely important part of any program of healing and prevention. Some PWAs are following macrobiotic diets to build up their health.

REFRAINING FROM SMOKING: *All* health practitioners—Western doctors and holistic alike—strongly recommend that people who are HIV-infected stop smoking.

YOGA: At the core of yoga is the development of awareness—awareness of how we move, stand, sit, feel, and think, and most important, of who we are. Through yoga, we exercise our internal organs, as well as stretch our muscles, straighten the spine, and use deep breathing to energize our minds and bodies. Yoga provides a means to deep relaxation and relief from stress. Meditation and visualization exercises are effective in relieving pain and other symptoms of many chronic illnesses and are widely used by PWAs.

The Role of the Nonexpert in Treatment Issues

The issues of medical research and treatment of HIV/AIDS may seem so complicated that only scientists and doctors seem able to play a role in them. But actually, there are important roles for people who are not experts. While some decisions depend on expert knowledge, other decisions are made out of people's values, biases, and individual preferences. PWAs have played a major role in affecting the course of medical research and treatment, because they have recognized that even though they are nonexperts, their views mattered, since it was they who needed the treatment. This section will examine areas in which the layperson's beliefs and actions make a difference. It will look at decisions about treatment, issues related to drug trials, the cost of drugs, and women and medical issues.

DECISIONS ABOUT TREATMENT

HIV/AIDS does not yet have a prevention or cure. Some drugs appear to be effective for certain conditions related to HIV/AIDS; other drugs appear to work for some people and not for others. The toxic effects of certain drugs must be weighed against the benefits, and some drugs work for a limited period of time and then lose their effectiveness. Doctors differ in their opinions on options about a certain course of treatment. This means that choices have to be made about what course of treatment to take. Some people rely on holistic measures, others combine holistic measures with more traditional medical measures.

It is important to have a doctor and/or health practitioner whom you can trust, because expert knowledge is necessary for understanding the way drugs and other treatments and the virus itself impact on the body. But most people defer to experts and are not used to playing a role in their own health management when they get sick. It is rare to find doctors who accept and encourage a patient to play an active role in helping define a course of treatment. Most doctors see themselves as having all the knowledge and the patient as incapable of knowing enough to play a role. And most patients actually feel that way about themselves. In addition, patients feel very vulnerable and scared, and this can easily lead to passivity in the face of the experts: "Just tell me what to do and I'll do it."

Yet, studies in health psychology and behavioral medicine show that a good relationship between medical practitioner and patient significantly improves a person's treatment prognosis. Because of the absence of a definitive prevention or cure for HIV/AIDS, choices need to be made by each person needing medical help. To begin to participate in one's own medical strategy requires both becoming educated and acquiring an attitude that one has a right to help determine the direction of one's own treatment.

Needless to say, you may be in a situation in which you can't choose a doctor with an attitude that fits your needs. The main thing is to be aware of how you want to be working in relationship to your health providers and to struggle for that kind of a relationship.

Some people do not trust doctors and modern medicine. This may be based on their individual values and experience and/or on their particular culture. These beliefs are also part of creating a treatment plan that will work for the particular person.

People in prison, as well as many people on the streets who must rely on public health facilities, face the problems of inadequate, overloaded health care facilities and personnel who are not personally involved with their patients. At Bedford, we have begun to use health advocates from among ACE members to overcome some of these problems.

ACE members and PWAs who have educated themselves about treatment options work with others to share information, answer questions, and help people prepare for medical appointments by defining questions they need answers to and the choices they must make. They also sit in on medical consultations to support the patient's ability to articulate questions and to help explain information presented by the medical practitioner in layperson's terms. We also encourage medical personnel to utilize us to enhance their relationships with patients. We identify problems in the health care delivery system and negotiate with the medical department to remedy them, and we work with individuals to enhance their ability to negotiate the system. Here are some of the stories of the choices ACE members made about their treatment; some of the voices you will read are those of the first open PWAs in ACE, who inspired the women in Bedford with their courage and commitment as they struggled personally to survive and thrive.

* * *

From the very beginning, a lot of my opinions were formed from reading material by people who were anti-AZT. From these readings I related to their feelings. It didn't make sense putting something so toxic in your body, supposedly to prolong your life for six months with no question. This was the first decision that I made—I wouldn't go on an antiretrovirus drug. It's not important to give me six more months to live—rather give me six more months of living well.

My approach, and also the approach of my doctor, Dr. Sonnenbend, is to have prophylactics. The reason is that what you die of is opportunistic infections, and the prophylactics are aimed at preventing and treating them. So even though a lot are experimental, I go on his advice and on the information that I read and discuss with him.

I also try to make some efforts around nutritional values. I know it's important, and sometimes I do well, but I have to admit I don't do great.

I've found my acupuncture to be very helpful in bringing my state of being into balance with self. I really feel it works. There's no scientific evidence, but I really feel a difference when I walk out of a treatment.

Finally, for me, the caring of an individual has made me stay happier and healthier.

—CARMEN ROYSTER

* * *

One close friend of ours, Carmen Rivera, who died, said she didn't want any medical treatment. She always argued with the doctors, throwing them out of her room, discharging herself from the hospital to come back to Bedford, not taking her medicine. She fought with all of us when we tried to struggle with her. She called us "retards" when we bugged her. She was herself, totally herself, a spirited, funny, strong-willed person. I used to say to myself, "Damn, if only she had taken her medicine, she would have lived longer." And then I said to myself, "No, she didn't believe in medicine or doctors. She loved her mother, she loved her friends, love was her medicine, and she lived according to who she was and no one could change her." Being true to herself gave her strength to live, as long as she could, being totally herself. And that was her approach to treatment. She made us accept it. It was about accepting her and we loved her.

* * *

Necessary treatments that have helped me a great deal with my illness:

AZT: It helped me for a period of time. In the beginning, though, the dosages the doctors gave me were too strong. It resulted in my anemia, which was alleviated with blood transfusions. Today, I do not take AZT anymore but I think it's a good medicine.

Toxo: I have tumors in my brain. Because of this I got a lot of headaches, and the right side of my body feels like it's asleep and heavy. The treatment I receive for this is a derivative of sulfur, pentamidine, and folic acid. The combination of these medications helps to stop the progression of this disease.

PCP: This infection is a permanent threat that I have in my chest and lungs. The treatment I receive for PCP is a monthly dosage of aerosol pentamidine.

CMV: This is an infection in the eyes. It has left me blind in one eye and is a constant danger to the other. For this infection, I receive DHPG (Ganciclovir) every night for five nights in a row through an IV unit.

All of these treatments have been very good for me. I recommend these treatments for anyone who has had similar cases to mine. Above all you must have a positive attitude and avoid depression, because it does not help.

There is one thing that gave me much strength, and that is helping others. In IPC I would help the women bathe themselves, wash their clothes, and clean their rooms, and I usually would do the cooking for them. I would also counsel the women who were depressed. They usually felt like they only had a few days to live. I was the one who cried with them, since I, too, was suffering with them. I used to let them know that if they took care of themselves and used the treatment available, they could live a few years longer. I also helped during my stay at St. Clare's Hospital. I helped feed and clothe the men who were sick and also inmates. Above all, I counseled them to take care of themselves and take their medications. Many of them took my counseling, and today they feel better and are happier. The help I give to others is the best medicine I could receive.

—SONIA PEREZ

* * *

MY AZT EXPERIENCE

When I think of the numerous debates that surround AZT, I think about its toxicity, its ability or inability to prolong life, its costs, the fact that it is the only FDA-approved antiviral drug for HIV/AIDS illnesses, and the whole social problem that AZT brings with it. Because I am an individual with HIV infection, AZT has also become a personal, internal debate for me. I had read so much information about AZT, simply because I knew we needed something desperately to help fight off progression. So I learned about its toxicity and its ability to slow down progression of HIV infection.

Yet, knowing the pros/cons of AZT's effects, I still underwent tremendous emotional/psychological turmoil in deciding to use something (AZT) that was supposed to slow down my HIV progression. Why was there this conflict? Why did I cry for the first several weeks, five times a day, every time I took this blue/white capsule that was supposed to help me? Why was there this pressing internal conflict? Was I concerned about its toxicity? Did I believe that it would prolong my life irrespective of what my quality of life would become? These were the numerous questions that I asked myself each time that I medicated myself with AZT.

This confrontation with AZT came approximately eighteen months after my diagnosis. I guess I had never really believed that AZT would do for me what it had allegedly done for less that half the HIV/AIDS population (slow down progression), even when my doctors told me it was crucial that I take it. I never quite overcame that first impression that AZT had made upon me. But in spite of that first impression, I agreed to take AZT for a six-month period, because of a drastic drop in my T cell counts—to forty. I felt chemically out of balance, and I truly felt experimental. I walked around, for the most part, in a state of lethargy and nauseated limbo. I broke out with several rashes, which particularly disfigured my body. I continued to ask my physician if these symptoms were signs of intolerance or toxicity. I knew they were, but my physician continued to try and convince me that these symptoms did not outweigh AZT's benefits, much to my confusion. I hoped that he was right. After several long months of laying this out, I decided that I no longer wanted to be a walking, chemical, lethargic fool, willing to undergo anything (regardless of my quality of life) for the sake of slowing down progression. I am off AZT now—an informed choice that I do understand—and not nauseated or drunk. My skin problems are trying to clear up, and in spite of my physician's belief, I feel wonderful and more like me. I do not see physical signs of progression, and I no longer feel like I'm chemically off-balance. I tried AZT, and the pros do not outweigh the cons for me. As I expected, it was not the miracle drug for me. So, DDI here I come . . . off and onward to another experiment.

—KATRINA HASLIP

* * *

When Cathy first came back from the outside hospital, I was scared to death to touch her. I mean, she looked like she was dead, or perhaps dying right then and there! I said to myself, "Why did they (the doctors at the outside hospital) send her back?" I even went so far as to ask the nurses on duty the same thing. They told me that she was sent back because there was nothing else that could be done for her there.

Cathy was sent to the outside hospital in July 1989. At that time we discovered that she had cancer, but I didn't know to what extent. Neither did anyone else at that time. In any event, she was back. And part of my job (I was a nurse's aide) was to help her recover and regain her strength and courage and to actually join the living again. What a job!

Unbeknownst to me, Cathy had had a mastectomy, so the medication kept her drugged and basically in and out of reality. After leaving work, I informed everyone who knew Cathy that she was back and to come down to IPC to see her.

I was afraid to go to work the next morning, for fear that Cathy had died in her sleep, but, thank God, she hadn't. I prepared to wash her and brush her teeth, when she told me that she wanted to do this herself. She tired very easily and needed to lie down in between her chores.

ACE members started to come down to cook for her (her appetite went completely to hell during her long illness). A long-standing friend of hers was there for her damn near "Twenty-four-Seven," along with other people she had met while she was here before and when she returned.

A few days later I came to work, and I'll be damned if Cathy wasn't up and standing over the sink, brushing her own teeth. She was holding on to a chair for support, but she was standing on her own without the assistance of anyone! Needless to say I was shocked and scared for her at the same time. Shocked because one day she was looking death in the eyes, and scared because I was afraid for her.

Bush (a very close, old friend of hers) cooked for her diligently, and always salmon cakes. We used to tease Cathy and say that she had expensive taste. I mean salmon is at least $2.99 a can, but whatever Cathy said she wanted to eat, regardless of what it was, we fed it to her. We even got one of the nurses to bring in some crab legs for her one day. But who could blame us? When she came back to us, she didn't even want to look at food, let alone eat it. So whatever Cathy wanted, Cathy got.

Kathy B. and Judy C. often came down to IPC to give Cathy massages, read to her, talk with her, or just plain sit with her in the quiet and listen to the sounds around them.

At times, there were so many visitors in Cathy's room that I sometimes thought that she would tire from so much going on around her, but she never tired of the attention and love that was given to her.

When the doctors said that there was nothing else that could be done for her, we—ACE and a host of loving friends—brought Cathy back with lots of TLC: a prescription that is accessible over the counter but is not utilized quite enough.

When she died, we all got together and discussed all of what I've written above, and we came to the conclusion that Love gave Cathy back to us for just a little. If not forever, for a little while.

Drug Trials for Treatment

In order to develop possible drugs to fight HIV infection, scientists/doctors have to run "trials." These are studies where the drugs for HIV/AIDS and related illnesses are tested for three main purposes: to determine safety, effectiveness, and proper dosage. Drug trials are traditionally conducted by the government and research hospitals, and by private drug companies. The Food and Drug Administration (FDA) is responsible for regulating the entire process of testing experimental drugs in humans. By law, the FDA must approve all drugs sold on the open market as both safe and effective.

For thousands of men, women, and children with HIV-related conditions, drug trials used to represent the only access to effective treatment available, either because private treatment was too expensive or because already approved drugs had been ineffective for them. There are a number of issues about drug trials that have been the subject of enormous struggle, social pressure, and debate. Who has access to drug trials? Who conducts the drug-trial process and how long does it take? By what methods are the drug trials conducted?

WHO HAS ACCESS TO DRUG TRIALS?

One issue in drug trials is *who* is included in these trials. This is crucial, since most of the drugs used to fight HIV-related opportunistic infections are experimental, and very often one must be in a drug trial to obtain the drug. Yet, HIV-related drug trials have excluded many of those who are infected. Below is a review of the key groups historically excluded from most trials, with the reasons for their exclusion. Increasingly, newer drug trials include these diverse population groups, as the scientific community has recognized the need to study the effects of new drugs on different subgroups.

Originally, drug trials were conducted with adult males. Women were normally excluded except in trials for contraceptive devices, breast cancer, or gynecological conditions. At this time, women, including female adolescents and pediatric patients, constitute 18 percent of the participants in the federally funded AIDS Clinical Trials Group. The exclusion was partly the result of the disaster resulting from the use of thalidomide, a sedative that was marketed to prevent miscarriages but led to terrible birth defects. Excluding women from drug trials was partly motivated by a desire to protect the health of future children. Yet, if drugs are marketed before they are tested on women, there is no way to evaluate the impact of drugs on the particular hormonal system of women or to know if the drug's impact, dosage level, and other variables are different for women than for men. In addition, it means that women are denied access to possible treatment therapies for HIV/AIDS through these drug trials.

Even when not explicitly excluded by protocols, women have less access to drug trials because they have less access to the research hospitals where trials are usually conducted. Medical institutions typically make no provision for child care and transportation costs.

Black and Hispanic people are severely underrepresented in drug trials. Until the recent expansions in drug-trial populations, for example, statistics showed that blacks and Hispanics accounted for only 18 percent of the total enrollment in drug trials, yet in New York they represent the vast majority of the total of diagnosed cases. In the federally funded AIDS Clinical Trials Group, 61 percent are white, 21 percent are black, 16 percent are Latino. Among women in drug trials, 69 percent are white, 18 percent are black, and 13 percent are Hispanic.[1]

Drug research has generally excluded IV drug users. Often the reason given is that IV drug users are not reliable, either because they may take other drugs or because they will miss appointments. These assumptions lead to excluding all former IV drug users from some HIV trials, or requiring, as in the case of testing the drug Ampligen, that they be drug-free for seven years.

Prisoners are excluded from clinical trials and often from getting experimental drugs. This is because for many years prisoners were used essentially as guinea pigs for many studies involving physical and psychological experimentation. There was a long history of struggle against this practice, and the federal government and local governments now forbid research on prisoners.

Poor people have rarely been included in drug trials. Researchers have argued that they are not reliable participants because they miss appointments. Poor people usually get medical care in municipal hospitals, while drug trials are usually conducted in academic medical centers that do not accept patients who lack insurance coverage. People without resources are so marginalized that they have little or no awareness that drug trials exist.

Without undercutting the important protections that were won against research abuse, ways must continue to be developed to safely include the excluded groups in drug trials.

WHO RUNS THE DRUG TRIAL PROCESS AND HOW LONG DOES IT TAKE?

The current drug approval process can involve eight to ten years for a three-stage testing process. This extensive process was developed to protect people. There is a history of doing experiments in which the safety of people as subjects was not taken into account. There is a history of abuse by drug companies in promoting drugs that were either unsafe or did not have the promised effect. The strict approval process developed out of this

---

1. This information came from the AIDS Clinical Trials Information Services on March 17, 1995.

history. Yet this eight-to-ten-year testing and approval process is more time than many PWAs and other HIV-infected people have.

There has been a great deal of struggle and discussion about how to create a testing-and-approval process that opens up trials and speeds up the process by which people get access to possible new drugs, without jeopardizing the important rules and regulations designed to protect the public.

One recent development is the "parallel track" policy, adopted by the FDA after much struggle by community health organizations such as Community Research Initiative on AIDS (CRI) in New York, County Community Consortium (CCC) in California, and ACT UP. Under this policy, those who cannot get into trials can be prescribed experimental drugs still in the effectiveness-testing stage, once they are known to have passed the test for safety. The parallel-track patients are followed by their doctors, who report back to the Food and Drug Administration or the drug companies on how the patients are faring. This data, though not as scientifically useful as that obtained in a clinical trial, can be included in the final analysis of how effective the experimental drug might be. It will give many more people access to experimental drugs.

How Are the Drug Trials Conducted?

Traditionally, in drug trials half the participants are given the drug to be tested and the other half (without their knowledge) are given either the regular drug treatment for the condition or a sugar pill, or placebo. Comparisons between the two groups permit scientists to evaluate the effectiveness of the new drug. Many people believe that when one is dealing with a deadly disease, it is unethical to deny treatment by giving people placebos. This is particularly serious, because usually a person entering a drug trial has to agree not to take other potentially beneficial drugs.

Community-based clinical trials (as opposed to trials conducted by the FDA and drug companies) have developed drug trials and treatment research that address the needs of PWAs. They have attempted to reach out to those generally excluded from drug trials and have been more willing to test holistic treatments as well as drugs. They are not geared toward making money, as are private drug companies, but toward providing desperately needed new treatments and drugs. Instead of using placebos, they use an alternative drug such as AZT, whose effectiveness is already known. The decision-making boards of CBCTs are composed of PWAs and others involved in HIV/AIDS advocacy, as well as doctors and researchers.

Even the government's agencies—such as NIAID, the National Institute for Allergy and Infectious Diseases—have acknowledged the effectiveness and reliability of CBCTs. In fact, aerosol pentamidine—used to prevent and treat PCP—was the first medication approved by the FDA that was tested solely by a CBCT.

WHICH DRUGS ARE DEVELOPED AND TESTED IN THE DRUG TRIALS?

Choices are constantly being made as to what drugs will be tested in the drug trials. This is determined by the priorities and directions in research, which in turn are affected by who is able to get research grants and for what drugs. There are ongoing debates as to how much emphasis in research should be placed on researching antiretrovirals as opposed to an emphasis on developing medicines to fight the opportunistic infections or on research in other directions. One ongoing issue is how much emphasis continues to be placed on AZT research and whether the benefits thus far continue to support the emphasis.[2]

Women and Treatment

There are very few studies on the particular ways that HIV affects women. Yet women are the fastest-growing group of people contracting the virus. In what ways are women's symptoms for HIV infection the same and/or different from men's? We know that men and women have different symptoms for certain STDs (sexually transmitted diseases). Men show symptoms much sooner, and by the time a woman realizes that she has contracted an STD, it's already ascended to more vital organs, such as her uterus or tubes. During a woman's menstrual cycle, she is also more susceptible to infections than at any other time. Also, during menstruation a woman's hormones fluctuate, which results in recognizable changes in weight, fatigue, and sexual desire. Because these changes take place normally in a woman, she may not realize that something abnormal is also happening inside her body, therefore leaving the illness undiagnosed and with room to progress.

---

2. John S. James, "AZT, Early Intervention, and the Concorde Controversy," *AIDS Treatment News*, April 23, 1993, 1–6; Editorial, "After Concorde," *Treatment Issues*, May 1993, pp. 6–7.

It is important to know whether there are particular symptoms or illnesses associated with the HIV virus that women get. This will help determine treatment for women and any particular development of the disease.

The vast majority of HIV-infected people in this country are men. The majority of women affected by HIV/AIDS are black and Hispanic; many are poor and involved directly or indirectly with IV drug use. In addition, medical providers often do not take women's health complaints seriously. Women who express health problems are often told that their problems are psychological. When women go for treatment for sexually transmitted diseases, health clinics do not always do follow-ups to find out if there are other underlying problems.

Race and sex biases in this country play a role in the lack of attention that women are getting as a group in research around HIV/AIDS. This is an area in which social action could make a difference. For example, ACT UP in Chicago organized a demonstration in 1990, demanding more services for women. The day after the demonstration, the first woman was admitted to the AIDS ward at Cook County Hospital. In December 1990, women and HIV/AIDS activists from all over gathered in Washington, D.C., to meet with federal officials to demand that government agencies address the particular impact of HIV on women. Pressure is a continuing necessity.

* * *

I feel one of the reasons women are dying at such an alarming rate is that they are not taken seriously in this society. Unfortunately, women have always been viewed generally as caretakers or childbearers and nothing more. Another unfortunate fact is that most women have readily accepted this role, which consequently causes and allows them to reject themselves. The main problem with this is that by the time most women even seek treatment, the virus has progressed to a point where early intervention is not possible. There is also stigma as far as how medical staff view women and our medical problems. In short, women and their illnesses are not taken seriously. If a women goes to the doctor complaining about weight loss, nine times out of ten she will be told how good she looks instead of being questioned about whether it could be because of some health problem. On the other hand, if a man went to the same doctor complaining about weight loss, steps would be taken immediately to find out why.

The media contributes to the way women have subconsciously learned to stigmatize themselves. I'm sure you have seen the commercials advertising douches—"Do you feel unclean during this time of the month?"—

which consequently causes many women to automatically run to the corner store and purchase a douche. In actuality, there is nothing unclean or nasty about a woman's menstruation. It is our body's natural way of cleansing itself. Most women are not aware that an abundance of douching strips the body of its natural defenses, leaving it vulnerable to infections. Because of shame and a lack of education, most women are either unaware of what goes on with their bodies or ignore all the signs telling them something is wrong.

* * *

A WOMEN'S TREATMENT AGENDA

—RISA DENENBERG

We need primary, universal health care for all people, including women and children, at all stages of HIV infection, that incorporates all of the following:

- Treatment facilities that meet all of women's needs, including transportation, child care, substance-use detoxification programs, psychological support services, peer group support, safe sex education, and nutritional counseling.
- Adequate, on-site comprehensive gynecological and obstetrical services.
- Access to experimental drugs at the site where health care is received.
- Comprehensive information and informed consent, so each woman can make her own best decision regarding experimental drugs and treatments.

We need a research agenda that incorporates women's issues and includes:

- Comprehensive research into the unique aspects, natural course, and progression of HIV illness in women and children.
- Research into the effects of new drugs on women's and children's bodies, with an emphasis on the effects on women's reproductive systems.
- Research on the use of new drugs during pregnancy and their effect on both women and fetuses.

• Research into alternative, holistic models of treatment, as they affect women and children.

We need policies that promote wellness and choice in our lives as women with HIV illness, including:

• No directed counseling about HIV-antibody testing, pregnancy, or medical therapies. Women need information and must be allowed and encouraged to make their own decisions.
• No coercive sterilizations, abortions, or other reproductive imperatives. A full spectrum of medical services, which must include obstetrics, gynecology, and abortion.
• Informed consent for experimental drugs and treatment that are specific to women.
• Government agencies, including institutional review boards that oversee drug protocols, must be charged with the responsibility to determine how women will be included in all approved drug trials.
• No risk of loss of child custody due to HIV illness.
• Services such as child care, home health care, and home maintenance must be part of the comprehensive health services available to women with AIDS and HIV illness.[3]

The Cost of Drugs

The pharmaceutical companies that produce the drugs are monopolies, in a sense, because they patent the drugs that their labs develop. Consequently, the cost of the drugs is controlled, often at an artificially high level. The cost of drugs such as AZT and aerosol pentamidine is so high that most PWAs who have no insurance or cannot receive Medicaid cannot afford them. There has been an outcry against this, and pressures have forced the companies to agree to lower prices and/or provide drugs cost-free to those in need.

The AIDS Drug Assistance Program (ADAP) is a federally funded program that makes certain medicines related to AIDS available free of

---

3. Risa Denenberg, "Treatment and Trials," in the ACT UP/NY Women & AIDS Book Group, eds., *Women, AIDS, and Activism* (Boston: South End Press, 1990), pp. 78–79. The entire Women's Treatment Agenda is reproduced here as written by the above-named author.

charge to medically and financially eligible residents of New York State. U.S. citizenship is not required. ADAP has just expanded to include fourteen drugs for AIDS and clinical symptomatic HIV illness. To request information or an application, you can call a toll free number: 800-542-2437.

The drugs that ADAP covers include:

NEW YORK STATE DEPARTMENT OF HEALTH
AIDS DRUG ASSISTANCE PROGRAM (ADAP)
FORMULARY — PAGE 1
AUGUST 1, 1994

ANTIRETROVIRALS

didanosine (ddl, Videx)
stavudine (d4T, Zerit)
zalcitabine (ddC, HIVID)
zidovudine (AZT, Retrovir)

PCP PROPHYLAXIS AND TREATMENT

atovaquone
dapsone
leucovorin
pentamidine
sulfadoxine/pyrimethamine
trimethoprim
trimethoprim/sulfamethoxazole (TMP/SMZ)

NEOPLASMS

alpha interferon
bleomycin
cyclophosphamide
cytarabine
dexamethasone
doxorubicin
etoposide
lomustine
methotrexate
prednisone
procarbazine
vinblastine
vincristine

OPPORTUNISTIC INFECTIONS

ANTIVIRALS
acyclovir
foscarnet
ganciclovir

ANTIFUNGALS
amphotericin B
clotrimazole
fluconazole
itraconazole
ketoconazone
nystatin
terconazole

TOXOPLASMOSIS
azithromycin
clindamycin
leucovorin
pyrimethamine
sulfadiazine
sulfamethoxazole
triple sulfa

CRYPTOSPORIDIOSIS
paromomycin

MYCOBACTERIAL INFECTIONS
amikacin
azithromycin
capreomycin
ciprofloxacin
clarithromycin
clofazimine
cycloserine
ethambutol
ethionamide
isoniazid

kanamycin
ofloxacin
para–amino
  salicyclic acid
pyrazinamide
rifabutin
rifampin
streptomycin

BACTERIAL INFECTIONS
intravenous immune
  globulin (IVIG)

OTHER

cyproheptadine HCl (Periactin)	For treatment of anorexia or cachexia.
epoetin alfa (Procrit)	For AIDS-related anemia, with Hct < 30% and endogenous erythropoietin levels < 500mU/ml. A free serum erthropoietin test is available through local Ortho Biotech Product Specialists (800-325-7504).
dronabinol (Marinol)	For treatment of anorexia associated with weight loss.
filgrastim (G–CSF)	For severe neutropenia due to drug toxicity.
octreotide acetate (Sandostatin)	For treatment of AIDS-related diarrhea.
megestrol acetate (megace)	Potential treatment for HIV-related wasting syndrome, when other causes of weight loss have been excluded.

NEW YORK STATE DEPARTMENT OF HEALTH
AIDS DRUG ASSISTANCE PROGRAM (ADAP)
FORMULARY — PAGE 2
AUGUST 1, 1994

ANTIBIOTICS
amoxicillin
amoxicillin + clavulanate
ampicillin
aztreonam
bacitracin
cefaclor
cefadroxil
cefazolin
cefixime
cefoxitin
cefpodoxime
cefprozil
ceftzaidime
ceftriaxone
cefuroxime
cephalexin
cephradine
chloramphenicol
chlorhexidine gluconate
cloxacillin
dicloxacillin
doxycycline
erthromycin
erthromycin ethylsuccinate
erthromycin ethylsuccinate
    and sulfisoxazole acetyl
flucytosine
furazolidone
gentamicin
griseofulvin
imipenem — cilastatin
loracarbef
metronidazole
miconazole
minocycline
nitrofurantoin
penicillin G
penicillin VK
probenecid
spectinomycin
tetracycline
ticarcillin K + clavulante
tobramycin
vancomycin

ANALGESICS
butalbital combination w/wo/
    codeine
codeine w/wo ASA, APAP
diclofenac
diflunisal
fenopofen
fentanyl
flurbiprofen
hydrocodone w/ ASA, APAP
hydromorphone
ibuprofen
indomethacin
ketoprofen
ketorolac tromethamine
levorphanol tartrate
methadone hydrochloride
morphine sulfate
naproxen
oxycodone w/wo/ ASA,
    APAP
proxicam
sulindac
tolmetin

PSYCHOTROPICS
alprazolam
amitriptyline
bupropion
buspirone
butabarbital
carbamazepine
chloral hydrate
chlordiazepoxide w/wo
    clidinium
chlorpromazine
clomipramine
clonazepam
clorazepate
clozapine
desipramine
dextroamphetamine sulfate
diazepam
divalproex sodium
doxepin hcl

PSYCHOTROPICS (cont.)
fluoxetine
fluphenazine
flurazepam
halazepam
haloperidol
imipramine
lithium carbonate
lithium citrate
lorazepam
loxapine
magnesium sulfate
mesoridazine
methylphenidate
molindone
nortriptyline
oxazepam
paroxetine
pemoline
pentobarbital
perphenazine
phenytoin
prazepam
primidone
prochlorperazine
risperidone
secobarbital
sertraline
temazepam
thioridazine
thiothixene
trazodone
triazolam
trifluoprazine
trimipramine
valproic acid
venlafaxine
zolpidem

NOTES: ADAP covers all forms and all brands of the medications included in the Formulary. Additional antibiotics are listed for HIV/AIDS indications on the Formulary – Page 1.

REFERENCE MATERIALS

AIDS Intervention Management System (AIMS), under the auspices of the AIDS Institute New York State Department of Health. *Criteria Manual for the Treatment of AIDS*. New York: New York Statewide Professional Standards Review Council, 1988.

Burroughs Wellcome Co. *Management of HIV Disease Treatment Team Workshop Handbook*. New York: World Health Communications, 1991.

Feist, Jess, and Linda Brannon. *Health Psychology*. Belmont, CA: Wadsworth, 1988.

Grimes, Deanna E., and Richard M. Grimes. *AIDS and HIV Infection*. St. Louis, MO: Mosby-Year Book, 1994.

Haseltine, William A., and Flossie Wong-Staal. "The Molecular Biology of the AIDS Virus." *Scientific American*, October 1988.

HIV/AIDS and Children: Answers for Caregivers. New York State Department of Social Services. SUNY Research Foundation/Center for Development. Buffalo, NY: 1994.

Massachusetts Department of Public Health and Massachusetts Department of Education. *Learn and Live: A Teaching Guide on AIDS Prevention*. Massachusetts, 1987.

Mass, Lawrence, M.D. *Medical Answers About AIDS*. New York: Gay Men's Health Crisis, 1989.

Mid-Hudson Valley AIDS Task Force, Information Packet, ARCS, 1988.

TEACHING PLAN

A. Role-Play: Empowering Ourselves for Getting Medical Treatment

Open the workshop with some quick role-plays of patients seeking medical treatment and their interactions with the doctor and a health advocate.

ROLE-PLAY 1:

A patient and a health advocate ask questions of a doctor. The doctor objects to the presence of the health advocate and answers questions superficially, saying it is not important for the patient to know because the doctor is the one that has to make decisions.

ROLE-PLAY 2:

A Hispanic patient attempts to communicate with the doctor. The doctor says that it isn't important that she can't understand everything, because the doctor has the information.

ROLE-PLAY 3:

The patient is now educated and goes in to see the doctor on her own. The doctor makes a recommendation, and the patient suggests an alternative treatment, which the doctor acknowledges makes more sense (use an example from your own experience). The doctor acknowledges the strength of the patient's education.

These role-plays help set the theme of this entire workshop: the possibility of people becoming educated about HIV/AIDS treatments and the importance of this.

B. Understanding Strategies for Treatment

1. Review the *main points* of the "What is HIV/AIDS" Workshop.
   a. The immune system is one aspect of what defends the body against disease. It is made up of the defenders—different types of cells and chemicals that work together.
   b. The HIV virus invades the immune system cells. It especially attacks two key white blood cells: the T4 cell and the macrophage cell.
   c. It gets into the T4 cell by a lock/key relationship in which the protein "coat" of the virus fits the particular protein section on the T4 cell and the virus blueprint slides inside the T4 cell.
   d. At some point, the HIV begins to multiply and spread throughout the immune system.
   e. Scientists are looking at cofactors that appear to affect the speed with which the virus multiplies.
   f. Certain disease-causing agents—viruses, bacteria, fungi, and so forth—take advantage of the weakened immune system and cause diseases.
2. Then ask: If you were scientists trying to develop a way to deal with HIV/AIDS, what different strategies might you use? Gen-

erate a brainstorm. (Every time we have done this workshop, people's responses to this question have covered the five strategies!)

Using the charts that were used last week and people's responses to the brainstorm, develop an understanding of the main strategies scientists are pursuing to deal with HIV/AIDS (see background materials).

3. Talk about the strategies and about the existing treatments. Use examples from PWAs who have utilized the different approaches, such as those described in the boxes or from PWAs in your group who are open about talking about themselves. Let people talk about the pros and cons of different approaches. Emphasize the real advances and the difference each approach is making in people's lives.

4. In the discussion about holistic health care, do some breathing or relaxation or visualization exercises to give people an idea about one type of holistic technique.

C. Dealing with Doctors and Treatment Choices:

1. Ask: What are the problems people have in dealing with doctors?

Generate a brainstorm, making two lists:

• Problems in ourselves—our attitudes, feelings, and so on
• Problems with doctors and other medical people

Possible answers generated:

• As soon as I see the doctor, I forget all my questions.
• The doctor rushes and doesn't take any time to talk.
• I don't ask because I don't want to know the answer.
• I'm intimidated.
• He doesn't take me seriously because I'm a woman.
• I don't know what to ask.
• I'd rather just let the doctor make decisions.
• He gets annoyed if I speak up.
• I don't go to doctors. I don't believe in Western medicine.
• I get frustrated and pissed off at the doctor and I leave.

2. Ask: What can we do about some of these problems?

Generate a brainstorm, with possible responses being:

- Prepare a list of questions before going.
- Take a friend with you.
- Have a medical advocate with you.
- Look for a doctor with whom you can work (if possible).
- Educate yourself. Knowledge is power!

3. Encourage people in the workshop to talk about their own treatment choices and experiences. Read some of the excerpts from the background materials or other personal histories of PWAs.

NOTE: We suggest breaking up into small groups for the following role-play and discussions. Pick those of the following that are most relevant to your group, or define some of your own.

1. ROLE-PLAY: TAKING INITIATIVE

Angie is going for a breast exam because her breasts are leaking fluid. She is worried that she may have breast cancer. She has an appointment with a doctor whom she has seen only once before. She wants to establish a relationship with the doctor so that she/he speaks to her about what is happening, discusses treatment choices, and works cooperatively with her. But the doctor is used to directing the process totally and assuming that the patient does not need to know everything. Angie tries her best to open the doctor to a new kind of patient/doctor relationship. (When preparing the two people for this role-play, ask the one playing the doctor to act like a "typical doctor" who doesn't expect to have to talk with the patient as an equal.)

2. DRUG TRIALS FOR TREATMENT

Possible discussion questions:

A. Do you think women should be included in drug trials, and if so, why? How would you institute protection against the potential damage to the unborn fetus so that disasters such as the thalidomide experience will not occur?

B. What is your opinion about scientists' evaluation that IV drug users should be excluded from drug trials because they are not reliable? What kind of stipulation/rules would you set up that does not totally exclude drug users but that takes potential problems into account?

C. What kind of system could be developed that would protect prisoners from abuse in drug experimentation and testing, yet would open up access to drug trials for those prisoners who want it?

D. What can be done to try to involve more poor people and more black and Latin people in the drug trials for HIV/AIDS?

3. WOMEN AND TREATMENT

A. Possible discussion topics in small groups:
Why are women overlooked in terms of treatment needs?
Our experiences of sexism in dealing with medical needs.
Questions about particular health concerns for women.
Important: Men should talk about these issues of women and treatment too!

B. We are a community of women with a high level of HIV infection. Are there suggestions for how studies done in our community could make a contribution to the overall understanding of HIV's impact on women? Could such a study be done without violating prisoners' rights or subjecting women to any abuse or danger? If so, how could we play a role in implementing such studies?

4. ETHICAL ISSUES IN DRUG TRIALS

There are many ethical issues and debates surrounding the conduct of drug trials by both community-based groups and the medical establishment. Workshop facilitators can choose a current debate, utilizing newspaper articles to draw this out.

For example:

What do people think about using placebos in drug trials? How can the effectiveness of experimental drugs be scientifically determined without using placebos? What are the pros and cons?

Efforts by CBCTs to conduct streamlined trials of experimental drugs, such as Compound Q, have led to criticisms by medical experts for not providing enough protection for those involved in the trials and for not being rigorous enough in their testing procedures. How do you weigh the advantages and disadvantages of "streamlined" trials that may subject participants to greater risk?

REFERENCE MATERIALS

Books

The ACT UP/NY Women & AIDS Book Group, eds., *Women, AIDS & Activism*. Boston: South End Press, 1990.

Alternative and Holistic Treatment Subcommittee prepared by ACT UP. *Alternative Holistic Treatment*. New York: 1989.

Burroughs Wellcome Co. *Management of HIV Disease Treatment Team Workshop Handbook*. World Health Communications, 1991.

Callen, Michael, ed., *Surviving and Thriving with AIDS: Collective Wisdom Vol II*. New York: People With AIDS Coalition, 1988.

Community Research Initiative, New York and County Community Consortium (San Francisco). A conference called "Organized Community-Based Clinical Trials: Models for the AIDS Epidemic." The National Institute for Allergy and Infectious Diseases (NIAID), July 7-9, 1989, New York City.

Criteria for the Medical Care of Adults with HIV Infection. AIDS Institute, New York State Department of Health, 1993.

Matthews, Thomas J., and Dani Bolognesi. "AIDS Vaccines." *Scientific American*. October 1988.

"Special Edition Women's Treatment Issues," in Mary Beth Caschetta and Garance Franke-Ruta, eds., *Treatment Issues* 6 (Summer/Fall 1992).

Yarchoan, Robert, Hiroaki Mitsuya, and Samuel Broder. "AIDS Therapies." *Scientific American*. October 1988.

Periodicals

AIDS Treatment News
John S. James
P.O. Box 411256
San Francisco, CA 94141

PWAC NY Newsline
50 West 17th St., 8th Floor
New York, NY 10011

PWA Support
PWA Legal Assistance Newsletter
Prisoners Legal Services
2 Catherine St.
Poughkeepsie, NY 12601

SIDA AHORA
50 West 17th St., 8th Floor
New York, NY 10011

The Body Positive
2095 Broadway
New York, NY 10023

Treatment Issues
Gay Men's Health Crisis
129 West 20th St.
New York, NY 10011

WORLD
Women Organized to Respond to Life-Threatening Diseases
A newsletter by, for, and about women facing HIV disease
P.O. Box 11535
Oakland, CA 94611

Workshop #5
HIV/AIDS: Transmission and Risk-Reduction Activities

* * *

My friend used to borrow all of my clothes from me, especially my shoes, but when she found out I was HIV-positive she wouldn't even ask to borrow my brand new things with tickets on them.

* * *

Even if you know the information, you still can get scared. Like, I had a close friend who was HIV-positive and we shared everything. One day I made some broccoli and I took a bite of it and then I offered her the rest. I thought that she was going to eat the whole piece, but she took a bite and pushed the rest toward me. Even though I was teaching people that you cannot get AIDS from food, I hesitated, feeling fear. My mind told me that there was nothing to be afraid of, and I ate it, but we both felt that hesitation. That experience taught me how one could know but still have the fears.

* * *

When I was on the streets, I was always doing drugs. I didn't want to think about how messed up my family is, or about all the terrible things that had happened to me. I really wanted someone to love me. But . . . I just couldn't believe that anyone ever would. So I decided nothing mattered, and I stayed high. Eventually, I had a baby. A little girl who was so sweet and precious and so very beautiful. I really think we could have loved each other, but by then I had stopped believing, stopped feeling.

I'm no longer doing drugs and I'm trying to learn about what it feels like to live and love and to be loved. If you're doing drugs, you need to stop, you deserve to. For me, no matter how positive I live, no matter how long I live, drugs will never do anything for me again. There just isn't a drug around that can get me high enough that I can't still look down and see that my little girl died from the HIV virus I gave her, before I even had a chance to learn how to love her. What is it like to live with HIV? For me, it is like learning to love myself and live for the first time, but doing it a little too late.

OVERVIEW

For two weeks, we are going to be talking about how the HIV virus is transmitted and exploring how we can and can't put ourselves at risk of infection. In the years since the AIDS epidemic became a visible crisis in the United States, the shape of the epidemic has changed. Of those who were probably infected in the early to mid–1980s, about half were gay men and a little more than a quarter were IV drug users; fewer than 10 percent were heterosexuals. Yet in 1994, a quarter of new infections were among gay men; almost half of the new infections were among IV drug users who shared needles, and about a quarter were heterosexually transmitted.

Several factors are involved in changing behaviors to prevent the spread of HIV. First, facts and information are important tools for changing behaviors. Second, our individual needs, values, and personalities all play a role in how we weigh that information and arrive at decisions about what to do. Third, only by changing *group* values, attitudes, and norms in our various communities will we be able to change individual behaviors enough to successfully stop the spread of HIV/AIDS. We are learning to come together as a community, struggling for the rights and needs of PWAs, and through that building our sense of self-respect. We are learning to care about ourselves and one another *enough* to actually go through the changes we need to, in order to promote the prevention of infection.

This first workshop on HIV transmission will examine the impact of drugs—both IV drugs and others, such as crack—on transmission of HIV. It will look at mother-to-child transmission and transmission through blood products. We will also focus on understanding how HIV/AIDS *isn't* transmitted in order to look at the deeper roots of stigma and isolation of people with HIV/AIDS. All the energy of avoiding what is not a danger is energy robbed from our real struggles to change our behaviors that do put us at risk. All our feelings that make PWAs (people with AIDS) different— "others"—feeds our denial of our own potential vulnerability.[1]

GOALS

1. To understand how HIV is and is not transmitted: developing a basic knowledge of both the myths and realities concerning HIV

---

1. Gina Kolata, "New Picture of Who Will Get AIDS Is Dominated by Addicts," *The New York Times*, February 28, 1995, Section C, p. 3.

and its transmission. How do we get the real facts, and how do we deal with the flurry of information and misinformation?

2. To understand the role of needles, drugs, blood, and pregnancy in HIV transmission.
3. To become aware of individual and group values and attitudes that impact on decision making about HIV transmission in order to reduce risks.
4. To deepen the discussion of combating stigma by exploring our common fears that remain untouched by facts about HIV/AIDS.

ISSUES TO EXAMINE

1. HIV/AIDS is not spread by casual contact.
2. HIV infection can be spread through the sharing of needles with infected blood.
3. All drugs can place people at risk for HIV infection.
4. A mother who is HIV-positive can pass the HIV virus to her unborn child; breast milk can pass the virus to an infant.
5. Infected blood products can infect an individual with HIV.
6. There is a relationship between ignorance about how HIV is transmitted and stigma.

BACKGROUND MATERIAL

HIV Is Not Transmitted by Casual Contact

HIV/AIDS is not easily transmitted. Studies show that it is transmitted mostly by infected blood and infected semen. HIV infection can also be transmitted by infected vaginal/cervical fluids. HIV has sometimes been found in saliva and breast milk of individuals with HIV infection but at much lower concentrations than in blood, semen, or vaginal secretions. Theoretically, transmission from saliva *may* be possible, but there are no known cases of transmission in this way.

Let's look first at how it is *not* transmitted: HIV/AIDS is not spread through *casual contact* with an infected person: the HIV/AIDS virus *cannot* be transmitted by:

• Being around people infected with the virus, even on a daily basis (for example, talking to, eating with, sitting next to, or working with them).

- Sleeping in the same bed.
- Handshakes, hugs, kissing on cheek.
- Sharing bathtubs, showers, or toilet seats.
- Sharing dishes, utensils, or linens.
- Smoking after someone.
- Eating food prepared by an infected person.
- Sneezing or coughing.
- Drinking from the same soda can.

How Do We Know?

1. SCIENTIFIC KNOWLEDGE ABOUT THE VIRUS: HIV is not an airborne virus. It cannot be transmitted through the air like the common cold or flu. It loses its potency and within minutes dies in the air, food, or water. It is killed by bleach, rubbing alcohol, Betadine solution. It's a *fragile* virus that needs a protected, warm, moist channel to be transmitted from one person to another. The skin is the body's first line of defense. HIV is impossible to transmit unless blood or semen or vaginal secretions come into contact with open areas of the skin. It is a *dangerous* virus, but *fragile*.

2. HOUSEHOLD STUDIES: Several studies of the families of infected adults and children evaluated the risk of HIV transmission through casual contact. In one study done at Montefiore Hospital, *not one of 400* family members was infected with HIV through household contacts, except for sexual partners of the infected person and children born to infected mothers.

Summary: The risk of household transmission was zero.

3. COMMON SENSE: If the HIV/AIDS virus spread through casual contact, we would see a different pattern of infection. For example, people living in the same household with people infected with HIV would become infected. People living in public institutions, such as prisons or schools, would become infected. If it were an airborne virus, people might get it from riding on public transportation or eating in restaurants. If you could get it by smoking the same cigarette or sharing a soda, it would have spread widely through schools and the workplace.

Two other studies have helped to deepen our understanding of how HIV/AIDS is not transmitted:

1. BELLE GLADE, FLORIDA MOSQUITO STUDY: This farming community showed a high incidence of HIV infection. It also had a lot of mosquitoes. The purpose of the study was to see if mosquitoes transmitted HIV. Results showed that the only people who got HIV were those with other

risk factors, such as IV drug use and unsafe sexual practices. People who got many mosquito bites but had no risk activities did not get HIV. For example, children and elderly people had a lot of mosquito bites, but they did not get HIV infection. This is only one of a number of studies done in communities affected by HIV/AIDS in which there were also mosquitoes.

- The study in Belle Glade, Florida, is one important piece of data showing that mosquitoes do not transmit the virus.
- While mosquitoes draw blood *from* people, they do not exchange blood between people.

Summary: There was no evidence that mosquitoes transmitted HIV/AIDS.
2. STUDIES OF HEALTH CARE WORKERS: In the United States, it is estimated that 800,000 to 1 million punctures and other occupational exposures occur annually in health care settings. Of these exposures, approximately 2 percent are likely to involve HIV-infected blood.[2] According to the CDC, as of 1994, there have been thirty-seven documented cases of HIV transmission from patients to health care professionals, with an additional seventy-eight possible cases.[3]
Summary: Occupational risk of acquiring HIV infection in health care settings is most often associated with needle-stick injuries, and strict guidelines should be followed to prevent direct exposure to potentially infectious body fluids.

PERSONAL HYGIENE IS IMPORTANT

Although HIV/AIDS is not spread through casual contact, there are commonsense things that are important in terms of general personal hygiene. For example, although there are so far no cases of HIV/AIDS linked to sharing razors or toothbrushes, it would be smarter not to share these things. Razors or toothbrushes could have a little blood on them, which you might not see. They also could carry other types of germs. Don't leave sanitary napkins around; keep your body clean. Sharing cigarettes and drinking out of the same soda can expose a person not to HIV/AIDS but to other germs. So far, no AIDS cases have been linked

---

2. New York State Department of Health, *100 Questions and Answers* (April 1994), New York: New York State Department of Health, 1994.
3. Federal Centers for Disease Control, *HIV/AIDS Surveillance Report* (October 1994), Atlanta, GA: Federal Centers for Disease Control, 1994.

with the piercing of any body part or with tattooing. To guard against possible infection, however, all needles or equipment used for these procedures should be sterilized between uses.[4] These are commonsense habits of cleanliness to protect us from other germs that are more easily spread than HIV.

SOME COMMONLY ASKED QUESTIONS:

Does biting transmit HIV or AIDS?

This is a question that comes up in such contexts as prison and for mothers with young children.

The only documented, known means of transmission is intimate contact with blood, semen, or vaginal excretions and breast milk. Thus, only if the person doing the biting is bleeding through the mouth *and* seriously breaks into the flesh of the other person, creating a bleeding area, could there even theoretically be transmission.

Usually when a person bites someone, her saliva is what comes into contact with the other person. Although saliva may have the HIV in it, the concentration is much lower than in blood, and there is no known case of saliva transmitting HIV. If it is even theoretically possible, it would require quarts of saliva coming into contact with a direct route of blood in another person. This doesn't happen when an individual bites someone.

The people doing the biting are actually in more danger of getting HIV. If they bite someone who is HIV-infected and they draw their blood into their mouth, and if they have open sores in the mouth, theoretically the blood-to-blood contact could transmit the HIV.

Summary: There is no known case of biting transmitting HIV.

Is coming into contact with blood dangerous?

As long as our skin is intact, it is a good line of defense (see background material on Studies of Health Care Workers). If you're helping someone who is bleeding, however, it is recommended that you use a plastic glove if available or that you put a cloth over the bleeding rather than use your hand. If your hand is exposed to blood, wash with soap and water as soon as possible. If you know that you have open sores and cuts on your hands, then be sure to use a cloth to cover the person's bleeding area.

---

4. New York State Department of Health, *100 Questions and Answers: AIDS*, April 1994.

What if two children want to be blood brothers/sisters and they press their fingers against each other after pricking them? Or what if two children are playing on a playground and one gets scraped and her friend wants to kiss it or hold it to make it better?

There is a possibility of transmission, yet there have been no documented cases of HIV infection from such incidents. Documented cases exist involving the direct entry of blood into the bloodstream, which occurs in a blood transfusion or in drug-abuse needle sharing. This is why New York State recommends that children with AIDS or HIV infection should be allowed to attend school and classes and to participate in activities if physically able. We should, however, advise our children to be careful with blood and to wash after coming into contact with blood.

How HIV Is Transmitted and How We Can Protect Ourselves

SHARING NEEDLES

IV drug abusers often share needles and syringes, cotton, cookers, and other equipment used for injecting drugs. This can result in small amounts of blood from an infected person being injected into the bloodstream of the next user. This is one main way that the HIV virus is spreading now.

A used needle or syringe may look clean but can still contain germs or another person's blood, even if it cannot be seen with the naked eye. Washing and rinsing works with soap and water will not adequately remove germs and traces of blood. Also, buying a "clean" needle on the street does not assure that it is sterile. If you cannot stop shooting drugs, then make certain to flush needles with fresh bleach first and then water.

Any needle-sharing activity with a person infected with HIV is a high-risk activity. This includes needles used for IV drug use, intramuscular injection such as steroids, skin popping, piercing, and tattooing.[5]

HOW TO CLEAN WORKS TO REDUCE THE RISK OF HIV[6]

1. Rinse out the blood in the syringe with cold water three times. Draw the water in and then shake or tap the syringe before pushing it out. This will loosen any blood that has clotted.

---

5. Ibid.
6. Beck Young, "News on Bleach," *LAP NOTES,* Spring 1994, Gay Men's Health Crisis, pp. 6–7.

2. Clean the syringe with fresh, *undiluted* bleach three times: Draw in, shake the syringe, and push out three times. If you can, let the bleach remain in the syringe for at least thirty seconds.

3. Rinse out the bleach with clean water: Draw in, shake the syringe, and push out three times. (Be sure you don't shoot or drink the bleach.) Do not reuse the water, cotton, or other filter materials.

* * *

THE COOKER: swish clean water around in it;
swish bleach around in it and then dump it out;
swish more bleach around and leave it in the cooker for at least thirty seconds;
empty the bleach and rinse the cooker with clean water.

THE COTTON: throw cotton away after shooting up or cleaning needles, works, or cookers.

* * *

IF YOU SHOOT DRUGS,
DO NOT SHARE NEEDLES,
WORKS, OR COOKERS

Q. How likely is it that people will really use bleach?

D. When I was on drugs, I didn't have time to think about cleaning something, especially when I felt I was really sick. Shooting galleries don't think about having to spend money on anything like bleach or alcohol, even as inexpensive as they are. They are thinking about using money for drugs.

L. I believe that the love for either children or spouse can motivate one to take lifesaving precautions like using bleach, because with children, they may wonder who is going to take care of my children if I die.

* * *

Needle-exchange programs have been developed in numerous cities, including New York, as one approach to slowing down the spread of HIV infection among IV drug users who are addicted. The rationale behind such programs is that providing addicts with clean syringes and supplies will cut down on the sharing of needles that are possibly infected with HIV. These programs have raised controversy: those opposed to them have argued that they will encourage drug addiction by providing clean needles. The most recent statistics from the New York City needle-exchange program had two important findings: (1) only 1 to 2 percent of those enrolled in the program became infected with the HIV virus each year, compared with 4 to 5 percent of high-frequency IV drug users who were not enrolled; (2) there was no evidence that needle exchanges increased the rate of drug injection by participants or attracted new people to become involved in IV drug use.[7]

ALL DRUGS—EVEN NON-IV DRUGS—ARE RISKY IN HIV INFECTION

The impact of the use of drugs in the HIV/AIDS epidemic goes beyond the actual use of needles. Drugs of any kind, including alcohol, and especially crack, make us less likely to use the judgment that we need to have safer sex. Drugs can also make us desperate for money, so that we will be willing to engage in unsafe sex for the money.

The CDC has found that nearly three-quarters of the 40,000 new infections with HIV in 1994 were among addicts. And although many were among IV drug users who shared infected needles, an estimated half of these numbers were crack addicts who were contracting the virus through unprotected sex, often with multiple partners. Both men and women go on binges, having sex with many partners in exchange for crack or money to buy it.[8]

MOTHER TO CHILD

Recent studies show that in the United States there is a 20 to 30 percent average chance that an HIV-positive woman will pass the virus to her unborn child. It is believed that a mother can transmit the HIV virus to her unborn child either while the fetus is in the uterus (transplacental transmission) or during the labor and delivery (perinatal transmission) by

---

7. Felicia R. Lee, "Data Show Needle Exchange Curbs HIV Among Addicts," *New York Times,* November 26, 1994.

8. Kolata, "New Picture of Who Will Get AIDS."

exposure to maternal blood and perinatal fluids. A mother is most likely to transmit the virus to her child immediately after she is infected or when she has more advanced HIV infection.

A baby can become infected from a woman's breast milk. Therefore, doctors recommend that if a woman knows she is HIV-positive, she not breast-feed her infant, or if she is going to allow another woman to breast-feed her child (a wet nurse), she should make certain that the woman is not HIV-positive.

(Note: All babies of HIV-positive mothers will test positive for the antibodies for the HIV virus after birth. This is because all mothers who are HIV-positive will pass HIV antibodies to their infants. You can't be sure if the baby is infected with the virus until it begins to produce its own antibodies. It takes a baby on the average 8 to 18 months to develop its own antibodies, and sometimes up to 30 months. Only when a baby has begun to produce its own antibodies is it possible to use the HIV-antibody test to know if the baby itself has the virus. Doctors have to observe symptoms of young babies as a way of diagnosing HIV infection. Increasingly, doctors are using a PCR test on infants to determine whether the virus is present. See Workshop Number 7, on Testing, for more details about the HIV-antibody test.)

AZT AND PREGNANT WOMEN: The National Institutes of Health (NIH) released a report in the spring of 1994 that AZT can reduce transmission of HIV from mother to unborn baby. In the study, AZT was given to some HIV-positive women during their pregnancy, while they were giving birth, and to their babies during the first six weeks after they were born. The study found that only 8 percent of the babies whose mothers took AZT were born with HIV infection, while 25.5 percent of the babies whose mothers did not take AZT had HIV infection. The results were considered so significant that the drug trial was stopped and all participants were offered AZT.

There are many questions that scientists are now studying. Some of these include: What are the long-term effects of giving AZT to a baby? Which therapy was responsible for lowering the rate of transmission: AZT during pregnancy, AZT during birth, or giving AZT to the baby? Since the women enrolled in the study had a T4–cell count of over 200, what are the benefits of giving the therapy to a pregnant woman with a low T4–cell count?[9]

---

9. Dave Gilden, "Study Finds AZT Reduces Mother-to-Child Transmission," *Treatment Issues* 8 (March 1994): 15–16; Lawrence K. Altman, "In Major Finding, Drug Limits H.I.V. Infection in Newborns," *New York Times*, February 21, 1994, p. 9.

Should all pregnant HIV-positive women take AZT?

Here are some factors that a woman may want to consider when facing such a decision:

- How does she feel about taking AZT for herself?
- How does she feel about exposing her fetus to AZT, since the long-term effects of this are unknown?
- How does she feel about giving AZT to her baby after it is born? (The long-term effects of this are also unknown.)
- How does she weigh the possible problems with taking AZT for herself or for her child born with the HIV virus (for which there is a 25 percent chance) or for her child born without the virus (for which there is a 75 percent chance), versus being able to reduce that chance to 8 percent?[10]
- How would she feel if her child is born HIV-positive and she realizes that she *might* have been able to prevent that by taking the AZT treatment?

These are the issues that women whom we have talked with at Bedford Hills have considered.

BLOOD PRODUCTS

Before 1985, the blood supply was not screened for HIV, and many people contracted HIV when receiving blood products. This was of particular danger for hemophiliacs. Since 1985, the HIV-antibody test has been performed on donated blood and organs. As a result of this test and health history screening, the rate of infection from blood transfusions has been reduced dramatically, and the risk of HIV infection is now extremely remote.

Although the risk of infection from a blood transfusion is extremely low, some people are donating their own blood for an operation if they are able to plan ahead.

The blood supply in foreign countries may not be tested. Thus if a person is considering receiving medical care in another country, it is important to investigate the safety of that country's blood supply.

---

10. Rebecca Denison, "Update: AZT & Pregnant Women," *World,* April 1994, Oakland, California.

TEACHING PLAN

Introduction

This workshop should be one that gives information, but feelings are very important too, because they affect how people deal with the information. Asking about the fears that people have has helped the interaction in previous workshops. Role-plays are important, and we suggest that they be done with a sense of humor, because we find that people then become more involved.

Discussions, Presentations, and Explanations

1. DISCUSSION:

What are people's feelings about whether they believe they can protect themselves against getting the HIV/AIDS virus?

Present the following to begin discussion:
Many people feel that there's nothing they can do to avoid getting HIV/AIDS. *Why do people feel that way?*
Let's look at the experience of the gay men's community. During the early 1980s, HIV/AIDS spread frighteningly through that community. And people felt powerless to stop it.
Certain specific behaviors promoted that spread:

- unprotected anal sex
- anonymous sex
- recreational drugs

Along with a growing movement and community consciousness that gay men had to and could take responsibility for fighting HIV/AIDS, they changed some of their group norms and attitudes and behaviors. This significantly helped to reduce the rate of new HIV infections.

Do we believe that other communities can do this?

Often the media and establishment promote the idea that poor people, young people, and people who have used drugs cannot be educated and cannot change. Do we believe that?

2. DISCUSSION: ASSESSING PEOPLE'S KNOWLEDGE ABOUT HIV TRANSMISSION

Ask: "What have you heard about how HIV/AIDS is spread? You can mention what you think are facts, what you think are myths, and what are things that you have questions about." (Write down these answers on the blackboard.)

PRESENTATION

Describe the main ways HIV is transmitted and explain that casual contact does not transmit it. Give many examples of casual contact that people would wonder about. Give the three main kinds of evidence that show casual contact does not transmit HIV/AIDS (*scientific knowledge* about the virus; *household studies; common sense*).

Ask: "What would it be like if HIV/AIDS were spread through casual contact? Would children and old people be getting it in the same numbers as sexually active adults and IV drug users?"

Ask people what their questions are and ask the group to try and answer the questions, based on what they have learned.

3. PRESENTATION: THE IMPORTANCE OF PERSONAL HYGIENE

4. DISCUSSION: MOSQUITOES, BITING, AND HANDLING BLOOD

Ask people for their answers, based on what they have learned, about the following commonly asked questions (see background material for information):

a. *Do mosquitoes transmit HIV?*

b. *Does biting transmit HIV?*

c. *Is handling blood dangerous?*

5. PRESENTATION: IV DRUGS, TATTOO NEEDLES, AND TRANSMISSION OF HIV

Discussion of HIV and IV drug use: (This can either be a small-group or large-group discussion.)

At this time, HIV is spreading among IV drug users. There is great concern that education does not yet seem to be having an effect on prevention.

   a. What are the difficulties in carrying out effective HIV/AIDS prevention education among IV drug users?

   b. What do you think about the potential of the needle exchange program?

   c. What do you think about the potential of making bleach part of the routine?

   d. What are your ideas about how to best educate people who use IV drugs about HIV/AIDS prevention so that lives can be saved?

   e. What are some of the ideas and methods people have about how to keep needles clean when they don't use bleach?

6. *PRESENTATION:* THE EFFECT OF CRACK AND OTHER DRUGS ON TRANSMISSION OF HIV

Ask participants to share from their own experiences about crack and other drugs and how they are tied to the spread of HIV.

7. *PRESENTATION AND DISCUSSION:* MOTHER-TO-CHILD TRANSMISSION OF HIV

Ask participants about their thoughts and feelings about the use of AZT to reduce transmission of the virus between a mother and her unborn child.

8. *PRESENTATION:* BLOOD PRODUCTS AND TRANSMISSION OF HIV

9. *SMALL GROUP DISCUSSIONS:* STIGMA AND CASUAL CONTACT

At this time the large group should break into smaller groups of five to eight people. Small group discussions will facilitate talking about feelings. They are also useful for developing a role-play and discussing a dilemma.

All small groups should discuss the following issue:

Why do we react out of fear of getting HIV/AIDS, even if we have information that should eliminate that fear? It is helpful if the group leader can give an example from her/his own life, because that helps to make people feel more open about discussing their own fears. Why do we pull back or even ostracize someone who is HIV-positive even if we know that she or he is not a danger to us?

Answers that emerged in one brainstorming session:

- Fear of death.
- Fear of the unknown.
- We've been lied to so much, why believe them now?
- I think of how colds can be contracted, so I associate it with how I could get HIV/AIDS.
- Peer pressure.
- It is hard to let myself get close to someone who is very sick.

The following are four examples of dilemmas that can be worked out through role-plays. One approach is to let each small group do one role-play and then present it to the whole group.

Situation #1: Your local beauty parlor is refusing to cut the hair of several women who are HIV-positive. What would you do if you heard about this?

a. How would you explain the facts to them?
b. Do you think explaining the facts would change their minds? And if not, how would you deepen the discussion with them to help them change their minds?
c. Do you think the beauty parlor should be forced by a non-discrimination law to cut their hair?

Situation #2: You have taken a two-year-old foster child into your household. You have three other children of elementary school age. Shortly after you take the child into your household, you discover she is HIV-positive.

a. Would you keep the child or not? What might your concerns be? What would your feelings be?
b. If you kept the child, what measures would you take within the household?

Situation #3: You are going home from prison on parole. You are HIV-positive. You are trying to decide when to tell your family to whom you will be paroled that you are HIV-positive.

    a. Would you tell them before you leave or after, and what are the reasons for your choice?

    b. What are the things you would want to say to them about an HIV-positive person living with their family? What are the issues about HIV transmission? What are the issues about support? What do you think their questions would be?

    c. How would you handle the emotional and factual issues in a conversation?

(The above situation depends a lot on the different personalities and the kind of relationship that exists. When you are doing an actual role-play, there will be many different possible approaches and outcomes.)

Situation #4: You will be paroled to your household, where your brother, who is HIV-positive, is living.

    a. What are your feelings about this?

    b. What are your questions about being with him in the same household?

REFERENCE MATERIALS

Heyward, William and James W. Curran. "The Epidemiology of AIDS in the U.S." *Scientific American.* October 1988.

Mass, Lawrence. *Medical Answers About AIDS.* Gay Men's Health Crisis, 1989.

New York State: Mario Cuomo, Governor; David Axelrod, Medical Comissioner. *A Physician's Guide to AIDS Issues in the Medical Office.* March 1988.

New York State Department of Health AIDS Institute, *Overview of HIV Infection and AIDS,* Training Manual. New York: New York State Department of Health AIDS Institute, 1994.

New York State Department of Health. *100 Questions and Answers: AIDS.* April 1994.

Patton, Cindy, and Janis Kelly. *Making It: A Woman's Guide to Sex in the Age of AIDS.* Ithaca, NY: Firebrand Books, 1990.

Workshop #6
HIV/AIDS: Sexual Transmission

* * *

While we are educated to understand that safe sex is important, practicing safe sex is not that easy when it comes right down to it. A lot of us who teach about safe sex don't even practice it ourselves.

* * *

It is necessary that we send a message out to the people, not in
such a technical manner, but in a more realistic way
as only someone living with AIDS can express.
It's always the issue of AIDS the disease,
Never the issue of the person with AIDS.
Statistics are too formal. They make people feel as if they're
being labeled something horrible.
PWAs sometimes tend to eliminate themselves from life because
of the rejection given by society.
Let's stop pushing away and turning our back on PWAs
but help them and in return let them help society.
Our main concern here is how to get people to protect themselves.
If only more people would remember that this can also happen to a
sister, brother or someone they love.
In my opinion, as someone affected and infected by this highly
common disease—that shows no discrimination—
it is necessary to protect ourselves as well as others
by using the proper contraceptives.

—A PWA

OVERVIEW

Despite all the information that we have about the dangers of unsafe sex, statistics have shown that many people are not practicing safer sex.

Our experience shows us that changes in people's sexual behavior are very slow and difficult. And even once changes are made, there is no guarantee that they will be permanent. There are alarming statistics that show that even among gay men who did adopt safer sexual behaviors, many are now reverting back to prior unsafe habits.

Much more than information is involved. We need to talk about our feelings. We need to recognize our responsibility to make choices. We need to open up discussion about the ways we are not free—or do not feel empowered—to change our behaviors. Some of the factors are our dependency on or domination by men, our addiction/dependencies on drugs, religious attitudes about condoms, peer pressure, and ways that the particular environment can block access to the concrete means for safe sex. For example, in some countries, especially in rural areas, condoms are too expensive for people or not easily accessible. It's one thing to know what must be done; it's another to find the ways to do that. Individual awareness and choice are crucial, but we are going to be a lot more successful when we have group support and peer solidarity to make these choices.

We do not expect to change behaviors through one workshop. The most important thing in such a workshop is for people to feel free to say what they really think and feel. In any group situation, when people are told what is safe and unsafe behavior, they are going to feel some pressure to say, "I'll do the right thing." In many of our workshops, women have said things like "If you love yourself, of course you will not put yourself at risk," or "I just have to be strong and I'll stay safe." But that doesn't mean they actually change their behaviors when the workshop is over. The very act of saying, "I don't know if I can or want to change my behavior" appears to be a more positive step toward actual change than asserting a false sense of certainty.

GOALS

1. To communicate the facts about sexual transmission of HIV.
2. To create an open atmosphere for people to express their true feelings about changing sexual behaviors.
3. To become aware of different factors that impede the change to safer sexual behavior.

ISSUES TO EXAMINE

- What is considered unsafe, safer, and responsible sex in both heterosexual and homosexual activities?
- What are the psychological, social, and physical factors that make it difficult to change our sexual behavior?

BACKGROUND MATERIAL

Some Basic Facts About HIV and Sex

- HIV is found in semen. Semen transmits the virus between a man and a woman and between two men during sex.
- HIV is found in blood. Blood can transmit the virus during sex.
- HIV is found in vaginal/cervical secretions, and these secretions can transmit the virus from a woman to a man or between two women during sex.
- HIV appears to be less concentrated in vaginal/cervical secretions than in semen and blood.
- The danger of transmission increases when a man or a woman has another sexually transmitted disease, because sores are a place of entry for the virus.
- The danger of transmission increases when a woman has a vaginal infection, because of the greater number of white blood cells in the vaginal area; white blood cells carry HIV.
- Menstrual blood, like all blood, carries HIV and can transmit HIV.
- Some individuals with HIV infection have HIV in their saliva; it is in very low concentrations. There are no known cases of transmission of HIV via saliva, but scientists at this time cannot say with absolute certainty that saliva can't transmit HIV. It is theoretically possible, although very low-risk. Blood in saliva increases the risk of transmission of HIV.
- In the United States, there are fewer documented cases of transmission from a woman to a man than from a man to a woman. But in Africa, woman-to-man transmission is almost equal to man-to-woman transmission.

Heterosexual Transmission:
Sex Between a Man and a Woman

Unsafe Sex

1.
   a. Vaginal and anal intercourse *without a condom* are both unsafe, because infected semen transmits the virus.
   b. Oral sex is also a risk without a condom, because infected semen can find an opening in the mouth, such as a sore, or gums that bleed or have been recently brushed or flossed.
   c. Transmission of the virus from a man to a woman is a growing means of transmission of HIV infection.
2.
   a. The risk of woman-to-man transmission from intercourse increases if a man has STDs (sexually transmitted diseases), such as sores on his penis.
   b. It is risky for a man to perform unprotected oral sex on a woman. The danger increases in the presence of menstrual blood and vaginal infection; it increases even more if he has sores in his mouth.
3. Fisting (hand in rectum or vagina) is risky, because it can tear the vaginal or rectal walls and cause bleeding.
4. Sharing sex toys that have contact with body fluids can be a risk.

How can I have sex and protect myself and partners from HIV?

We offer you this information so that you can make a conscious decision as to what choices you and your partner(s) are willing to take. Unsafe sex is having sex without even thinking about the risks involved. Responsible sex begins with thinking, talking, and making conscious choices. A major step toward responsible sex is being able to *talk* to your partner, to feel comfortable enough to raise fears, and to present choices *you* know you want to follow in order to make sex safe and fun. Sometimes, if you don't really know your partner, it's harder to work out these decisions and avoid feeling pressured into something you wouldn't *choose* to do.

Here are some options:

SAFER SEX

In vaginal, anal, and oral sex, the key to safer sex is *using barriers* (condoms/dental dams/finger cots). This is not absolutely safe sex, since a condom or dental dam can leak or break, but if it works, then it protects you from the infected semen or vaginal fluids.

An additional protection is to use the spermicide nonoxynol–9, which is known to kill the HIV/AIDS virus (either in the condom or on the side of the dental dam that touches the vulva area). The spermicide alone is not considered adequate protection. Some women may have an allergic reaction to nonoxynol, and it is important to be aware of how the spermicide is affecting you, since small irritations or sores in the vagina from such a reaction could make a woman more vulnerable to HIV infection.

SAFER-SEX ACTIVITIES

- Vaginal intercourse with a male wearing a condom.
- Oral sex with a man wearing a condom.
- Oral-genital contact using a thin piece of latex placed between the vulva and tongue.
- Hand or finger and genital contact, or vaginal or anal penetration with finger(s), using a disposable glove or finger cots. (This is particularly important if your hands are blistered and if there is a chance you will come in touch with body fluids or feces.)
- French (wet) kissing (when you do not have open sores or bleeding gums, and not immediately after brushing or flossing teeth).
- External urine contact.
- Anal-oral contact (rimming) with a latex barrier.

Anal intercourse, even with a male wearing a condom, is considered risky by the New York State Department of Health, because of the incidence of condom breakage; also, the risk of tearing delicate rectal tissues is high, thereby putting semen directly in touch with blood. Water-soluble lubricant in a squeeze bottle or tube, such as KY jelly, should be used to minimize tearing of rectal walls.

EXTREMELY SAFE SEX

Some people want to try to eliminate all risk from sex. They want to make certain that there is no exchange of or contact with semen, vaginal or cervical fluids, or blood. (Note: this does not include sweat and tears, which carry no risk of transmission.) Possible activities include:

KISSING ON LIPS AND BODY: Although saliva does not have enough HIV to transmit the virus, if you have open sores or cuts in your mouth it is advisable not to deep-kiss. Also, your gums could bleed after brushing your teeth.

GENTLE TOUCHING: Massaging, hugging, nibbling, taking baths, kissing on nipples and dry parts of the skin (such as the cheek, hand, or skin that does not have cuts or wounds), body-to-body rubbing and cuddling.

PLAYING WITH SEX TOYS: Always clean shared toys with bleach or alcohol and rinse with water.

MASTURBATION: Use latex gloves.

VISUAL AND MENTAL STIMULATION: Use your imagination, exhibitionism, fantasy movies, erotic talk, mirrors. Share your fantasies.[1]

CONDOMS

(Also known as rubbers, prophylactics, bags, skins, raincoats, sheaths, hats. . .)

When to wear a condom:

- Wear a condom when you have sex, and semen could get inside the mouth, vagina, or rectum (in oral, vaginal, or anal sex).
- Put the rubber on as soon as the penis gets hard. The virus that causes AIDS could be present in pre-seminal fluid.

HOW TO USE A CONDOM PROPERLY

1. Carefully tear open the package with your fingers. Handle the condom with care, so you don't cut it with your fingernails, teeth, or other sharp objects.
2. Hold the tip of the condom to squeeze out the air. This leaves some room for the semen when the man ejaculates.
3. Put the condom on the end of the erect penis.
4. Keep holding the tip of the condom. Smooth it on with your fingers. Be sure to keep air bubbles from forming.
5. Unroll it all the way down the shaft of the penis, making sure to leave an air pocket at the end.

---

1. Denise Ribble, *Women Loving Women,* brochure, Gay Men's Health Crisis, 1991.

REMOVING A CONDOM

1. Pull out while the penis is still hard, and while you are pulling out, hold on to the condom at the base of the penis so that the condom doesn't fall off or leak.
2. Be careful when you take the condom off so that the semen doesn't spill.

IMPORTANT FACTS ABOUT CONDOMS

- Use latex condoms, because the virus cannot go through the rubber. Don't use natural condoms, such as those made out of lambskin—the virus can go through them.
- Use a generous amount of water-based lubricant such as K-Y, Foreplay, or contraceptive gel. *Do not use* oil-based lubricants such as Vaseline or Crisco or anything else you have to dip out of a jar. The risk of breakage is higher and the risk of tearing of the rectal lining and contact with blood is greater.
- Use a condom only once and then throw it away.
- Don't store condoms for a long time in your wallet or near heat.[2]

IS THIS ALL POSSIBLE?

Realistically, changing our sexual practices means changing ourselves and our relationships. Men have traditionally been the ones who have initiated sex. *Talking* is the critical factor, yet that in itself can be very difficult. Talking about items that relate to sex is usually more difficult for women than for men. It can even be slightly uncomfortable to walk into a drugstore and buy sanitary napkins. And if a woman wants to take initiative in protection and have a condom to give to the man, she probably will feel awkward buying a condom. On some college campuses, people have struggled to install condom machines—to avoid having to go into a store and talk about it with anyone. The fact that talking about sex can be uncomfortable makes it difficult for a woman to raise the issue with her man. Yet, there are lessons from the struggle for birth control. It has been a long, hard struggle, and in the end it is

---

2. For more information about condoms, see *The Safer Sex Condom Guide for Men and Women*, brochure, Gay Men's Health Crisis, 1992.

women who have to care about themselves and control whether they get pregnant or not.

It is frequently difficult or impossible to get men to wear condoms. Many men will say that they don't want to wear condoms. Many feel that it is not as pleasurable or that they may have more trouble getting an erection. A man may feel that wearing a condom implies or suggests that he might be infected with HIV/AIDS, which he would find insulting. Power dynamics between men and woman leave many women unable to even raise the issue of safe sex, let alone to implement it. Women are often economically dependent, physically weaker and subject to threats or force, and controlled by social expectations, such as "It is up to the man to initiate and be in control sexually." These power dynamics between an individual man and woman reflect and are reinforced by broader societal inequalities between men and women in the economic, political, and social spheres.

Financial factors also play a role in whether a woman is more or less likely to rely on a condom. For example, a prostitute's client may offer to pay more for sex without a condom, and she may feel desperate for the extra money. And teenagers may not have access to condoms or the financial means to get them.

In our experience, many women also do not like condoms. They don't want to use condoms because it feels less spontaneous or because it doesn't feel as intimate or pleasurable. They have mixed feelings about trying to get a man to use one, because on the one hand they know it is important protection, and on the other hand they don't like how it affects sex.

Many women will assume that their man is not going to have the virus if he isn't an IV drug user. Even if they suspect him of having affairs, they will feel safe, because in the United States it is less likely for a woman to pass the virus to the man, even though it does happen. But many men have had sex with another man and don't define themselves as bisexual. This is true in male prisons, and it is true in most cultures.[3] Either the social stigma or the prevailing cultural assumptions make it difficult to talk about a man having sex with another man.

* * *

A woman who went home after seven years in prison shares her experience:

---

3. Yannick Durand, "Cultural Sensitivity in Practice," in The ACT UP/NY Women and AIDS Book Group, eds., *Women, AIDS, & Activism* (Boston: 1990).

I was in prison, and after six years I had my first furlough. I wanted to be with a man fast! I missed it. A friend of mine introduced me to a guy who had done a little time in prison, and we got along. I had sex with him. I didn't think about a condom, because he looked great. He worked out at the gym. He was built, he looked not just healthy but really fit. When I got back to prison I talked with friends, and they asked me if I had used a condom. I said, "No. He looked fine and he was in good health and he told me he wasn't gay." My friends got really upset with me. They were in ACE, and they said that I had to use a condom.

The next time I went out on a furlough, I got together again with him. I asked him a little more about his history. It turned out that he had actually been in the hospital and he was a little worried. We used a condom and we talked most of the night. I spent that whole first night trying to help him make up his mind to take the HIV test. He agreed to, and then I went with him. The whole furlough ended up focusing on his fear of being HIV-positive and helping him deal with it. Then my next six weeks back at Bedford I spent worrying about what his results would be and what it would mean for me if he was HIV-positive. I didn't even have the emotional space to look forward to my next furlough, all the joy was gone.

Then I remember that day when I called him, the day he was getting his results: he was HIV-positive. I thought I would die. I had children and grandchildren that I was looking forward to being with. Now I had to wait six months and see if I was HIV-positive. Instead of this being a joyous time in my life—furloughs, work release—I was miserable. Finally, I went out on work release, and a few months later I took the test. Thank God I was HIV-negative. But I will never forget. He looked good; he said he wasn't gay. He probably had sex with men. I'm sure he did, at least in prison. I'll never know. I just know I was lucky, and I hope other women don't make the same mistake.

* * *

There are no easy answers. We have to care about ourselves and take more control of making decisions. We have to support one another as women. We have to change our attitudes that lead to passivity. And we also have to struggle with men about their image of a woman's and a man's role in sex.

In ACE we discuss the need to talk about the issue of AIDS and sex before you are in bed with someone. If you're in prison and you are going home to a particular man, it means beginning to raise it with your partner before you're suddenly home.

* * *

I decided to raise the issue of safe sex with my husband before I came home. I had a visit with my husband and his two sisters, and we got into talking about AIDS. In the course of the conversation, my husband mentioned to his sisters that I had requested that he wear a condom when I get out. His sisters took offense to that. They asked why he had to wear a condom if he wasn't doing anything sexually. They were angry, but my husband said he would do it for me. I'll have been away from him for two years when I get out. I say he has to wear a condom because I'm not in his back pocket, and he's a human being. He's not a saint, he's just a human being.

* * *

And if you are beginning to date a man, try to figure out ways to talk about safer sex before you are faced with the situation of having sex, because at that moment it is very difficult to raise. Many partners are getting into condoms as part of the sexual acts: buying them together, talking about what kinds, putting them on together.

Another important way is to find support among friends. In prison, we talk about these issues and draw support from one another. Women often say, "When I go home, I'm definitely going to use a condom," or "If he won't use a condom, he won't get none." Yet, we know that saying it from prison is easy compared with the feelings and pressures of the real situations. We suggest taking the experience of women-supporting-women wherever you are. Talk about it with friends, learn everything you can, talk about your feelings, talk with one another about sex, and encourage one another to protect yourselves. Wherever you are, at home or at work, women can support one another.

Finally, you can become part of a safer-sex campaign in your own community, whether through a church or a community center or a clinic or a local AIDS task force. In our own experience and the experience of community activists around the world, a safer-sex campaign has to be very culturally specific or else it will not reach people. Different ACE members have different opinions about what this means.

Two opinions about the African-American community:

* * *

In the African-American community, I think that the safe-sex campaign might have been more successful if it had come into the African-American community with a different approach to men. They have said that African-American men have already been battered by this system—its racism, its unemployment, its drugs and poverty. African-American families have been struggling to survive. Then there is the safe-sex campaign, which makes it seem as if men are the problem. This safe-sex campaign threatens their masculinity by asking black women to take control of their men and make them use condoms. They suggest it would have been better if black men were approached as protectors. The safe-sex campaign should have talked of HIV/AIDS the way it is, genocide on African-American people, and talked to the men as being responsible for stopping genocide of African-American women, of African-American children. Then the men would feel a sense of responsibility as African-American men to help stop HIV/AIDS, instead of them being defined as the problem.

* * *

I think as long as we place the emphasis either on "black men" or "black women," we're going to be in trouble as a community. We always seem to point the finger, either to blame or to name responsibility at *either* the black man or the black woman. Until we take responsibility together—black men and black women—we will not be able to deal with the problem of AIDS, or any other problem.

* * *

An opinion about the Hispanic community:

* * *

You have to be more cautious about how you talk about sex and AIDS to Hispanic women. You can't be as open as when you talk to an English community, because the women were raised in a different way. They believe that only certain kinds of women have sex with a lot of men, even if they themselves have had sex with more than one man, which many have. They aren't going to say it, because they were raised to think it is wrong. And, if they have more than one man, they aren't going to tell me, they aren't going to talk about it, because they feel ashamed of it. They feel that only certain women are going to get gonorrhea or other STDs, and they don't want to say they have it. When we talk about AIDS it's important to say that you can get it even if you only have one partner, one lover, because your partner might have it from a previous relationship or another relationship now. That way they are willing to accept the idea that they might need to protect themselves.

Sex Between Women

We talk about "sex between women" or "woman-to-woman" sex in this section instead of "lesbians." Many women have sex with other women but do not think of themselves as lesbians. And many lesbians have sex with men. When we speak of "lesbians" we will be talking about an *identity* that some women have. In this chapter we are talking about an *activity*—sex between women—and the risk of transmitting the HIV virus.

Can a woman get the HIV virus from another woman with whom she is having sex?

There is a scientific basis for a woman transmitting the HIV virus to another woman during sex. An HIV-positive woman's vaginal and cervical fluids have the HIV virus in them, as does blood, both of which can be exchanged during sex between women. When a woman has an infection, white blood cells flow to the area and increase the amount of HIV virus in the area—because the HIV virus lives in certain white blood cells—even when the woman does not know that she has an infection. Finally, menstrual blood carries the virus, and blood cells may be present in our fluids for several days before and after our menstrual period without our knowing it. We know that other STDs are transmitted by woman-to-woman sex, though at a lower rate than either heterosexual or man-to-man sex.

What is the data regarding the transmission of the HIV virus during woman-to-woman sex?

After much criticism and pressure, the CDC conducted two studies on woman-to-woman transmission, and these two studies found that there were no documented cases of woman-to-woman sexual transmission. On the other hand, there have been questions raised about the methodology and accuracy of these and other studies for a number of reasons. For example, if a woman had any other identifiable risk factor, such as heterosexual activities or IV drug use, it was assumed that one of those was the route of transmission, regardless of the relative frequency or other specific details. The studies were based on a hierarchical set of categories, and it was assumed that the most effective/risky transmission route was the route by which transmission occurred, not woman-to-woman sex.[4]

_____

4. S. Y. Chu, T. H. Hammett, and J. W. Buehler, "Update: Epidemiology of Reported Cases of AIDS in Women who Report Sex Only with Other Women, United States, 1980–1990," *AIDS* 6 (1992):

There are a number of anecdotal cases of women saying that they were infected through woman-to-woman sex. All of these cases involved the exchange of blood.

We know that it is far less likely for a woman to transmit the virus through sex to another woman. Some reasons for this include:

1. Less concentration of the virus in vaginal/cervical secretions as opposed to semen and blood.
2. Sex between two women does not involve penetration, with release of a sexual fluid, such as when a man ejaculates during intercourse in a woman's vagina. Yet, we need more data. The people gathering statistics (CDC, epidemiologists, and so forth) need to do more and better studies, and there always must be a category asking the question about woman-to-woman transmission.

Even though the existing information is not sufficient, both scientific reasoning and the existing data mean that women having sex with other women need to be concerned, talk about it, and make conscious choices. Some of the choices are discussed below.

How can I have sex with a woman and not get HIV infection?

Some women are trying to develop "safer sex."

SAFER WOMAN-TO-WOMAN SEX

The key is using barriers. Barriers are important in oral sex. It can be a risk for a woman to perform oral sex on another woman without a barrier. The danger increases in the presence of menstrual blood, and this includes the days just before and after menstruation, when blood exists even if it is not visible. The danger also increases with vaginal infections, such as yeast infections, and sexually transmitted diseases, such as chlamydia, herpes, gonorrhea, and syphilis. The risk increases even more if there are cuts and sores in the mouth of the one performing the oral sex act.

(Continued from previous page.) 518–19; Rebecca M. Young, Gloria Weissman, and Judith B. Cohen, "Assessing Risk in the Absence of Information: HIV Risk Among Women Injection-Drug Users Who Have Sex with Women," *AIDS & Public Policy Journal* 7 (Fall 1992): 175–83.

One type of barrier is a dental dam. This is a piece of latex about five inches square. Some women are using a piece of latex rubber as the center of their underpants.

It is also advised that when touching your partner with your fingers, either in her vaginal or anal area, that you use latex gloves or finger cots. An opening in the cuticle area gives a direct opening to the woman's bloodstream for HIV transmission, as does any other kind of cut or blister on the fingers.

SUMMARY OF SAFER-SEX ACTIVITIES BETWEEN TWO WOMEN:

- Oral-genital contact using a thin piece of latex placed on the vulva and tongue.
- Hand/finger-to-genital contact or vaginal or anal penetration with fingers, using a disposable glove or finger cots.
- French (wet) kissing (when there are no open sores in the mouth and no bleeding gums and not directly after brushing or flossing teeth).
- Anal-oral contact (rimming) with a latex barrier.

EXTREMELY SAFE SEX BETWEEN WOMEN

Some women do not want to take any risk, and they therefore prefer "extremely safe sex," meaning no exchange of vaginal fluids or blood. Possible activities include:

KISSING ON LIPS AND BODY: Although saliva does not have enough HIV to transmit the virus, if you have open sores or cuts in your mouth, it is advisable to not deep-kiss. Also, your gums could bleed after brushing your teeth.

GENTLE TOUCHING: Massaging, hugging, nibbling, taking baths, kissing on nipples and dry parts of the skin (such as the cheek, the hand, or other skin that does not have cuts or wounds), body-to-body rubbing and cuddling.

PLAYING WITH SEX TOYS: Always clean shared toys with bleach or alcohol, rinse with water.

MASTURBATION: Use latex gloves.

VISUAL AND MENTAL STIMULATION: Use your imagination, exhibitionism, fantasy movies, erotic talk, mirrors. Share your fantasies.[5]

---

5. Ribble, "Women Loving Women."

Are women practicing safer sex with one another?

Women are usually not practicing safer sex with one another. Many women do not believe woman-to-woman sex is really a risk. They feel that there is not enough risk involved to go through the hassles of practicing safer sex. In addition, many of the same emotional issues are involved between two women in a relationship as between women and men: insecurity, dependency, power, control, need to prove love, need to feel loved. And these needs can make practicing safer sex difficult even when people really know the facts. In cases where it is known that one of the women is HIV-positive, there is a greater likelihood that there will be some consciousness about safer sex. There is a wide spectrum of opinions among women as to what kind of precautions it is necessary to take.

* * *

I am HIV-positive, and I found out before I came to prison. When I was first involved with a woman, we talked about safe sex. She didn't want to go down on me without a dental dam, and I agreed that it wasn't safe. But I found I couldn't deal with a dental dam. It made me think about being sick. It brought attention to the fact that I was infected, and it took away from my feeling normal and happy. Even though she really wanted to use it, I couldn't take it. So I just said let's not do that. It meant eliminating a part of sex that was very important, but I chose that instead of using the dental dam. Maybe someday I'll change, but that's where I've been.

* * *

A Dialogue: Different Feelings About Practicing Safe Sex in a Relationship Between Women

D: I can't say I would take that risk of putting someone else at risk. I couldn't take that possibility.

V: If the person doesn't have sores in their mouth and the HIV woman doesn't have an infection or have her menstrual, the risk isn't there. Because in deep kissing the enzymes kill the virus. Then the virus can't be transmitted.

D: It's not true that enzymes kill the virus. It's just that it isn't concentrated enough. We don't even know for sure how much virus is concentrated; I can't know if I have an infection for sure. I am not always aware of my medical situation, so how can I put someone at risk?

V: If two women have been together for quite some time, then they should know each other's bodies well enough to feel the changes in body odor, feel, smell, and differences in wetness and aroma.

J: How does it affect you teaching someone to use a dental dam when you don't believe it?

V: Well, I teach it, I give the facts, but I try to not recommend it, because my opinion is different.

D: I hate this subject, because it has emotionally hindered me even on whether to be involved. If a person is going to care about me, I feel they would use the barriers. With me knowing that my illness is progressing, I have to take precaution with more things, and because there is a change, how can you be sure how infectious we are? I also feel if a person is recently diagnosed and they are HIV, they may be more or less infectious.

J: Even though I think that someday we might find out that the risk of woman-to-woman infection is almost nonexistent, at this point we don't know, and we do know that the virus is in our fluids. I know when I present the material about dental dams that most of the people I'm talking to won't follow the information I'm giving, because there are so few statistics about women giving it to women. So I try to raise the choices for people and also try to say what is the most dangerous according to what we know—i.e., menstrual blood, or if a person has a vaginal infection.

C: I feel a woman can get it from another woman, but it is a personal choice as to whether she wants to use rubber gloves or a dental dam. And a woman is most at risk around blood—rough sex, or a tooth pulled, or menstruation. As far as presenting it, I can present the safety techniques, but I know in the past in my own relationship I didn't practice it, but I knew we were both HIV-negative. If I were involved with someone who was HIV-positive, I wouldn't take precautions unless we were into rough sex or a person was having her period. I think it is a personal decision and a decision between the two people.

D: If a person is HIV, like me, and my partner doesn't want to use protection, I still feel I have to insist on protection.

V: Maybe it's easier if you are just beginning a relationship to make that choice. But I was once involved with this person before I knew my status, and she didn't want to start using precautions, so we didn't use any precautions.

D: I just don't want to see anybody else go through what I am going through.

V: I feel that our partners have a say-so. Just because we are HIV-positive, I don't feel that we run the relationship.

D: When I decided that it was appropriate to look for information about safe sex, I came into contact with pairs of women having sex, and in one case, no one got infected, and in the other case, the person did infect her partner. So 50 percent was a pretty high ratio.

D: Would you, C, practice safe sex when you first meet someone?

C: Yes.

D: Case proved. We're talking about woman-to-woman transmission, for one night or a relationship.

C: I feel it is different for a one-night stand; if I am in a relationship, it would be different, because I would know her.

V: My reality would be between me and my partner.

D: I could never risk someone going through what I am going through.

* * *

Sex Between Men

We are women, writing about our experiences and knowledge about sex with men and about sex with women. Yet, the HIV/AIDS epidemic has devastated the gay men's community; sexual transmission between two men has been a central route of transmission for the virus, and we know that many men who are having sex with other men will read this book. We present below some basic facts about sex between men. We also know that men who are having sex with men will continue to create and produce their own materials to stop the spread of the virus.

UNSAFE SEX

- The virus that causes AIDS is present in the semen and in the blood of an HIV-positive man. It is unsafe to allow either semen or blood to enter your body.

SAFER SEX

The key is to use condoms.

- Condoms must always be used for anal sex.
- Oral sex is far safer when you use a condom. If you are not using a condom, you are safer when you lick the shaft of the penis. The risk of becoming infected with the virus increases when you lick the head of the penis, because you may come into contact with semen. (For information about condoms, see above section on Heterosexual Sex.)

EXTREMELY SAFE SEX

Some men do not want to take any risk and they prefer "extremely safe sex," meaning no exchange of fluids or blood. Again, possible activities include:

KISSING ON LIPS AND BODY: Although saliva does not have enough HIV to transmit the virus, if you have open sores or cuts in your mouth, it is advisable not to deep-kiss. Also, your gums could bleed after brushing your teeth.

GENTLE TOUCHING: Massaging, hugging, nibbling, taking baths, kissing on nipples and dry parts of the skin (such as the cheek, the hand, or other skin that does not have cuts or wounds), body-to-body rubbing and cuddling.

PLAYING WITH SEX TOYS: Always clean shared toys with bleach or alcohol and rinse with water.

MASTURBATION: Use latex gloves.

VISUAL AND MENTAL STIMULATION: Use your imagination, exhibitionism, fantasy movies, erotic talk, mirrors. Share your fantasies.[6]

LOOKING AT THE WHOLE PICTURE

Whether we look at sexual relationships between a woman and a man, a woman and a woman, or a man and a man, deep emotional and psychological factors will affect whether or not they practice safe sex. These will include both universal qualities and particular cultural factors, as well as specific dynamics between men and women, or women and women, or men and men. Here are some examples of situations that reveal these factors.

---

6. Ibid.

* * *

I knew of a woman who knew that her husband was HIV-positive and she did not want him to use a condom; she is willing to die with him. And she and he have kids. Maybe she wants to prove her love to him, either out of her own need or his demands. Maybe she feels guilty about being healthy and living and watching him die. Maybe she doesn't have her own sense of identity and can't imagine living without him. Or maybe marriage means to her total commitment and union and she is living out her deepest personal values.

* * *

My friend is HIV-positive, and she is also an AIDS educator outside in the community. One day she cut herself, and her lover, a woman who is not HIV-positive, licked her blood, both of them knowing that HIV is very concentrated in the blood. She told me about it, half boasting and half acting guilty. When we talked about it, she told me it made her feel that her lover really accepted her, loved her, and wouldn't feel any different even though she had tested positive. Her lover said she wanted to prove to her that she really loved her, and taking a risk is a way of showing that you will sacrifice yourself for love. Licking a wound is a way of showing caring. Being willing to take on the same illness represents being totally one with your lover.

* * *

In the gay men's community, safer sex is decreasing after a period of increase. Why? Different reasons are given: One important one is "survivor's guilt"—the feeling that so many close friends have died, that the whole community has been devastated. The guilt of surviving drives people to feel that trying to protect themselves makes them less worthy as a person.

* * *

We know that simply having a fact—such as what *safer* sex is—does not alone dictate what a person will do. We know from the "no smoking" campaigns that people do self-destructive things all the time. People's need for security, for proving their commitment and love, for becoming one with the person whom they love are deep feelings and needs. Individual counseling or support and "safer sex" campaigns will be limited if they don't account for these issues.

But as difficult as it is for individuals and communities to change sexual behaviors, *change is possible!* We can look to the example of the gay men's community, which was one of the first hit by the epidemic in the United States. In the early 1980s, the rate of sexual transmission of the virus among gay men was staggering. In the face of a rising death toll and many others infected and sick, gay men began to question deeply cherished sexual habits. Along with building a community of support for PWAs, they educated themselves, promoted safe behaviors, and began to use condoms and other safer-sex behaviors. It took an entire community's mobilization, mutual support, frank discussions, and commitment. Safe sex became an affirmation of identity and love, just as the "sexual freedoms" had for an earlier generation of gay men. And the difference was seen in the significant lowering of the infection rates among gay men by the late 1980s.

But even this success story ends with a cautionary note. There are alarming statistics that show that even among gay men who did adopt safer sexual behaviors, many are now reverting back to prior unsafe habits. Younger gay men who have not yet seen their peers die are not using condoms as much as older gay men. So we learn that education, support, and cultural awareness must be continual and in touch with changing conditions.

Tips for Teaching and Counseling About Sex and HIV/AIDS

I. *Be clear about which activities pose the greatest risk. This gives a person who wants to change some activities a way to choose, or to negotiate with her or his partner.*

- Vaginal and anal intercourse between a man and a woman or between two men is high-risk without a condom. People may be willing to use a condom for intercourse even if they don't want to use it for oral sex or won't use latex gloves or finger cots.
- Two women may believe that they really are not at risk for HIV infection, yet they may be willing to use barriers during a woman's menstruation or when they are aware of a vaginal infection, because they can understand the danger of blood.
- STDs can cause open sores which make viral infection easier. If protection can be used when there are open sores, this would be an important first step.

II. *Do not present safer sex as an all-or-nothing choice. Doing anything is better than doing nothing, and using protection sometimes is better than never using protection.*

When you are counseling an individual, it is important not to expect immediate change. Sexual choices are the result of many complicated factors. For many people, just beginning to talk about sexual choices with their partner is a difficult and important step.

III. *As a counselor, be aware of your own feelings, biases, and choices.*

This will help you keep from imposing your own attitudes on another person, and it will also help you to be more realistic about other people's choices. For example, as educators, many women teach about the use of dental dams in woman-to-woman sex, yet they do not use them themselves. Becoming aware of our own feelings can help us to connect to the real and not-so-real suggestions that we teach, and together we can perhaps develop more effective approaches to HIV/AIDS prevention work.

Common Questions

1. What are my chances of becoming infected after I have come in contact with someone who is HIV-positive?

Some information is known to help answer this question.

1. HIV is transmitted more easily during two periods of the infection: when a person first contracts the virus and many years later, as many as ten, when the immune system is collapsing.
2. A woman is at much greater risk having sex just once with a man who is in the infectious stage than having sex many times with a man who is in the least infectious, or "latent," stage.
3. This suggests that it is particularly risky to have sex with many partners, because statistically it is likely that some of them will be particularly infectious.[7]

Individual differences also play a role.

---

7. Gina Kolata, "New Picture of Who Will Get AIDS Is Dominated by Addicts," *The New York Times*, February 28, 1995, Section C, p. 3.

- Depending on your actual physical state/health, you can be exposed once, twice, and more and not become infected. But if your health is failing, then your chances may be greater.
- There are known cases where an infected IV drug user didn't know his status and had unsafe sexual contacts with his spouse for numerous years. When she was tested, it turned out that she never became infected. But after knowledge of the man's diagnosis, they then converted to practicing safer sex to prevent the woman from ever becoming infected.

Every time you have *unsafe* sex, you are exposing yourself to every sex partner your lover has ever had. Being into casual sex, one-night stands, bar pickups, and the like can create problems. Such situations make it harder and less likely to negotiate responsible sex.

2. How safe is deep, prolonged (French) kissing?

There are no known cases of AIDS transmitted through deep kissing. The virus appears in lower concentrations in saliva; some studies indicate that enzymes in the saliva kill the HIV/AIDS virus.

The virus is in the saliva of some HIV-positive individuals, however, and therefore prolonged, deep kissing is not considered absolutely safe, according to the present state of medical knowledge.

Two things to consider that pose risk:

a. If there is blood in the salvia of the infected person.
b. If openings exist—such as open sores, bleeding gums, tooth extractions—that create possible routes for transmission.

You have to weigh the facts and make your own choice about what level of risk you and your partner(s) want to take.

3. If I am already HIV-infected, do I have to practice safe sex?

Many people who are infected with HIV feel that they do not have to practice safe sex because they are already infected. This is not the case for the following reasons:

a. Because of the many strains of the virus, a person who is already infected with the virus can become reinfected and become

sicker even faster. It is important to realize that safe sex should be practiced at all times, whether you are HIV-positive or not.
b. Any time the virus enters the body, it makes the immune system work harder, and the virus count will multiply faster.

4. Is artificial insemination safe?

It is important to screen the donor for HIV antibodies. Women inseminated with HIV-positive semen are at risk of getting the infection and passing it on to their babies. Recommendations for safer donations include:

a. Test the donor at the time of donation for HIV infection.
b. Freeze the donor semen for at least six months and then retest the semen before using it.[8]

Sexually Transmitted Diseases (STDs)

The first time I contracted an STD, it was gonorrhea. After a shot of penicillin, it was gone. But several months later I got syphilis, and even though it was treated, I was told it would always be in my blood and that it could become active again. Some time later, I started having bad pains in my lower left abdomen. After going to a GYN doctor, I was informed that I had PID (pelvic inflammatory disease). While being treated for PID, it was discovered that the syphilis I contracted was penicillin-resistant. So after administering another form of medication, the doctor told me that the syphilis would always be in my blood.

Being that I had numerous STDs and continued having unprotected sex, I was susceptible to all kinds of viruses, because my immune system was already weakened because of the STDs and drug use. I never gave my body a chance to recover from one infection before I contracted something else. Therefore, when I was exposed to the HIV virus years later, there was nothing left to fight it.

A sexually transmitted disease (STD) does *not* turn into HIV infection or AIDS, but having STDs makes you more likely to get the HIV virus. This is true because your immune system is already weakened. Also, many STDs cause open sores, and that gives the HIV virus an easy way to enter into the bloodstream.

---

8. Ribble, "Women Loving Women."

An individual who is HIV-positive is more likely to transmit the HIV virus when he/she has an STD. This is because the white blood cells, which fight infection, are also the cells that carry the HIV virus. So when people have an STD, they will have a higher concentration of cells with the virus in them.

VAGINAL DISCHARGE

A vaginal discharge is a normal thing for a woman to have. It helps keep a vagina clean and damp. The discharge will take on different appearances. The normal discharge is clear or white, and it may have a slight odor. When it dries, it may be a yellow color on underwear. About halfway between periods, the discharge may become extra heavy, slippery, or stretchy, because this is when the ovary releases the ripe egg, and the discharge helps the sperm reach the egg.

A *change* in vaginal discharge may be a sign of a sexually transmitted illness.

- Odor: foul or strong.
- Color: greenish, grayish, or bloody.
- Amount: heavy discharge and itching and/or burning around the opening of the vagina.

Other symptoms of STD infections *might* include:

- Pain or unusual bleeding, during or after sexual intercourse.
- Chills or fever, diarrhea, or vomiting with fever during or just after your fever.
- Burning when you urinate.

For more details about specific STDs, see the Appendix to the Workshop on Sexual Transmission.

TEACHING PLAN

Our main goal in this workshop, along with communicating the information, is to create a nonjudgmental, open, exploratory atmosphere that encourages frank discussion about what people really feel, what they think the obstacles are, and what they think would most help create behavior change. The only way for this workshop to be successful is if the facilitators themselves really feel comfortable discussing sex. People may sign up for facilitating the workshop yet not really feel comfortable. Part of preparing to lead the workshop should involve discussion among the team facilitators about their own feelings on the issues.

1. Brainstorm with Words Relating to Sexual Transmission

Using newsprint, brainstorm for different words that people use for sexual parts of the body: e.g., penis, dick, cock, hammer, etc. This exercise will help loosen up or break the barriers for being able to talk about safe sex.

2. Discussion

List the different categories—Unsafe Sex, Safer Sex, Extremely Safe Sex—and ask people what some of the activities are and where they should be listed. This is to see just how much your audience knows before you begin your presentation and to create a process of involvement, as opposed to pure presentation.

Inform your audience that you are going to give them the facts and tools for safer sex so that they will be able to make a conscious choice (use background materials).

After giving the facts once again, open up to the group by asking for questions for those who might need more clarification.

Negotiating Safer and Extremely Safe Sex: Before breaking into small groups for discussion and role-plays about negotiating safer sex, do the following role-play for the large group:

SCENARIO: TWO FEMALE FRIENDS TALKING

Anne is getting ready for a date with a hunk whom she has been seeing, and she knows that *Sex* is going to happen tonight. Sharon is raising the discussion around safer sex—a condom—protection from HIV.

ASK: WHAT COMES OUT OF THE ROLE-PLAY?

- The fear of contracting HIV/AIDS if having unsafe sex.
- You cannot tell if someone is infected just by looking at him/her.
- Open the thought of asking him to use a condom. You can even say this is your means of preventing pregnancy (if you are not quite ready to discuss HIV/AIDS openly yet).
- If he says no, then you know that he isn't practicing safer sex, and then you might wonder if you even want to have sex with someone with that behavior.

BREAK INTO SMALL GROUPS:

This part of the workshop should be the longer section. It is the time in which people can actually talk about what they feel, and it is crucial if behavior change is to take place. There are many possible role-plays. Trainers should define them ahead of time and write them on paper for the group to read, discuss, and then role-play.

SUGGESTIONS FOR ROLE-PLAYING:

- HIV-positive individual tells her lover (man or woman) about being HIV-positive.
- Talking to your teenagers.
- Woman comes home from prison to the man who has been supporting her while she was in prison (or goes on trailer visit, or furlough).
- Woman is out at a party and is planning to go home with a man she has just been getting to know.
- A PWA is talking to her friend about her date. Her friend reminds her to practice safe sex. She tells her friend that she has the virus already and that there is nothing more that could happen to her. Her friend then goes on to explain how she can infect others and become reinfected.
- Ask the women in the group to come up with a scenario that they are worried about.

Now have several groups do the same one and come up with alternative ways it could go down.

- The man gets abusive.
- The partner refuses and walks out.
- The woman is insistent and firm.
- The woman uses flirtation and humor.
- The man says no. What do *you* do?

SMALL-GROUP DISCUSSION: DO A BRAINSTORM ON THE FOLLOWING QUESTION:

What makes it so hard to establish safe sex (with men or between women)?

- I'm too shy.
- Men think they run it.
- It creates distrust or raises the possibility of one of you cheating.
- I just don't *talk* about sex.
- Condoms don't allow total pleasure.
- I'm afraid of violence.
- It's economics.
- It's traditional sexual roles.

SMALL-GROUP DISCUSSION: EXPLORE SOCIAL FACTORS THAT INFLUENCE SEXUAL BEHAVIOR:

- Religion
- Hispanic, black, white cultures
- Class background

SMALL-GROUP DISCUSSION: WHAT IS GOING TO MAKE IT EASIER TO STRUGGLE FOR SAFE SEX?

SMALL-GROUP DISCUSSION: HOW DO YOU FEEL ABOUT CONDOMS, DENTAL DAMS, EXTREMELY SAFE SEX?

Putting on a Soap Opera

An alternative approach to this workshop is for the facilitators to prepare a soap opera in which characters interact with one another, raising the emotional and practical issues of sex and AIDS. The workshop participants can interact with the characters, arguing or struggling with them and asking them questions. In this approach, there is no separate formal presentation of facts. Instead, the information comes out during the interaction between the actors and the audience. We found that this approach was a lot of fun and people were very engaged. And if you are doing a series of workshops, the characters can come back in their next situation, building on the events of the previous one, creating interest in "What's going to happen next?"

REFERENCE MATERIALS

The ACT UP/NY Women & AIDS Book Group. *Women, AIDS & Activism.* Boston: South End Press, 1990.

A.M.A. Family Medical Guide. New York: Random House, 1992.

"GIRLS' NIGHT OUT": A Safer Sex Workshop for Women, Manual for Peer Leaders. Chicago: Chicago Women's AIDS Project, 1990.

The Boston Women's Health Book Collective. *The New Our Bodies, Ourselves.* New York: Simon & Schuster, 1992.

The New Complete Medical and Health Encyclopedia, vol. 2. J. G. Ferguson, 1992.

New York State Department of Health. *A Guide to AIDS Issues in the Medical Office.* Albany: New York State Department of Health, February 1988.

New York State Department of Health. *100 Questions and Answers: AIDS.* April 1994.

Patton, Cindy, and Janis Kelly. *Making It: A Woman's Guide to Sex in the Age of AIDS.* Ithaca, NY: Firebrand Books, 1990.

APPENDIX TO WORKSHOP #6: SEXUALLY TRANSMITTED DISEASES (STDS)

Veneral disease (VD) is an infection contracted and transmitted during sexual contact. VD organisms cannot survive for any length of time outside the body. Air, light, lack of moisture, and slight variations in temperature will destroy *most* VD organisms.

VD cannot be contracted from inanimate objects such as toilet seats, bed linen, or clothes. It is transmitted directly by the organisms entering the body, where tissues provide a favorable environment (dark, moist, and warm). These tissues are the mucous membranes of female and male genitalia, the mouth, eyes, and anus.

The early signs of VD are usually obvious in the male, while often neither felt nor seen in the female. The woman can become an unwitting carrier, transmitting the disease to others. Venereal diseases include:

Syphilis

Syphilis is caused by a bacterium (one of a type called spirochetes), can be diagnosed by a blood test, and is curable with antibiotic injections unless damage has already been done to the blood vessels and brain.

The symptoms of syphilis come in three stages:

1. First stage: A small, red, solid sore or ulcer (chancre) appears anytime between nine and ninety days after infection. This chancre *usually* appears in the genital area and may not be noticed if it occurs within the vagina or cervix. It may also occur on the mouth or rectum. The chancre heals in one to five weeks, leaving a thin scar. It is during this first stage that the spirochetes are circulating in the blood throughout the body.
2. The secondary stage starts anywhere from a week to six months after the chancre has healed. A fever may develop and/or the person may experience aching joints, sore throat, a sore in the mouth, headaches, and loss of appetite. There may be swollen glands in the neck, armpits, or groin area. A skin rash of small, red, non-itching bumps may appear, either generalized or only on the palms of the hands and the soles of the feet. During this stage the disease can be spread by simple physical

contact, including kissing, because the bacteria are present in the open sores that may appear on any part of the body.

3. The third, or tertiary, stage starts with the latent stage, which may last from ten to twenty years, during which there are no outward signs of the disease. In this stage the inner organs may be invaded, including the heart, brain, and spinal column. After the first few years, the disease is not infectious. The disease may suddenly flare up without warning. Loss of equilibrium, paralysis, insanity, senility, and, rarely, blindness may occur, as well as serious heart disease.

Syphilis can be passed from mother to fetus, especially during stage one or stage two. It attacks the baby just as it attacks an adult.

Gonorrhea (commonly called "the Clap")

Gonorrhea is caused by a bacterium (gonococcus) transmitted through sexual contact. It may infect your eyes if they are touched with a hand that is moist with infected discharge. It can be passed to a baby during birth. Donor semen used for artificial insemination can carry gonorrhea.

Gonorrhea is more apt to spread and persist in women than in men. If untreated, pelvic inflammatory disease (PID) can develop, as well as proctitis (inflammation of the rectum). Blindness can occur if the eyes become infected. Rare but serious infection occurs when bacteria travel through the bloodstream and cause infection of the heart valves or arthritic meningitis. Joints are the most common extragenital sites affected.

The symptoms of gonorrhea in women are often not noticed or are confused with other conditions. They usually appear from two days to three weeks after exposure. Often there are no symptoms in the early stages. The cervix is the most common site of infection, developing a discharge caused by an irritant released by the gonococci when they die. As the disease spreads, the urethra may become infected, causing painful urination and burning. The rectum can be infected by a vaginal discharge and/or anal intercourse, causing anal irritation, discharge, and painful bowel movements. If the disease spreads up into the uterus and fallopian tubes, pain occurs on one or both sides of the lower abdomen, as well as fever, vomiting, and/or irregular menstrual periods. The Skene's and Bartholin's glands may become infected, producing swelling and great discomfort. Gonorrhea can be spread from the penis to the throat, producing no symptoms or a sore throat and/or swollen glands.

Men's symptoms usually include a thick, milky discharge from the penis and painful, burning urination. It is often confused with NGU (nongonococcal urethritis, also called nonspecific urethritis, or NSU). Since NGU requires a different antibiotic for treatment, a lab test is necessary.

Treatment of gonorrhea is mostly by high dosage injections of penicillin. An IUD may make cure more difficult, as it helps spread infection and increases the chances of getting PID. It should be removed before treatment. Tetracycline is recommended by some doctors because there is less risk of an allergic reaction. Its disadvantage is that it must be taken for two weeks or so, and has a high failure rate in cases of anal and rectal gonorrhea. Unfortunately, new strains of gonorrhea keep appearing, requiring longer and stronger doses of antibiotics.

Herpes Genitalis (HSV2)

This virus can produce a painful infection of the genitals, called herpes genitalis, which is transmitted through sexual intercourse, through oral and anal sexual activity, and through contaminated hands.

Groups of blisters develop on one or several areas. These blisters eventually rupture and become shallow ulcers or sores.

In women the sores may appear anywhere about the external genitalia (labia minora or labia majora outside the vagina), along the inner thighs, and within and about the urethra.

In some women a single lesion may appear, while others may have continuous lesions from the urethra to the anus.

Females frequently complain of severe pain while urinating, being unable to direct their stream away from the sensitive ulcers.

Females may get *internal* lesions—in the vagina or on the cervix. Like the external sores, the internal lesions vary in severity and may be surface ulcers or deep and extensive.

A severe infection may occur on the cervix, which might at first be confused in appearance with cancer during lab testing.

It is possible to acquire genital herpes *without* sexual intercourse. Oral sex can transmit an oral herpes infection to the genital area. Also with "autoinoculation," a herpes sufferer spreads the virus from one part of her own body to another. For example, a person with a fever blister may during sleep touch her lip lesion and then inadvertently touch her genitals, spreading the virus.

Herpes is not a reportable disease: doctors are not legally required to report cases, as they are with gonorrhea and syphilis. Therefore, it is not known how many individuals, including pregnant women, have herpes.

Most of the infants who acquire this disease do so from their mothers, who do not know they have an active infection.

Nonspecific Urethritis (NSU)

Nonspecific urethritis (NSU), sometimes referred to as nongonococcal urethritis, is an infection of the urethra, the tube urine goes through to pass from the bladder to outside the body.

The group of organisms that cause NSU are transmitted through sexual activity but are considered to be less dangerous than syphilis or gonorrhea, since they are thought to produce no serious long-term illnesses.

In about half the cases, the disorder is caused by a type of organism called *chlamydia*.

Men and women who have NSU have no symptoms but can pass the infection to their sexual partners. In men who have symptoms, the symptoms often resemble gonorrhea, with painful urinating and a cloudy mucous discharge from the penis. Analysis of this discharge can determine which of these diseases it is.

Women with symptoms generally have symptoms resembling a urinary tract infection (cystitis, which is inflammation of the bladder). These symptoms include a painful, burning urination and the need to urinate frequently without expelling much urine.

Lymphogranuloma Venereum (LGU)

Chlamydia, as mentioned, is an organism. Certain strains of chlamydia produce lymphogranuloma venereum, another disease transmitted through sexual intercourse.

The initial sign of infection is a painless pimple or blister that develops on the penis or the outer labia or lips of the vagina, five to twenty days after exposure. About two to twelve weeks later, the lymph nodes in the groin painfully enlarge, mat together, redden, and drain pus.

The infection sometimes seems to improve without treatment, but ugly ulcers or sores may appear on the genitals. Later complications include scarring, which causes strictures in the urethra, vagina, or rectum. Strictures are small bridges of tissue that narrow the size of the body opening.

Chlamydia disorders are usually identified by a blood test in which the levels of certain antibodies (the substances the body produces to combat infections) are measured. Antibiotics will usually clear up the infection.

Genital Warts (Human papilloma virus, or HPV)

These are caused by a virus similar to the type that causes common skin warts. When these HPV-caused lesions occur on the cervix, the woman probably has a higher-than-normal risk for developing cervical cancer.

Symptoms usually appear from three weeks to three months after exposure. They are highly contagious even before any symptoms are visible. They look like regular warts, starting as small, painless, hard spots, which usually appear on the bottom of the vaginal opening. Warts also appear on the vaginal lips, inside the vagina, on the cervix, or around the anus, where they can be mistaken for hemorrhoids.

Treatment of genital warts is now usually by laser beams that do not affect normal tissue or cause scarring.

During pregnancy, warts tend to grow large, probably because of the increasing levels of progesterone. When numerous and large, they may cause the vagina to become less elastic, making delivery difficult.

Other Sexually Transmitted Diseases

These include chancroid, granuloma inguinale, intestinal sexually transmitted diseases, and hepatitis B. These are rare, or tend to affect men more than women.

YEAST INFECTIONS

So-called yeast infections are believed to be caused by a yeastlike fungus belonging to a species known as *Candida albicans*. Some people in authority believe that other similar microorganisms could be responsible for other forms of the disease. The organism is known to be passed by sexual intercourse, woman-to-man being more common than man-to-woman. Also, nonsexual means of transfer—such as douche nozzles and wash-cloths—can introduce the organism into the vagina. It can also be found in the feces of between 17 and 40 percent of all people. Care should be taken in wiping, as this may spread infection to the vagina. Candida is apparently a normal inhabitant in many women's vaginas. It doesn't cause problems unless the environment of the vagina changes. They do not multiply out of control in the acidity of a normal vagina—they prefer an alkaline, or base, environment. Conditions that will change the acidity of the vaginal environ-ment are the taking of antibiotics, douching, increase in carbohydrate intake, diabetes, pregnancy, and oral contraceptives. Cancer treatments, such as chemotherapy and radiation, may increase a woman's susceptibility, as they weaken the body's immune system. Women who have deficient immune systems tend to be more prone to yeast infections.

TRICHOMONIASIS

Trichomoniasis is one of the most common vaginal conditions. It is caused by a simple one-celled mobile organism known as *Trichomonas vaginalis*. A woman may not know she has this until a pap smear is done, as it can be asymptomatic. In most cases, however, women infected will notice a frothy yellowish-green vaginal discharge, with itching and an unpleasant odor, within four to twenty-eight days after exposure. Irritation and redness of the vulva are frequently caused by the discharge, and blood may also be in the discharge. Small red dots, known commonly as "strawberry marks," may be revealed in the mucous membranes and cervix during a vaginal examination. Lymph glands may become enlarged in the groin. Symptoms of urinary frequency and urgency may mean that the infection has spread to the urinary tract. Frequently associated with other STDs, trichomoniasis may mask their symptoms. A specific cure for trichomoniasis is metronidazole. If metro-nidazole is prescribed, alcoholic beverages must be avoided, and furthermore it mustn't be taken during the first four months of pregnancy. All sex partners should be treated simultaneously. Vaginal creams, suppositories, and douches, although they relieve symptoms, are not cures.

PELVIC INFLAMMATORY DISEASE (PID)

PID is an infection of the ovaries and tubes, and among its many causes are STDs. Among the PID-causing microorganisms, some of the most common are chlamydia, tuberculosis, *Neisseria gonorrhoea,* Strep-tococcus, and *E. coli.* It's now known that some IUD users with no past history of STDs are contracting PID. If the infection doesn't respond immediately to treatment, in these cases the IUD should be removed. Infectious organisms journey up through the cervix to the uterus, causing inflammation and in some case abscesses of the fallopian tubes, ovaries, and pelvis. A woman who has PID usually is acutely ill with lower abdominal pain and fever. Approximately 13 percent of women after their first attack of PID are infertile. The ratio is as high as 75 percent after three attacks.

To reduce your risk of reinfection, make sure that your sexual partner isn't an asymptomatic carrier of an STD. PID diagnosis is accomplished by past history, pelvic and abdominal examinations, and lab testing. The interior of the abdomen is at times viewed with the laparoscope to distin-guish between appendicitis, PID, ectopic pregnancy, and other intra-abdominal emergencies—these all require surgery, while PID usually doesn't. A combination of orally or intravenously ingested antibiotics is the usual treatment. Surgery may be required if abscesses have been found that cannot be cured by antibiotics. If this is the case, the chance of sterility resulting is higher, as in many cases the uterus, both tubes, and the ovaries must be removed to ensure a cure. Laser surgery, however, may preserve fertility in some cases.

Workshop #7
HIV/AIDS: Testing

* * *

Finding out about being HIV-positive was the most frightening experience I've had to deal with. As I began to educate myself, the fear didn't lessen. My greatest fear was that others would perhaps reject me and mark my person. How was I suppose to deal with this feeling in a prison? Being HIV-positive in a prison, with all kinds of women who at times have fears, and being in such close quarters, would make my struggle twice as hard. I was determined to use my fear as my strength.

I heard about the ACE program. I began to educate myself, and I also began to establish new relationships with people who really cared. My friends from ACE allowed me my own personal space for anger, fear, and pain. Yet they were at my space with much love and concern. I began to develop reasons for my survival. And as I grew emotionally, my hope grew too. When I became an ACE member, sharing and identifying with others were my strength.

When I look back on my life, I recognize that nothing was able to stop me from destroying myself with drugs and other abuses. And now my HIV-positive status has become my will to survive and to live. I only hope and pray that others will recognize that AIDS is not death but the beginning of quality living.

So if you can't decide what to do or you have a suspicion that you might be HIV-positive, just come to ACE, and there you'll find the support you've been searching for. If the information turns out bad, don't give up. You still have ACE to fill in the space we might think was so empty.

* * *

OVERVIEW

Testing for HIV is a very anxiety-producing issue for people. This workshop is a place for people both to learn concrete information and to express individual experiences and needs. It also focuses on peer support in order to give workshop members the tools to help one another in their community. Finally, because there are important social debates about HIV testing, the workshop discusses some of the broader social issues.

GOAL

To provide information about the medical, psychological, and social issues related to HIV testing.

ISSUES TO EXAMINE

- To understand what the HIV-antibody test tells you and what it does not tell you.
- To understand the process of HIV-antibody testing.
- To understand what a positive test result or negative result means.
- To understand social, psychological, and medical issues involved in the personal decision about taking the test.
- To discuss issues surrounding confidentiality.
- To understand the necessity for pre- and post-test counseling.
- To discuss the particular issues of testing for a pregnant woman.

BACKGROUND MATERIAL

What Is the HIV Antibody Test?

The HIV-antibody test looks for the presence of antibodies to the HIV virus in the blood. If an individual tests positive, it means that antibodies to the HIV virus are present in the person's blood. If antibodies are present, it must be assumed that the person has been infected with the HIV virus and is capable of infecting others.

A positive HIV-antibody test does not necessarily mean that the individual will develop AIDS. Reports now show, however, that the vast majority of people infected with HIV will eventually progress to AIDS.

What Tests Will Be Done?

A blood sample will be taken and analyzed in a laboratory, using a test called ELISA (enzyme-linked immunosorbent assay). This test is done twice on the same blood sample. If both ELISA tests are negative, then no further tests are done, and the individual receives a piece of paper saying she is HIV-negative, meaning that no antibodies to HIV were found. If the ELISA test is positive or not clear, a second, more specific test is done called the Western Blot test. If it, too, comes out positive, then the individual will be told that antibodies for the HIV virus were present in the blood. If the Western Blot comes out negative, then the individual will be told she is HIV-negative, meaning no antibodies to the HIV were found.

Both the ELISA and the Western Blot tests are done on the same sample of blood that the individual has given.

The HIV-antibody testing procedure is quite accurate, but like other medical tests there will be some false negatives (the person *does* have antibodies to the HIV, but the tests show up negative). There are very few false positives (the person does *not* have antibodies, but the tests show up positive). A false positive may be the result of health problems or infections other than HIV, medications, or unknown causes.

There is also a test called the PCR (polymerase chain reaction), which, unlike the HIV-antibody test, tests for the virus itself, instead of for antibodies to the virus. This test is still being developed for greater reliability. Because it is not completely reliable and is also very expensive, it is not used on a large scale at this time, except with newborn infants.

What Does a Positive Test Result Mean?

A positive result to the HIV-antibody test means that HIV antibodies are present in the person's blood. It also means that it can be assumed that the person has been infected with HIV.

The person is capable of infecting other people with HIV, through unsafe activities.

Some people with HIV eventually develop AIDS.

Testing for HIV antibodies cannot tell about the state of an individual's health, either now or in the future.

A person who is HIV-positive should:

- Eat well, avoid stress, and seek early medical intervention.
- Seek counseling prior to becoming pregnant.
- Avoid donating blood, sperm, and organs.
- Practice safe sex.

What Does a Negative Test Result Mean?

A negative test result means that the antibody to HIV is absent. This means one of the following is true:

EITHER

the person *has not* been infected with HIV

OR

the person *has* been infected with HIV, but his/her body has not yet produced antibodies.

Research indicates that most people will produce antibodies within six months of infection; **however,** a small number of people may not produce antibodies for several years, and it is possible that some may never produce antibodies.

The period between the time of exposure/infection with the HIV and the time that the antibodies show up on the test is called the *window period.*

- -

EXPOSURE/INFECTION   6 MONTHS: ANTIBODIES SHOW UP

If an individual tests negative and he/she repeats unsafe behavior, then that negative result may no longer apply, and the person should consider retaking the test, to know if he/she has been infected. Although a negative test taken six months after the last risk activity most probably means that the individual is not infected with HIV, it is not an absolute certainty.

Confidentiality

The New York State HIV Testing and Confidentiality law establishes strict requirements for confidentiality, pre- and post-test counseling, and voluntary informed consent. The purpose of the law is to encourage individuals to come forward for voluntary anonymous or confidential HIV testing so that they can learn their health status, make decisions about appropriate treatment, and change the behavior that may have put themselves at risk for contracting or transmitting HIV.

The New York State policy is to ensure that HIV testing is available to all New Yorkers upon request. In New York State, individuals have the right to confidentiality about their HIV-antibody test. If the person who is HIV-infected chooses not to tell his/her partner(s), he/she may ask a physician or local STD clinic to notify sexual and/or needle-sharing partners. When contacts are notified, the name of the person infected with HIV is not given. Contacts are told only that they have been exposed to HIV infection.

This result of the HIV-antibody test is not automatically reported to the Board of Health, nor is it available upon request by employers, landlords, or others. According to the 1989 Confidentiality Law of New York, the HIV-antibody test result may, however, be given to the following:

- You or a person authorized by law who consented to the test for you (for example, this would apply for a child).
- Anyone whom you have specifically authorized by signing a written release to receive such information.
- A health care facility (such as a hospital, clinical laboratory, or blood bank) or a health care provider (such as physician, nurse, mental health counselor) providing care to you or your child and anyone working for such a facility or provider who reasonably needs the information to supervise, monitor, or administer a health service.
- A person who your doctor believes is at significant risk for HIV infection, if you do not notify that person after being counseled to do so (e.g., an identified spouse or sexual partner or an identified person sharing needles or other drug equipment with the infected individual).
- A federal, state, county, or local health officer when state or federal law requires disclosure.
- A government agency, when the agency needs the information to supervise, monitor, or administer a health or social service.

- An authorized foster-care or adoption agency.
- Insurance companies and other third-party payers, such as Medicaid, if necessary for the payment of services to you.
- Any person to whom a court orders disclosure under limited circumstances set forth by law. Except in an emergency situation, advance notice and an opportunity to oppose the release of such information would be given to you.
- The Division of Parole, the Division of Probation, the Commission of Corrections, or a medical director of a special correctional facility. This means that parole officers inside and outside prison will have this information. They are not legally allowed to disclose it to anyone, including families. Confidentiality laws do not, however, apply to laypeople who may know that someone is HIV-positive.

In sum, there are a lot of "exceptions" to pure confidentiality. The reason confidentiality is an issue is that people have experienced discrimination when it became known that they were HIV-positive. Discrimination has occurred in such areas as housing, employment, life insurance, schools, and personal relationships. If you get the confidential test through your private doctor or clinic, you might want to ask how they can safeguard your confidentiality.

If at any time you believe you might be experiencing discrimination due to a breach of confidentiality, contact either the City or State Human Rights Commission.

ANONYMOUS TESTING

There are a number of HIV testing sites established throughout the state for people who wish to be tested anonymously. This means your blood sample and test results are not identified with a person's name, just a number. (Note: As in the case of the anonymous HIV-antibody test blood sample, a confidential HIV-antibody test blood sample is also identified by number when it is sent to the lab. In a "confidential test," however, the person who gives you the result will know your name.) Anonymous testing allows individuals to learn what their HIV status is and have total control over the disclosure of that information. Even though the testing site does not know the individual's name, the individual still must be given both pre-

and post-test counseling. Anonymous testing can be set up through a phone call.

If a person has taken the anonymous test and his or her test result is positive, in order to receive treatment the person will then have to take a confidential HIV-antibody test to verify that he or she is HIV-positive. A doctor will not be able to give treatments unless the doctor has documentation that the person is HIV-positive.

CONFIDENTIALITY AND ANONYMITY AS THEY APPLY AT BEDFORD HILLS CORRECTIONAL FACILITY

There is no anonymous testing here in Bedford Hills. The New York State Department of Corrections is just beginning to develop possible anonymous testing procedures for prisons. There is, however, a facility policy of confidentiality. Nevertheless, there are many ways that confidentiality is not maintained. From experience, we have learned that people have a need to share difficult personal news, and frequently a friend will tell other friends and the word will spread. In addition, the HIV status is recorded in the health records, which may be visible to inmates, officers, and civilian personnel, who may talk. You may be identified through a particular hospital trip or seeing a particular doctor or receiving a particular prescription. All these factors mean that confidentiality is difficult to maintain, although it is not impossible. The test result will become part of your file that goes with you to the street, possibly affecting you when you go home.

In ACE, we support the right to confidentiality for each person. Even if that person is open about being HIV-positive, we do not take it upon ourselves to talk about her status to anyone without her consent. Yet, because it is so difficult to actually maintain confidentiality inside a small self-contained community like the prison, we believe a goal is the creation of a community of support within the facility so that confidentiality is not as important. Stigma is best dealt with through the development of a supportive environment.

Counseling

People who are deciding whether to take the test are advised to contact a knowledgeable health care professional or counselor for information or advice first. In New York State, as of February 1, 1989, it is mandatory that an individual be given pre- and post-test counseling. There are important medical, psychological, and social issues involved in being tested.

As of this writing, the New York State AIDS Institute policy is to encourage testing. It says, "If you have reason to believe that you have been exposed to the HIV virus, it is medically recommended to get tested. Research has shown that early intervention prolongs/improves the quality of life. Treatment is only available if you know your status."

ACE's Experience with the Role of Counseling

In Bedford Hills Correctional Facility, the prison medical staff do the formal state-mandated pre- and post-test counseling. Many ACE members are New York State certified HIV pre- and post-test counselors, and they do much of the ongoing psychological preparation and support for the testing and the follow-up testing.

ACE's experience is that counseling is crucial as part of the testing process, because it is a very emotionally difficult period of time. The decision to take the test, the period of waiting for the test result, the day of actually going to get the result, and the post-test period all require a great deal of support. Peer support is important, because one counseling session with an HIV test counselor cannot give individuals the kind of ongoing conversations they need. People may take a long time to decide whether or not to take the test, and they will need someone with whom to have an ongoing dialogue. It is important to develop during the decision-making period as strong a support system as possible.

ACE's policy about testing is that it is an individual choice. ACE recognizes the important positive reasons that exist for taking the test, but we also recognize that it may not be right for any particular individual at a particular time. It is for this reason that counseling and support are very important as a means of helping a person decide what is right for her or him.

* * *

I went through indecision about taking the test. I was trying to figure out whether it would be beneficial to me to take it. I told myself a million times that it wouldn't be. I didn't want to take it, because I was afraid I might be diagnosed as positive, and even though I knew it wasn't a death sentence, still a lot of people I knew on the outside are against people who are HIV-positive. I'm trying to educate my mother in general about it, but she fights me all the way. I couldn't imagine having to tell her if I were to be HIV-positive.

But I had two ex-lovers who were IV drug users and were in the prison system and were diagnosed as HIV-positive. That propelled me to go take the test. One of them looked fine and healthy, and I felt like if she could be feeling fine and she has it, then I could, too.

If it wasn't for my lover, I probably would not have had enough courage to take it. But when she told me, "I'll stick by you regardless of what the results are," I felt inside that it was authentic, that it wasn't just being said to appease me—and that gave me the extra strength.

* * *

How ACE Helps Women Prepare for the Test

- We explain the nature of AIDS and HIV-related illness.
- We explain the difference between confidential and anonymous testing.
- We provide information about discrimination problems that disclosure of the test result could cause and legal protection against such discrimination.
- We give information about the behavior that is known to pose risks for transmission and contraction of HIV infection.
- We explore with the women many personal issues, such as:

  - How would I feel if I learn that I'm infected?
  - How would others feel and act toward me?
  - Would I have to change my thoughts about having children?
  - Will it improve my medical possibilities?
  - What support system do I have?
  - Who should I tell?

How ACE Helps People Who Are Waiting for Test Results

Waiting is a period of enormous anxiety. Sometimes people have to wait as long as three months if there is a problem with staffing. During this time, people need someone to talk to, and we let them know that they can come and share their anxiety and questions that they may have.

* * *

WORRIED WELL

I've been waiting for six weeks now for the results of my HIV test, and the wait alone is about to drive me crazy. Not knowing or a possible positive reading is causing me a lot of stress and anxiety. One day I may feel like it's in God's hands and the next day feel like Okay, God, please let it be negative. I go through constant mood swings—up today, down tomorrow. If I get a pimple, I feel like I am doomed. If I start losing weight, I go crazy. Still other days I realize that psychologically I may be causing these symptoms to appear or playing mind games with myself.

AIDS is scary, and no one wants it, but in all reality I've done every behavior there is to actually have this disease. I'm now learning how to face as well as talk about my fears and worries, and I'm taking life one day at a time. If my result comes back positive, then I know that God will see me through and I also know that I am not alone, because the ACE office is always here for me, and I also have other ACE members that I live with. If ever I need to talk, be it day or night, someone is always there for me.

* * *

HOW ACE HELPS WOMEN COPE WITH THE TEST RESULT

- We help the individual cope with the emotional consequences of learning the result.
- We give information about how to change behavior to prevent becoming infected with HIV or passing the HIV virus to another person.
- We provide information about the potential discrimination problems that disclosure of the test result could create.
- We explain about the person's need to notify her contacts if she is HIV-infected.
- We explain the meaning of a negative result if the person has tested negative, and we explain the possible need to retest.

* * *

You know when they call you to the hospital and you don't have an appointment that it's probably to go with someone to get their HIV test results because they put your name down. So you walk down the hill and you say to yourself, "God, please don't let this one be positive."

As you walk into the hospital building, the person is waiting for you, and they have this nervous smile on their face, and the first thing they tell you is "I'm scared, what am I going to do if it's positive?" All you can do is try to calm the person down by talking to them: "Let's wait for the result and look at it from there. Either way it goes, you won't be alone. I'm here for you." You go into the doctor's office and you sit there with that person. And in some cases you hear the doctor saying, "It's negative." But you don't hear that—you need them to repeat it again. And the person just cries from the joy that they feel from finding out that they are not positive and that they have a new lease on life.

On the other hand, when they're told that they're positive, it's like all movement stops in your body. You just freeze, and the next thing you hear is the cry of that person, and you cry along with them and you tell them that you're going to be with them and will work it out with them. It's a chilling experience.

* * *

Advice From a PWA After Testing Positive

How Do I feel?

It is scary, but if you have friends, you can tell them. You can talk with them, cry with them. It's important to tell people so you don't keep it all inside. At first I didn't care about life in the same way. Now I care about everything. It's important to learn everything you can.

Advice to People Who Tested Positive:

Don't be scared people are going to reject you. They might, and it's hard, but you need some people who are your friends, and that will help. For me, really no one has rejected me. In fact, people got closer to me, tried to help me. That might be what happens to you, too.

You have to be very insistent with the medical department. You have to keep pushing. There are people, like people in ACE, who you can talk to and learn from. You have to educate yourself, too. And if anyone asks you to get high in this place, don't.

Advice to People Without AIDS:

Don't be afraid of people with AIDS. It's not easy to catch it. We won't hurt you. In a way you're more dangerous to us. Get education about AIDS! Play it safe, be careful!

* * *

The Social Issues of Mandatory Testing

There is ongoing public debate about mandatory testing. Mandatory testing refers to either a law or a policy that requires that an individual be tested for HIV-antibodies whether or not the individual wants to be. In New York State, there is no mandatory testing. This policy is founded on the assumption that mandatory testing would harm the general public, because it would drive the disease underground and make both treatment and education more difficult. New York State's policy assumes that mandatory testing will hurt those very individuals who most need help. Many people most afraid of testing positive will avoid contact with agencies administering mandatory testing out of fear either of discrimination or of psychological stress.

New York State policy is based on the assumption that education and voluntary mobilization of people are more effective than forcing people to test. There are those, however, who believe that mandatory testing of certain groups of people should be required in order to protect the health of other individuals or groups or the general public. This is reflected in the many bills requiring mandatory testing for different groups of people that have been proposed or signed into law in the past few years throughout the country. These bills and acts deal with testing in the following areas: marriage license applications; prisoners; hospitals; patients; restaurant/bar employees; people arrested for prostitution or assault; people arrested for rape; mental patients; rape victims; women seeking prenatal care or pregnancy tests; students; people immigrating to the United States or visiting. As of this writing, there is proposed legislation that all newborn babies would be mandatorily tested and that the test results would be given to their mothers. Most of these proposals require that positive results be reported to state officials.

PREGNANT WOMEN AND NEWBORN INFANTS

The most recent debates about mandatory testing have focused on the issues faced by pregnant women and newborn infants. Several issues have been raised:

1. Should the government require that all pregnant women be tested? This question is being raised because of the new AZT treatment for pregnant women and newborn infants that reduces

transmission of the HIV virus from a mother to her unborn infant. It is also being raised because if the mother knows she is HIV-positive, it can alert her to the possibility that her child may be HIV-infected.

2. Should all newborn infants be tested and the test results be given to the mothers? (In New York State at this time, all newborn infants are *anonymously* tested so that there can be an assessment of the percentage of reproductive-age women who are HIV-positive. Information about a particular infant is not passed on to the mother.)

NOTE: It is important to remember that if a baby tests HIV-positive, then the mother is definitely infected with the virus. On the other hand, approximately 75 percent of the infants of HIV-infected mothers will not be infected. Therefore, by testing all pregnant women or by giving the test results of the babies to the mothers, you are telling women who have not yet decided to take the HIV-antibody test that they are actually infected with the HIV virus, while approximately 75 percent of the children born to them will not be infected with the HIV virus.

Those in favor of mandatory testing of newborns and/or of pregnant mothers argue that the mother should know if her infant is HIV-positive because it will help her and her medical provider give the baby the best medical care possible if the infant later turns out to actually be infected with the HIV virus. Additionally, if she discovers that she is HIV-positive during pregnancy, she may decide to take the AZT treatment, which can help her reduce the likelihood of transmitting the virus to her unborn child.

Those opposed to mandatory testing believe equally strongly that it is very important for mothers to know whether their babies are HIV-positive, but they do not believe that *mandatory* testing is the most effective way to work with the mothers. They argue that the keys to the baby's health are a working relationship between health providers and the mother and the mother's own inner strength. They argue that the fears of HIV and of the stigma are so strong that a mandatory testing program would drive women away from prenatal care and from the health care system after the baby is born. They believe that developing a mandatory testing system will divert money and resources away from education, counseling, and treatment, which are the best insurance for the mother's being able to care for the child and herself if either she or the infant is, in fact, HIV-positive.

Often this debate is defined as between those in favor of protecting the baby versus those in favor of protecting a woman's right to confidentiality and her civil liberties. In actuality, most of those who are opposed to mandatory testing are also primarily concerned with the baby's health, but they view a continuation of present New York State policy of encouraging voluntary testing with counseling, education, and access to treatment as the most effective way to involve pregnant or new mothers in caring for themselves or their children.

The federal Centers for Disease Control have proposed guidelines for health care providers who are counseling pregnant women.

For pregnant women who may or may not be HIV-positive:

- Counseling.
- Encouraging testing.
- Providing voluntary testing for pregnant women and their infants.
- Access to HIV prevention and treatment services (e.g., drug treatment).

For HIV-positive pregnant women:

- Counseling.
- Provision of information about the AZT therapy, including the substantial benefits and short-term safety as well as the uncertainties of long-term risks. The information is to be provided in a noncoercive atmosphere and based on balancing risks and benefits.
- Provision of information about all reproductive options, to be provided in a nondirective manner.
- Advice to not breastfeed.[1]

(See the Appendix for a more detailed excerpt from the CDC proposed guidelines.)

---

1. Federal Centers for Disease Control, "Draft Guidelines: How Should Health Care Providers Counsel Pregnant Women?" excerpted in *World,* April 1995, pp. 4–5.

TEACHING PLAN

Introduction

The testing workshop is one of the most sensitive workshops. It touches on people's anxieties and helps many people decide whether or not to take the test. It may help to open the workshop with a brief role-play of a person trying to decide whether or not to take the test.

Discussions, Presentations, and Explanations

I. PRESENTATION OF FACTUAL INFORMATION:

Discuss what the HIV-antibody test is; the tests and procedures that are done; what positive and negative results mean. People will be confused about how a negative result is really positive and how a positive result is really negative. Be prepared to explain this.

II. SMALL-GROUP DISCUSSIONS ABOUT DECIDING WHETHER OR NOT TO TAKE THE HIV-ANTIBODY TEST:

Ask people to brainstorm on the pros and cons of testing, the positive and negative factors that would affect a decision. This issue will take up most of the discussion, because so many people have experiences with taking the test or trying to decide whether or not to take the test.

The following is a list of the pros and cons that have come out of our discussion about testing:

PROS:
- Peace of mind.
- Medical reasons.
- Can get AZT or other antiretroviral sooner.
- Can get Bactrim or other prophylactic medicines.
- Can interpret symptoms and get appropriate care.
- Can learn how to build up the body with holistic measures.
- Can talk with and prepare your family.

- Can protect others from getting HIV by taking safe measures.
- Can use your support system if you have one.
- Can use pregnancy planning.
- Can protect yourself against reinfection.

Cons
- Too much emotional stress.
- No support system.
- Rejection by friends or coworkers.
- Other discrimination.
- Test result might be wrong.
- Can't get adequate medical care anyway, so it won't make a difference medically.

III. PEER COUNSELING Break into pairs and do the following role-plays:

Janice is in prison. She has one year until she goes home to her mother and her six-year-old daughter. She just found out that a man she had been in a relationship with four years ago has AIDS. She is worried about herself, but she also is afraid to take the test. She comes to you for support about whether or not to take the test.

Anna is three months pregnant. Her boyfriend is an IV drug user who doesn't want to use a condom. He is also very proud that Anna will be having a baby. Anna is worried about whether she might be HIV-positive and she is worried about the baby. So she comes to you for counseling.

Bobbie is a close friend of yours. She has no children and is going to the parole board in two years. She is looking forward to having children when she goes home. She just got her test results and she is HIV-positive. She comes to you for comfort and support.

IV. DISCUSSION about the issues that a pregnant woman faces about HIV testing

V. SOCIAL ISSUES:

If there have been public issues recently in the news, we suggest that they be discussed in the smaller groups. Two issues that we have discussed are mandatory testing and contact tracing.

PANEL DISCUSSION OF MANDATORY TESTING

Set up a panel discussion on mandatory testing:

CHARACTERS IN SUPPORT OF SOME FORM OF MANDATORY TESTING

- A federal health official who thinks generalized mandatory testing of the population is the only way to control the spread of HIV infection.
- A representative of employers who argue that they should have the right to demand that their workers be tested before they are hired for a job.
- A health commissioner who argues that anyone seeking a marriage license should be tested.
- The director of a prenatal program who argues that any woman coming into a clinic for prenatal care should be mandatorily tested.
- A Department of Corrections official who argues for mandatory testing of all prisoners.
- A victim's-rights advocate who argues that anyone arrested for a sex-related crime such as rape (this includes sexual abuse) should be tested.
- A legislator who believes that all babies should be tested and the test results should be given to the mother.

CHARACTERS AGAINST MANDATORY TESTING

- A public official who believes it will drive people away from needed resources and counseling and that this will hurt both the individuals and the public welfare.
- A civil liberties lawyer who believes it will both infringe on individuals' rights and subject them to discrimination.
- A person who is HIV-positive who argues for voluntary testing because of the fear and stigma that an individual faces.
- An AIDS/HIV counselor who believes that there should be an increase in counseling for pregnant women and women who have just given birth about the risks of having a baby who is HIV-positive.

DISCUSSION: *CONTACT TRACING*

There has been a debate about the legitimacy of contact tracing. If a person refuses to inform her present or past sexual or IV drug partners about her HIV status, should the public authorities have the right to do so? What do you think about this issue?

REFERENCE MATERIALS

Education and Training Section, Bureau of HIV Prevention, AIDS Institute, New York State Department of Health, *HIV Counselor Training Participant Manual,* New York: AIDS Institute New York State Department of Health, 1991.

"How Should Health Care Providers Counsel Pregnant Women?" Excerpts from Proposed Guidelines from the CDC, *World,* April 1995, pp. 4–5.

New York State. *A Physician's Guide to AIDS: Issues in the Medical Office.* March 1988.

New York State. *A Guide to HIV Counseling and Testing.* February 1990.

New York State Department of Health. *100 Questions and Answers: AIDS.* April 1994.

Workshop #8
Women and HIV/AIDS

* * *

I was conscious of women before I came in here, but not on that level.
ACE has made it deeper. ACE made me realize that AIDS is bigger than
each individual woman, that it's going to take all of us coming together. I
never knew so many things affected just women. I had looked at issues as
a black woman—religious issues, being a single parent or not—but I had
never reflected on being a woman in society.

* * *

THE BEAUTY OF IT ALL

I've become a walking game of connect the dots, from the scars I've
accumulated from many ongoing viruses, fungi, and bacteria. My
tongue has become a mass production of cotton fields. Enough to
dress a few. I have an abundance of hair; jealous of my two
strands?
I was once called pretty, but now I'm called Beautiful.
                         Jealous, are you?
I was fast on my feet and great on my toes, now I let others do the
walking for me, just like the Yellow Pages. I've developed a
genuine sense of humor, and so I hide, I hide and wait.
                         Jealous, are you?
Even as I walk through the corridors at St. Clare's prison ward,
I see so many, yet they can't see me. They've lost their sight.
Where did it go?
                         Jealous, are you?

Just like me, we're on a permanent diet of anorexia.
                    Jealous, are you?
Don't be. I've just gained eleven pounds. I'm an overweight 96 pounds.
I'm the beauty of it all.
                    Jealous, are you?
I thought you might be. . . .

                                        —DORIS MOICES

OVERVIEW

Women are the fastest-growing group in the United States contracting HIV infection, and black and Hispanic women are affected in disproportionately larger numbers. Yet we were, for a long time, to a large degree, invisible. We have been hidden behind statistics that define us as "IV drug users and their partners." Or, even worse, we are seen primarily as a danger to others: pregnant women who pass the virus to their unborn children or prostitutes who might endanger their clients. Beyond the growing numbers of women who are infected, women also bear the burden of the social crisis surrounding the HIV/AIDS epidemic, because of our role in society as mothers and family providers, caregivers, and the lowest-paid service workers.

We carry the weight of our oppression as women, as well as the oppression of racism, poverty, shrinking social services, hopelessness, and the drug epidemic. Thus, when we talk about women and HIV/AIDS, we end up talking about every social problem faced by the most oppressed and marginalized people in this society.

GOALS

1. To examine the particular impact of HIV/AIDS on women, both
   a. women who are HIV-positive.
   b. women bearing the burden of the HIV/AIDS crisis.
2. To examine and raise consciousness about our oppression and role in society as women. To deepen our understanding of sexism and its interaction with racism and class oppression, by looking at the social impact of HIV/AIDS on women.
3. To incorporate our diverse experiences and perspectives as women who come from different racial, cultural, national, and class backgrounds.
4. To examine and encourage the ways we can strengthen our abilities as women on an individual and social level to confront the dangers of the HIV/AIDS crisis. To build solidarity as women.
5. To examine the issue of risk reduction and changing behaviors in light of a woman's consciousness.

ISSUES COVERED

1. The level of HIV infection risk for women.
2. The struggle to overcome our invisibility in the AIDS epidemic.
3. The vulnerability of women in heterosexual transmission.
4. The fact that women die faster of AIDS: possible reasons.
5. How the HIV/AIDS virus impacts on different groups of women: black and Hispanic women; prisoners; lesbians; teenagers.
6. Woman-to-woman sex and the risks involved.
7. Issues confronting women and pregnancy in the AIDS epidemic.
8. Women as caregivers.

BACKGROUND MATERIALS

Women and the Epidemic

WHY LOOK AT WOMEN WITH HIV/AIDS AS A SIGNIFICANT REALITY?

Although women still constitute a small minority of U.S. AIDS cases—about 13 percent—women and children make up the fastest-growing group of people with AIDS. AIDS is already the fourth-leading killer of women aged twenty-five to forty-four. And in a period when heterosexual transmission accounted for the largest proportionate increase in AIDS cases reported in 1993, about 70 to 80 percent of those new cases were women. If the international context is brought into the picture, the situation is even more drastic: in Africa, where the vast majority of AIDS cases in the world exist, almost half of those with AIDS are women, and women worldwide are being infected with the virus at almost the same rate as men.[1]

---

1. Federal Centers for Disease Control, *HIV/AIDS Surveillance Report*, October 1994; Lawrence K. Altman, "AIDS Cases Increase Among Heterosexuals," *The New York Times*, March 11, 1994; Gina Kolata, "New Picture of Who Will Get AIDS Is Dominated by Addicts," *The New York Times*, February 28, 1995, C3; World Health Organization, United Nations Development Program, *Women and AIDS Agenda for Action*, January 1995.

OVERCOMING INVISIBILITY

Recent newspaper stories have titles such as "HIV Found to Kill Women Faster Than Men"; "AIDS Risk Held Twice as High in Women"; "Sex and Needles Combine to Take a Devastating Toll"; "AIDS Cases Increase Among Heterosexuals."[2] All these articles point to the increasing impact and vulnerability of women and AIDS. Yet, AIDS has been seen for a long time as a "man's disease," and such attention on women in the AIDS epidemic is fairly recent.

Some of the examples of the "invisibility" of women in the AIDS epidemic include:

DOWNPLAYING THE SIGNIFICANCE OF HETEROSEXUAL TRANSMISSION: There was too slow a recognition of the dangers of heterosexual transmission of HIV from a man to a woman. The fastest-growing category of women contracting HIV is women who have had sex with an infected man. AIDS was defined first as a "gay male disease" and then as a disease of "IV drug users." It has taken many years to recognize the real danger women face from heterosexual transmission of the virus. Published opinions both reflected and contributed to this delay. One example was an article by a doctor in a 1988 *Cosmopolitan* magazine who said, "There is almost no danger of contracting AIDS through ordinary sexual intercourse." Another was a book published in 1989 entitled *The Myth of Heterosexual AIDS*.[3]

THE DEFINITION OF AIDS: Until January 1993, the Centers for Disease Control did not include important illnesses that women die from as part of their definition of AIDS. Because HIV infection affects women in ways that are particular to women, this meant that women were frequently misdiagnosed or underdiagnosed for HIV infection. It meant that women were denied access to the many supports that are needed to sustain a life— treatment, services, housing, drug trials, and disability and insurance benefits. The definition was expanded to include, along with an HIV diagnosis, advanced cervical cancer, two or more bouts of bacterial pneumonia, pulmonary TB, or less than 200 T4 cells.

---

2. "H.I.V. Found to Kill Women Faster Than Men," *The New York Times,* December 28, 1994, C10; "AIDS Risk Held Twice as High in Women," *The New York Times,* November 1, 1994, C5; Kolata, "New Picture of Who Will Get AIDS;" Altman, "AIDS Cases Increase Among Heterosexuals."

3. Robert E. Gould, "Reassuring News About AIDS: A Doctor Tells Why You May Not Be at Risk," *Cosmopolitan* magazine, January 1988, pp. 146–47; Michael Fumento, *The Myth of Heterosexual AIDS.*

MEDICAL RESEARCH AND DRUG TRIALS: Although women are now 18 percent of those enrolled in drug trials, early in the epidemic women were denied access to many drug trials. And race and poverty still play a role in participation: although nationally black and Hispanic women are 75 percent of the women with AIDS, they represent only 31 percent of those women who are participating in the drug trials.[4]

Earlier, FDA regulations allowed women of child bearing age to be automatically excluded from these trials. For example, this was true of testing AZT. But when these drugs are approved, they are prescribed for women too, with no medical knowledge of the different impact of these drugs on women. Women's bodies are different from men's in important ways, such as hormonally, and specific testing is important. Additionally, since most new therapies have been accessible to PWAs only through drug trials, this practice of excluding women has meant that women have been denied even the limited access to possibly lifesaving drugs that men have had. Patients wanting to enter drug trials often have to do so through private doctors, which poor women do not usually have.

Even now, few support systems are available. In many cases, women cannot keep regular appointments necessary for these drug trials because child care was not supplied and transportation costs are too high. Grassroots groups developed by PWAs—such as community research initiatives—have created their own trials open to women and have pressured companies and research hospitals to change their policies.

This exclusion of women from the focus in the AIDS epidemics has taken a toll. Only through enormous pressure of those committed to women and their health has the situation begun to improve. One important result is that the Centers for Disease Control has recently established an Office of Women's Health to study all significant health issues faced by women at every stage of life, including such issues as breast and cervical cancer, sexually transmitted diseases, and HIV/AIDS.[5]

WOMEN'S SPECIAL VULNERABILITY TO HIV AND AIDS

Women get HIV infection in the same ways as men: through sex, IV needle sharing, and blood transfusions. Yet there are important ways in

---

4. AIDS Clinical Trials Information Services, March 17, 1995.
5. Wanda K. Jones, "CDC Establishes Office for Women's Health," *World*, March 1995.

which women are particularly vulnerable to contracting HIV infection. And once infected, women seem to die faster.

Heterosexual Transmission

PHYSICAL FACTORS: Women are more than twice as likely to become infected with the virus during heterosexual sex, an Italian study found. This is partly attributed to differences in anatomy and biology:

- The surface of the area that is exposed to the virus is much larger for women—the vaginal area—than for men.
- Semen has higher concentrations of the virus than vaginal secretions.
- A man's exposure to the virus is limited to the time during sex, while semen remains in a woman's body after intercourse.[6]

DECISION MAKING: The decision-making process—who gets to decide about what happens during sex—is largely in the hands of men, including whether to use a condom or not. Some of the factors that reinforce this include social and cultural traditions that are internalized both by women and men, the economic realities of women's dependence on men, and the physical strength of men compared with that of women.

NONCONSENSUAL SEX AND VIOLENCE: Pressured sex, rape, molestation, and incest all have a deadly component in the age of HIV/AIDS. A woman or a child who has been raped must now go through the added terror of waiting to find out if she's been infected by the rapist.[7]

MARRIAGE AND SAFETY: Marriage suggests trust and fidelity, and it can be difficult, if not impossible, to raise the issue of using condoms within a marriage. And yet, in the United States, married women are at risk. A 1993 study by the CDC of women who were infected by heterosexual contact showed that nearly a quarter were married or in common-law relationships. And 35 percent of the women in the study had had only one sex partner in the previous five years. In Puerto Rico, during the past five years, most AIDS cases among women have come from heterosexual contact, and a vast majority of these cases involved women who were married or in common-law relationships and had no other risk factors than their partners, many of whom used intravenous drugs. Yet, married women

---

6. "AIDS Risk Held Twice as High in Women," *The New York Times.*
7. "Sexual Assault & HIV Silence = Death," *World,* June 1994.

tend to feel less vulnerable, and a woman's raising to her husband the idea that he use a condom can involve risks to her—he may abandon her or use violence.[8] And the use of condoms is very low, according to a recent survey reported in the *New York Times*. Only 16 percent of sexually active unmarried women use condoms, and only 15 percent of married women use them.

STIGMA AGAINST WOMEN FOR BEING SEXUAL: The social pressures against women can undermine women's attempts to get the health care they need. There still exists a double standard. For men to be promiscuous or sexually active is acceptable, a sign of masculinity; a woman carrying out the same activities is considered "loose," a bad woman. When women get a sexually transmitted disease—HIV/AIDS included—they suffer added stigma and loss of respect, because "women aren't supposed to do those kinds of things."

* * *

A woman told us that when she spoke to a doctor about trying to get the HIV test, the doctor said, "You seem like a good girl. You wouldn't need to have that test." The suggestion being that only "bad girls" would need to get the HIV test, only bad girls could get HIV/AIDS. This attitude will easily make some women hesitant to get tested or get the health care that they need.

* * *

Another form of stigma is when women have been projected as dangerous, as a potential conduit or "vector" for the HIV virus. The implication is that women will spread the virus from the IV-drug-using community to the "general population" (read: white, middle-class, straight men). This has particularly focused negative attention and repression against prostitutes, who became another scapegoat in the world of AIDS. Yet, men are central to the sexual decision making with a sex worker. Men make a choice not to protect themselves; some men also pressure women not to demand a condom by offering them more money. Prostitutes are affected by the same social and economic dynamics as all women: Those who are more affluent have more power to demand safe sex; those who are poorer and who are dependent on drugs will have less of an ability to control the terms of sex. When emphasis on the actual facts of heterosex-

---

8. Mireya Navarro, "Women in Puerto Rico Find Marriage Offers No Haven from AIDS," *The New York Times*, January 20, 1995.

ual transmission is downplayed or reversed, support and education for women are undermined.[9]

Women and Drugs

Women are very susceptible to HIV infection through drug use—IV drugs as well as drugs such as crack. Women use IV drugs and share infected needles. Many will have unsafe sex or resort to prostitution in order to support their drug habits. Many have partners who are IV drug users and who are infected with the virus.

The crack epidemic has intensified the relationship between drugs, sex, and HIV/AIDS. Women (as well as men) go on binges, having sex with many partners in exchange for crack or money to buy it. Younger and younger girls—and boys—are at risk, because they are supporting their habits by exchanging sex for crack. Also, many of them have sexually transmitted diseases which, it is believed, makes it easier to transmit the HIV virus. Although new HIV infections among women are moving fastest among those who have been infected through heterosexual relations, at least half of these women are also addicted to crack.[10]

How HIV Infection Affects Women Physically

Studies documenting survival after diagnosis show that women appear to become sicker faster and to die faster than men. Why?

- **Late diagnosis:** One possible explanation is that women are frequently diagnosed later than men are. Women often seek treatment later, because they are preoccupied with raising families and caring for other people's health. They often cannot get day care to free themselves of their children for a few hours so that they can take better care of themselves.
- **Misdiagnosis:** Misdiagnosis can be attributed to the fact that doctors do not take women's illnesses seriously. Misdiagnosis can also occur because health care providers are not trained to detect specific illnesses in women that could possibly be related to the HIV virus.

---

9. Mary Ide, with Wendy Sanford and Amy Alpern, "AIDS, HIV Infection and Women," in the Boston Women's Health Book Collective, eds., *The New Our Bodies, Ourselves* (New York: Simon & Schuster, 1992).

10. Kolata, "New Picture of Who Will Get AIDS."

- **Underdiagnosis:** The CDC definition of AIDS did not include the gynecological infections that women were getting that appear to be associated with HIV infection. Even now, the only GYN infection that is included in the AIDS diagnosis is invasive cervical cancer. This has led to an underdiagnosis for many women.

Early studies on AIDS were carried out within the predominantly white, middle-class, gay and bisexual male communities. Since most women with AIDS are from poor black and Hispanic communities and many of them have also used drugs, there are differences between the two groups in both health and access to health care. Poorer women are frequently less healthy, and their health has probably been further weakened if they have used drugs. They seek medical treatment later and receive worse medical care.[11]

How HIV/AIDS Affects Particular Groups of Women

Black and Hispanic Women Are Hit the Hardest

HIV/AIDS poses a particularly drastic threat for black and Hispanic women, especially for those who are poor and live in geographic areas of higher HIV/AIDS incidence. In New York City, as of July 1994, 53 percent of all women with AIDS were black and 33 percent were Hispanic; 13 percent were white. There is an interrelationship between HIV/AIDS and other social problems. For example, substance abuse is a major factor for women in contracting HIV. Yet, we know that substance abuse is tied to communities where poverty, lack of educational opportunities, unemployment, inadequate housing, and health care all prevail. It is impossible to separate race and race stratification from HIV/AIDS.

Black and Hispanic women who have HIV/AIDS are overwhelmingly poor and unable to have the same access to health care and treatment available to the more affluent groups of people who are sick. They often will put off getting the health care for themselves in order to take care of another family crisis. For example, the high level of violence that families

---

11. Risa Denenberg, "Unique Aspects of HIV Infection in Women," in the ACT UP/NY Women & AIDS Book Group, eds., *Women, AIDS & Activism*, Boston: The South End Press; "H.I.V. Found to Kill Women Faster Than Men," *The New York Times*.

in poor neighborhoods experience can force dealing with a long-term infection such as HIV/AIDS to take second place.[12]

The crisis of AIDS for black and Hispanic women is not just reflected in the high percentage of black and Hispanic women who have HIV/AIDS. These women are already struggling, frequently as heads of households, to meet the challenges of inadequate housing, lack of preventive health services, drug use, unemployment, poverty, and racism. AIDS, which is tied to these conditions, adds even more pressure and stress to women trying to support their families.

Finally, black and Hispanic women have to face stigma, prejudice, and insensitivities that are part of our society. This is true not only in individual encounters between medical or social service personnel but in the nation's spending priorities. Some researchers are concerned about the impact of the information that highlights the fact that HIV infection is concentrated in the inner cities; they fear that "the nation will turn its back on these infected groups," seeing them as not important.[13]

Teenagers

Teenagers, both girls and boys, are generally very vulnerable to HIV infection. Peer pressure, pressure from older men, family violence, ignorance about their own sexuality and about birth control, drugs—all increase their vulnerability. Adolescence is normally a time of greater sexual activity, yet teens are less able to deal with sexual pressure. It is harder to urge safer sex and drug practices, because teens have little or no fear of mortality.

* * *

I'm a mother of a teenage son and I am HIV-positive. The first problem with that is the fact that we are two different genders. The topic of sex has been embarrassing for him to talk about with me as he has become older and has experienced sexual encounters, although we've been quite open about sex from early childhood—for example, talking about sexual abuse, what's a good touch and what's a bad touch. They learn a lot from their peers in the street, but most of it is fantasy and rumors and little is experience. Dealing with AIDS has been very difficult, because he

---

12. New York City Department of Health, *AIDS Surveillance Update, October 1994;* Ide, with Sanford and Alpern, "AIDS, HIV Infection and Women."
13. Kolata, "New Picture of Who Will Get AIDS."

can't broaden his scope to imagine that a person that he's been dealing with sexually could have been exposed to the virus. I try to get him to understand that you can't tell by a person's appearance if she's been exposed to the virus. I try to get him to realize that a person had sexual relationships before him and he doesn't know what they've been like. But it's still difficult for him to believe that or think about that.

Condoms are a major issue. Out on the streets, kids are flaunting their condoms, but using them is another thing. So I worry about him as his mother. They have to prove to themselves that they don't need this as a way of showing faith both in the person and in their own invulnerability. On the one hand they are proving their manhood, and on the other hand they are trying to impress their peers. The boy says, "I don't need that, I can't feel anything," and the girl is about pleasing the boyfriend. And nobody is stopping to think about pregnancy or AIDS, and the combination is devastating.

* * *

Women in Prison

AIDS takes an immense toll on both men and women in prison. AIDS is the leading cause of death in New York State prisons and in prisons throughout the United States. And for prisoners who themselves may not be HIV-positive, most have experienced AIDS either through the death of one or more family members or through seeing friends or other inmates die in prison. As women, we can speak about some of the issues that we have focused on.[14]

The women in prison who suffer with AIDS are usually the same women in the community who are most vulnerable to HIV infection. They are overwhelmingly black or Hispanic, and they must cope with a combination of problems: drugs, homelessness, family violence, racism, and poverty, with the additional pressures that motherhood brings, especially that of being a single mother. When they come to prison, they bring enormous needs that have not been met in the outside society: education, preparation for employment, drug treatment, rebuilding families in crisis. AIDS is only one of many pressures they face.

---

14. New York State Department of Health AIDS Institute, *Focus on AIDS in New York State* (April 1994), ed. Miki Conn. Newsletter. Albany, N.Y.: New York State Department of Health AIDS Institute; Dennis Cauchon, "AIDS in Prison: Locked Up and Locked Out," *USA Today*, March 31, 1995.

AIDS then creates new and special pressures. As stated in the newsletter of the New York State Department of Health AIDS Institute, "HIV/AIDS has created a demand for medical, educational, and support services which the correctional system was not designed to provide."[15] Perhaps the overriding one is that of health care. Health care has always been an important concern of inmates, and the AIDS epidemic intensified those needs, creating a crisis not just for inmates but also for prison administrators. For women, there is the additional need for specialized gynecological care, since gynecological issues are so tied to HIV infection for many women.[16]

Support systems are necessary to meet the needs that prisoners have. Some of these are the need for emotional support when coping with an HIV-positive test result, facing the anxieties of becoming sick and unable to lead an independent life, and dealing with the fears of death. Self-help and peer support groups have been shown to be the most successful to give the needed support.

Support services are also needed to help make plans for leaving prison and rebuilding a life in the community. And there is a hope to leave prison alive. In New York State, a Medical Parole Law was signed in 1992. The law permits the Parole Board to release certain terminally ill inmates prior to the expiration of their minimum sentence. The law has strict guidelines, and many of those who receive medical parole die shortly after they leave prison; the law does not apply to many prisoners, who, therefore, die in prison.[17]

Most women in prison—80 percent—have children and are coping with child-related issues. Women who are HIV-positive have additional concerns. They have to:

- Plan for who will care for their children if they get sick or die.
- Arrange for the care for a child who is HIV-positive.
- Figure out how to talk to their children about being HIV-positive.

Not only has AIDS created a health crisis for individuals—there is also the social crisis of stigma. When prison administrators have built on the

---

15. *Focus on AIDS in New York State,* p. 7.

16. For more detailed discussions of HIV/AIDS health care issues, see Theodore M. Hammett, et al., *1992 Update: HIV/AIDS Prevention and Transmission in Correctional Facilities,* National Institute of Justice, January 1994; *Focus on AIDS in New York State;* Judy Greenspan, "Voices from Chowchilla Prison," *World,* December 1993, p. 6.

17. *Focus on AIDS in New York State,* pp. 18–19.

many resources in the prison—including civilian staff officers and inmates—and allowed for inmate peer education, positive changes have resulted.

In spite of the hardships that women face by being HIV-positive and in prison, some women have found more support at Bedford than in the outside community.

* * *

Being in jail and being HIV-positive is hard because so many things that I took for granted, I now see the beauty in them, and I just hope that I will find myself out there and that I will get to see them. But I feel that my treatment here is good, because if I was outside I wouldn't know where to go to get it or even what I should be getting. Most of what I learned I learned through ACE and other PWAs, whereas outside people don't go around broadcasting that they are PWAs, especially not women, and I don't know any gay men who I could discuss my gynecological problems with.

* * *

Lesbians

Lesbians face particular problems in the HIV/AIDS epidemic. The risk of HIV transmission through woman-to-woman sex has not been adequately studied, thereby leaving lesbians at a greater risk for infection and with less of an ability to make self-conscious educated choices.

But the vulnerability of lesbians to HIV/AIDS goes beyond the specific risk of woman-to-woman transmission. Lesbians have been defined as a "low-risk" group in the HIV/AIDS epidemic because the word "lesbian" has been defined as a woman who only has sex with another woman, and woman-to-woman sex appears to be low-risk. The term "lesbian," however, refers to an identity—it is not an adequate predictor of behavior. Lesbians are very much at risk for HIV infection, because many lesbians engage in behaviors that are high-risk. As one woman said, "Lesbianism is not a condom."[18]

The following are some of the reasons that lesbians are at risk for HIV-AIDS:

---

18. Amber Hollibaugh, "Lesbianism Is Not a Condom: Facing Our Risks for HIV in the Middle of An Epidemic," *The Lesbian AIDS Project Information Packet*, 1993/1994.

- Lesbians have sex with men. Several studies have reported that as many as half of all self-identified lesbians periodically have some sexual relations with men.[19]
- Lesbians may be IV drug users or use other drugs or alcohol, putting themselves at risk.
- Lesbians can be sexually assaulted.

One health advocate, herself a lesbian who is HIV-positive, writes:

Early in 1988 I decided to take the HIV-antibody tests. By that time I suspected I was positive, because of all the behaviors I had engaged in. I drank and used drugs for most of my adolescent and adult life, repeatedly sharing needles and practicing unsafe sex. . . . My biggest fear is that there exists a universal belief that lesbians don't get HIV or AIDS. We often forget that our behaviors vary. Many self-identified lesbians have sex—often unsafe sex—with men, or have unprotected sex with someone who used to share or still shares injection drugs. Lesbians believe that because these behaviors are only practiced on rare occasions, these behaviors pose no risk for HIV. We also forget that when we drink or use drugs, our judgment becomes impaired and we do many things that we wouldn't do otherwise. Also, our emotional state, feelings of vulnerability, loneliness, wanting to be accepted or loved put us at risk for HIV and other diseases.[20]

Verbal and physical attacks against gay people—including lesbians—have increased, often justified by the fear, ignorance, and stigma surrounding HIV/AIDS. In addition, lesbians have shouldered a major burden as caregivers and activists in fighting the epidemic.

WOMAN-TO-WOMAN TRANSMISSION

In this workshop, as in other workshops, we use the term "woman-to-woman" sex. Many women have sex with another woman but do not define

19. Rebecca M. Young, Gloria Weissman, and Judith B. Cohen, "Assessing Risk in the Absence of Information: HIV Risk Among Women Injection-Drug Users Who Have Sex with Women," *AIDS & Public Policy Journal* 7 (Fall 1992): 177. Some of the information in this article was drawn from a 1987 Kinsey Institute Study. Researchers found that 46 percent of self-identified lesbians had had sex with men since 1980; that 88 percent of those lesbians reported vaginal intercourse, and that only 8 percent of those used condoms; that 30 percent reported anal intercourse and that, of those, less than 5 percent used condoms.

20. Alice Terson, "Positively Lesbian," *Lap Notes* 1 (April 1993): 3.

themselves as lesbians. If we only use the word "lesbian" while talking about risks of sex between two women, then many women will not listen, because they will say "I'm not a lesbian."

When we explore the risks of woman-to-woman sex, we are talking about a risk activity, not a person's identity. We use the word "lesbian" when we are talking about an identity that some women choose and face homophobia and discrimination because of.

The CDC does not recognize sex between two women as a statistical category of possible transmission and has done only a few studies asking women questions about woman-to-woman sex. There is pressure on the CDC from women to take woman-to-woman sex more seriously and to begin collecting statistics. This absence of studies undermines the ability of women to be educated and to take responsibility for their sexual behavior (see Sexual Transmission, Workshop #6, for more detail).

* * *

As a woman who has relationships with other women, it really upsets me that there are not serious statistical studies about the risks of a woman giving HIV to another woman. It means I really don't have a way to evaluate how important it is to take precautions, and since the precautions are a drag, not knowing whether I really have to take them or not means sometimes I lean toward being extremely safe and sometimes I say, It really isn't dangerous, so I don't take any precautions.

* * *

MOTHER-TO-CHILD TRANSMISSION

Many important issues are raised for women who are HIV-positive and who either want to have a child or who are already pregnant. These issues exist because:

- A mother can pass the HIV virus to her unborn child.
- There is not yet a cure for AIDS.
- A recent study found that AZT can significantly lower the rate of transmission from a woman who is HIV-positive to her unborn child, yet the long-term side effects for the exposed, uninfected children, as well as infected children, are not known.

Personal Decision Making About Whether or Not to Have a Child

Women who are HIV-positive face the difficult question of whether to have children. Many personal issues go into the decision-making process.

Some women who are HIV-positive are deciding to have children. Some of the reasons they have given in discussions are:

- HIV-positive women without symptoms do not advance faster in their illness if they carry a child to term.
- The risk isn't that high.
- The facts aren't really known.
- The medical system can't be trusted.
- It's wrong to assume a death when it isn't for sure.
- The forced sterilization of black and Hispanic women is part of a genocide plan.
- Having a child is basic to her identity as a woman.
- Poor women's lives are full of constant risks and unknowns anyway.
- Abortion is against her religion.

Dr. Janet Mitchell, a black obstetrician/gynecologist who works at Harlem Hospital with women who are at high risk for HIV/AIDS, said about the women with whom she works: "They are survivors. They are smart. In a world that denies their existence, they struggle for some sense of self. Oftentimes that sense of self is intimately related to their ability to procreate and mother."[21]

Other HIV-positive women are deciding not to have children. Here are some of their reasons:

- They don't want to bring into the world a baby who might not live.
- They don't want to bring a healthy baby into a situation with a mother who may very well die.

---

21. Janet Mitchell, "What About the Mothers of HIV Infected Babies? National AIDS Network Multicultural Notes on AIDS," *Education & Service,* April 1, 1988, quoted in Risa Denenberg, "Pregnant Women and HIV," in the ACT UP/NY Women & AIDS Book Group, eds., *Women, AIDS & Activism,* (Boston: South End Press, 1990), p. 162.

- They don't have a dependable person in their life who could take care of the child if they were to die.

* * *

TEARS OF A BROKEN HEART

Then one night it really hit me, the realization that I will never be able to give birth to another child. The force of this reality and pain was so overwhelming that I got on my knees, tears running down my cheeks, and I started to bargain with God. I promised that I would be a better person. I promised that I would stop using drugs if only he would take this disease away so that I could conceive another child.

Now it's been five years since I've been diagnosed as having the HIV/AIDS virus, and although now I know more about this disease than I did then, I still find it hard to accept that this is really happening to me. . . . According to the CDC there is only a 30 percent chance that my unborn fetus will contract this disease from me, but I am not willing to take the chance to bring a child into this world who will suffer in the long run.

* * *

I've always wanted more children, and even though I'm still HIV-positive, I still want another baby. But now it's the fear that in an intimate relationship with a man, having to tell him I have the virus and wondering whether he would want the baby, knowing the baby might get sick, or his risking making love with me, knowing he could get sick. And then I also fear that if I have a baby and my baby converts and gets negative, then I get sick, then what happens to my baby? And for the two children I have now, ages ten and six, after all I put them through with my drugs, how do I tell them I might be leaving?

* * *

Social Attitudes About Pregnancy and Women Who Are HIV-Positive

Some people say that HIV-positive women should be involuntarily sterilized or pressured to have abortions. Support for these arguments includes these feelings:

- It's not right to take the risk of bringing an AIDS baby into the world.

- Whether or not the baby is HIV-infected, the mother will probably die, leaving the baby without a mother.

Negative attitudes toward women with AIDS have made it difficult to
get the abortions that some women choose.

- An HIV-positive woman may want to get an abortion, yet doctors may not be willing to perform the abortion for fear of contracting HIV infection.[22]
- Many women with HIV/AIDS may have difficulty affording an
  abortion. They may have lost their jobs and insurance coverage.
  Federal Medicaid coverage for abortion was eliminated in 1977,
  and thirty-seven state legislatures have also eliminated state
  Medicaid funding. So far, New York State continues to pay for
  the costs.

If an HIV-positive woman wants to bear a child, a support system—
including medical, psychological, and social help—may not be available.
Consequently, many HIV-positive babies are left in hospitals, abandoned
by parents too poor or ill to care for them.

Personal and Social Issues Raised
by the New AZT Treatment for Reduction of Transmission
of HIV Infection to the Unborn Child

A recent study has found that when a pregnant woman and her
newborn infant are given AZT, the rate of HIV transmission from a
woman who is HIV-positive to an unborn child can be reduced from
approximately 25 percent to 8 percent.[23] On the one hand, this is a
significant reduction, and on the other hand, there are many unanswered
questions relating to the long-term effects for a pregnant woman taking
AZT, as well as to the impact on the fetus and on a newborn infant.

The study raises a new set of decisions both for individuals and for
society:

---

22. New York City Commission on Human Rights, Law Enforcement Bureau, AIDS Discrimination Division, "HIV-Related Discrimination by Reproductive Health Care Providers in New York
City," October 20, 1990.

23. Dave Gilden, "Study Finds AZT Reduces Mother-to-Child Transmission," *Treatment Issues,*
March 1994, pp. 15–16.

- Does a pregnant woman who is HIV-positive want to take the AZT treatment for herself and her unborn child (see Workshop #5, Transmission, for more discussion on this issue)?
- How much does society pressure women who are pregnant to take the AZT treatment?
- How does this new information impact on the issue of voluntary versus mandatory testing for pregnant women (see Workshop #8, Testing, for more discussion on this issue)?

There is an increasing focus on pregnant women and HIV/AIDS. The most important things required by a woman who is trying to figure out the issues that HIV/AIDS raises about having children are information and counseling. In response to the importance of supporting pregnant women, the CDC has proposed guidelines for health providers in counseling pregnant women. These guidelines include:

For pregnant women who may or may not be HIV-positive

- Counseling.
- Encouraging testing.
- Providing voluntary testing for pregnant women and their infants.
- Access to HIV prevention and treatment services (e.g., drug treatment).

For HIV-Positive Pregnant Women

- Counseling.
- Provision of information about the AZT therapy, including the substantial benefits and short-term safety as well as the uncertainties of long-term risks. The information is to be provided in a noncoercive atmosphere and based on balancing risks and benefits.
- Provision of information about all reproductive options, to be provided in a nondirective manner.
- Advice to not breastfeed.[24]

(See the Appendix for the more detailed excerpt of CDC Proposed Guidelines.)

---

24. Centers for Disease Control, "Draft Guidelines: How Should Health Care Providers Counsel Pregnant Women?," excerpted in *World*, April 1995, pp. 4–5.

WOMEN AS CAREGIVERS

Women as Caregivers at Home

Women care for their families—their children, their husbands, their sisters and brothers, their mothers and fathers. Women are caring for loved ones who have AIDS. At Bedford, women have lost their babies, cared for their sisters and brothers, and buried their own mothers. The grandmothers at home have cared for their grandchildren while they nursed their own children who were sick. Families throughout the communities affected by the AIDS epidemic have taken care of the young who are sick or dying, and women have carried the central burden.

TO A SPECIAL SISTER AND A DEAR FRIEND, YVETTE

A million times we've missed you,
A million times we've cried,
If love could have saved you,
You never would have died. . . .

Things we feel most deeply are the
hardest things to say,
Our dearest one, we have loved you,
In a very special way. . . .

We often sit and think of you and
think of how you died. . . .

To think we couldn't say goodbye,
before you closed your eyes. . . .

No one can know our loneliness, and
no one can see us weeping. . . .
All our tears from our aching heart,
while others are sleeping. . . .

If we had one lifetime wish,
a dream that could come true,
We'd pray to God, with all our heart,
for yesterday and you. . . .

Thinking of and loving
you always,
your sister
AIDA

* * *

I was an IV drug user and I used to share needles—that's how I became HIV-positive. I found out July of 1990, and this is where the next stage comes in. My name is Jay and I am HIV-positive. I didn't know where to go or who to talk to until I came to Bedford Hills. Then I learned about ACE. The people there were loving and caring, and they gave me support and strength. So I would understand more about the virus. I also have a brother who has the virus and doesn't know how to get help. But when I go home I am going to help him and others who need help to know about it. But right now I need more information about it to do so.

Right now my brother feels like he's alone because he's been rejected by outsiders, but he's loved. But wherever he's at, I hope he be all right and someone helps him.

* * *

Women as Caregivers in Society

Women constitute the vast majority of nurses, social workers, primary and secondary school educators, home health aides, and attendants and orderlies in this country. Women are the more poorly paid of health workers and are frequently recruited from communities already severely affected by HIV/AIDS-related diseases. Often, after working at their jobs they must go home to care for family members who are ill. The lack of support, respect, and recognition for the work these women do increases stress, and they suffer burnout.

I worked as a home health aide, a nurse's aide. At first I didn't want to work around people with AIDS, but I still did because I needed the money. But now that I've learned about AIDS, I'm going to be working with people with AIDS because I want to, I want to let them know that it's all right, I want to be supportive. I'm not afraid, I just have to use safe precautions like a doctor and everything will be all right.

Worldwide, the burden of unpaid health services and care has always fallen to wives, mothers, grandmothers, sisters, aunts, and daughters. Women are the huge bulk of volunteers who have come forward to try to fill the void left by the government's lack of adequate social and medical resources for those facing HIV infection. Volunteerism is put forward by the government as the answer to the escalating costs of caring for those with AIDS. Unfortunately, the communities worst hit by HIV/AIDS already have the least support and resources from the health care system.

TEACHING PLAN

Workshop Design/Plan

A great deal of diverse background information is included in this workshop material. Although the background materials give us much information for use in the workshop, the experiences of the participants themselves are central to the workshop discussions. This is an important workshop for men as well as women. We suggest a number of possible formats for using the material of the workshop, depending on whether it is part of the nine-workshop series or it is being used alone.

FORMAT A: A TALK SHOW

If the Women and HIV/AIDS workshop follows the eight sessions before it, then participants will already have heard much of the information included in the background material. We have found a talk-show format to be a particularly successful way to involve participants in dealing with issues that women face. We have included in the talk show whatever recent topics have been in the newspaper that relate to women and the AIDS epidemic. Some of these have included: whether it is appropriate for a high school to distribute condoms; whether or not a lesbian has to be concerned about AIDS; whether prisoners who are HIV-positive should be given compassionate release; whether it should be mandatory for a pregnant woman to be given the HIV-antibody test. Different people take on the role of an individual representing a particular position. The talk show participants can either be the facilitators or someone from the workshop. The audience in the talk show is made up of the participants from the workshop. This kind of talk show is more successful if there is some practice, and if handouts are prepared that give information about the different issues—either handouts written by the staff or newspaper or magazine articles.

FORMAT B

If this workshop is to be used alone, outside of the context of the entire workshop series, then it will be important to spend more time becoming aware of the information in the background material. We suggest doing a lot of brainstorming, because much of the information is really part of people's own experience.

I. How HIV Infection Affects Us as Women

Ask the participants to brainstorm on the question: Why do we do a workshop just on women and HIV/AIDS? Here is a list that came out of one session we held:

- It's a man's world, so HIV/AIDS stigmatizes women more.
- HIV/AIDS affects our children.
- We have responsibilities as women.
- We need to take responsibility for our own health—and the health of others.
- Responsibility falls on us as caregivers and educators of children and spouses.
- We have to deal with male cheating and double standards.
- Our dependency on men makes us more vulnerable.
- Women are isolated and have to deal with all this individually and alone; we need to see it as a social problem so we can act together.

II. HIV Infection as It Affects Women

Introduce statistics: How women are contracting HIV, how HIV infection affects us physically, and who is most vulnerable. Brainstorm: What's the particular impact of the HIV/AIDS crisis on black, Latin, and poor women?

Here is one list that was generated by this question:

- It's one more strike against Latin and black women.
- It makes me angry. Nothing is being done. They are teaching whites but not teaching blacks and Hispanics.
- It's a poverty neighborhood with drugs. Whites come in to get what they want and then leave, but the problem stays with us.
- Health resources are terrible.
- The poor person is getting slapped.
- We're more susceptible to start with—we have less ability to fight it.
- We need to do workshops like this one in the community.

- I feel that the statistics are biased against black and Latin people. Statistics can be misused to stigmatize us, but they can also be used to bring in needed resources.
- Black people, Harlem people are looked at as expendable, so we won't be given the resources. We have to get them ourselves.

BRAINSTORM:

How are teenagers especially affected by HIV?
How are lesbians affected by HIV?
How are women prisoners affected by HIV?

BRAINSTORM:

How do our sexuality and sexism affect our vulnerability to HIV/AIDS? Cover the following areas of the background material using the discussion and examples to supplement the brainstorming:

- Women are supposed to be available as sexual objects for men.
- There's stigma against women for being sexual.
- Women are often pressured into having sex: rape, child molestation, date rape, unspoken pressure.
- There is neglect of woman-to-woman transmission—denial of risks, refusal to collect statistics, etc.

DISCUSSION TOPICS:

- The impact of HIV infection/AIDS on women as caregivers
- Mother-to-child transmission: decision making and personal issues; what issues might women who are HIV positive have to consider around having children?
- Social issues around reproductive rights relating to HIV infection and having children.
- Talking to our children about HIV/AIDS.
- Women organizing to fight for inclusion in drug trials.
- How to make the struggle for safer sex less individual and more a concern for our whole community.
- How do we develop solidarity/sisterhood and empowerment?

REFERENCE MATERIALS

The ACT UP/NY Women & AIDS Book Group. *Women, AIDS & Activism.*
Boston: South End Press, 1990.

The Boston Women's Health Book Collective, eds. *The New Our Bodies, Ourselves.* New York: Simon & Schuster, 1992.

Corea, Gina. *The Invisible Epidemic.* New York: HarperCollins, 1992.

Santee, Barbara. *Women and AIDS: The Silent Epidemic.* Women and AIDS Resource Network: New York, 1989.

White, Evelyn C., ed. *The Black Women's Health Book.* Seattle: Seal Press, 1990.

Periodicals

LAP Notes
Lesbian AIDS Project—GMHC
129 West 20th St.
New York, NY 10011

Sojourner: The Women's Forum
42 Seaverns Ave.
Jamaica Plain, MA 02130

The Positive Woman
A newsletter by, for, and about the HIV positive woman
P.O. Box 34372
Washington, DC 200434–372

WORLD
Women Organized to Respond to Life-Threatening Diseases
A newsletter by, for and about women facing HIV disease
P.O. Box 11535
Oakland, CA 94611

Workshop #9
Living with AIDS

It don't matter now, how or why or who.

It don't matter now when
  the year of the virus entered my life
    and my body
      and my bloodstream
      and my brain.

In the name of the indifference, who cares?

The life flow of my existence speaks loudly
in many tongues.

See me,
  Hear me,
    Hold me.

Now for a second I ponder,
  then I let it go.

In my world there is no time
  for idle thought
    nor space
      nor room to roam.

Only to gather as I go in a relentless
pursuit to the rhythm of my own pace
    is miracle indeed.

To hold my world—never to relinquish
my power
my presence,
my heart felt struggle with
conflict through change.

Until the end

Past tomorrow

Forever more

I am Gloria B.

—GLORIA BOYD

OVERVIEW

When we talk about living with AIDS, it is easy to identify the target toward which we direct our attention. Clearly, it is the individual who is HIV-positive. But we have learned that AIDS is a social problem from which no individual can escape. Whether we are angry, frightened, biased, or tired of, distant from, or fed-up with information or media coverage about this disease, we will still have to face another day in the life of AIDS.

AIDS finds a way of making its presence felt in almost any situation. It is the topic of conversation, the key subject of sexual education, the topic of the year, the most feared illness, the top women's issue, the top homosexual issue, and our young people's introduction to dating. It just will not go away. The number of us whose lives have been touched by this disease, or who will be touched, is indeed huge. If we include all the people related to those at high risk of getting this disease, the number is staggering. Each person with AIDS is someone's child, perhaps someone's brother, sister, husband, or wife. Someone's lover or friend, maybe even someone's parent. People are beginning to discover that something is going terribly wrong in their lives, or in the lives of someone they love.

People are beginning to care for PWAs or getting involved with AIDS issues and listening more intently to information about AIDS for their own survival. Society is being commanded to change its practices about sexual behavior and is being given instructions on how to cope in the age of AIDS.

Questions are being raised about how to live with this epidemic. What is necessary for our own survival? How can we reduce the pain, stigma, grief of AIDS? What do we contribute, how involved do we become? How can we be a friend? How do we live with AIDS, knowing that we are affected by it in one way or another? ACE has concluded that we are all living with AIDS in the broader sense of the word. We have taken on roles in which we are caregivers, friends, lovers, relatives, and in some cases strangers to PWAs.

Up to now, almost all attention and support has been focused on the people who are afflicted with this illness. It is comforting to know that there are people who are coping with and sharing their experiences with living with AIDS, even though they themselves are not infected. They have admitted to themselves that they, too, are indeed living with AIDS.

The workshop has some helpful hints for the newly diagnosed, and voices from both PWAs and those who are uninfected with but certainly affected by the epidemic, and are in fact living with AIDS.

This workshop is more focused on an emotional education than on an academic education, and the tone and language reflect this. A person can be brilliant and still be unable to display emotions. It's partly through sharing our emotions that ACE is no longer just a dream but a reality. This is a workshop where there are no longer any teachers—everyone is a student, and we learn through the sharing of our emotions. It is also a workshop where more people become open about their HIV status and where a transition is made from friends to family.

The goal of this final workshop is to strengthen a community of support and a commitment to struggling with the AIDS epidemic. We spend the workshop sharing the personal experiences of how AIDS has affected each of us who chooses to speak, how the workshops have changed us, and what we hope to do about AIDS. The workshop has no teaching plan. After we explain the purpose of the workshop, one of the ACE facilitators will talk personally about her experience of living with AIDS. A woman who is open about being HIV-positive often opens the workshop. Then we invite all the participants to speak about their experience of living with AIDS. The material for the workshop comes from the circle of participants who share their thoughts and feelings.

The background material comes from discussions that were held among PWAs in Bedford in the summers of 1989 and 1990, and from writings by other members of ACE who are living with AIDS in different ways. Your group may also want to begin to collect writings about how people within your community are living with AIDS.

BACKGROUND MATERIAL

During the summer of 1989, a group of us who are PWAs in ACE sat together to share and write down our experiences of living with AIDS. We looked at the following areas and wrote out of our own personal struggles:

1. Dealing, in a manner that is comfortable for the individual, with the stages of living with AIDS—for example, denial, anger, bargaining, depression, and acceptance.

2. Being informed about what you should know medically—for example, T4 counts, drugs available (approved or under clinical trials), treatments, and prophylactics (pros and cons).

3. Realizing that if a PWA has the knowledge of what goes on in her body, early detection can alleviate or slow the process of illness, through follow-up with good nutrition, exercise, relaxation, stress reduction, the do's and dont's.
4. Figuring out how to cope mentally; having a positive outlook:
   a. Not giving up on hope.
   b. Learning to love oneself and others again.
   c. Learning to let go of anger and fear.
   d. Making a commitment to health.
   e. Keeping a sense of humor.
   f. Forgiving yourself and others.
   g. Learning to accept that we cannot always have control but never giving up.
   h. Not looking back—no regrets. The past will only bring you backwards.
   i. *Keeping things simple, not overwhelming yourself, taking it one day at a time.*

Some Experiences We Have Had with Stages

DENIAL

Some examples of what people think/say/do in this stage:

- I can't be dying—I have to take care of my child.
- This can't be happening!
- The test is definitely wrong!
- I know I took a lot of risks, but this can't be happening to me!
- Only the junkies on the street get it—not me. I only get high socially!
- How did I get it? I don't practice high-risk behavior.
- Not me, the survivor, the superwoman.

All these and many more are things that may run through your head upon initial diagnosis. This is a stage that is necessary for everyone to play out. It is a helpful and needed part of the process. The length of time of denial varies from person to person, and often people revert back to it, but if you seek support and think positively, it will pass. The impact of the positive test result will lessen, and you will overcome denial.

You may fear giving AIDS to another person, or fear that you already have. If you continue to practice high-risk behavior during denial, the guilt of exposing others is compounded when you reach acceptance.

ANGER

Some examples of what people think/say/do in this stage:

- Scream and yell.
- Cry, cry, cry.
- Say, "I hate the world!"
- Become suicidal.
- Become vindictive (want to get even).
- Say, "I hate myself."
- Say, "Why me?"

Again, this is a stage that has to be played out. Anger can be one of the most dangerous stages. Being angry can make you feel vindictive, but do not take this out on the world. Learn not to react to this anger, because you will leave others vulnerable.

No one purposely sets out to get AIDS, but we have to accept the responsibility that the roles we played were possibly high-risk and realize that it is something that we can never change, but learn to forgive ourselves.

BARGAINING

Some examples of what people think or say in this stage:

- "I prayed five times a day, and you mean to tell me I got AIDS? God, you could fix this if you wanted to."
- "God, I swear I will never get high again and will go to church on Sunday if you take this back."
- "God, now that I have it, let me live for my daughter."
- "God, I want to be with my child—let me live."

Nothing we can exchange/sacrifice is going to alter our situation.

DEPRESSION

Some examples of what people think/say/do in this stage:

- "I feel like I have the cooties."
- When someone approaches and asks how you are, thinking or saying, "If you only knew."
- You think about your health twice.
- "No one can help me."
- "There is nothing to live for . . . no dreams. . . ."
- "I feel like an outsider, a misfit."

This stage seems never-ending, keeps coming back. It is an emotional roller coaster. We found that the best way of dealing with depression, when it comes, is not to dwell on it but to think positive. Try to surround yourself with as much love and support as possible. In this stage, you're more apt to push people away. Be conscious of this, because without love and support you will sink deeper into depression. Count your blessings. Express your feelings to someone supportive, and realize that like the other stages, this too shall pass.

ACCEPTANCE

Some examples of what people think/say/do in this stage:

- "Why do I make myself crazy? I can't change this, I want to live."
- "A sober death."
- "I'm strong. Life goes on."
- "I'm going to face this head on."

Believe it or not, this stage eventually comes and goes at times. Acceptance is like a yo-yo. Some days, you're powerful—you can deal with anything and everything that comes. Acceptance brings peace when it comes. The control is within yourself. Always keep in mind the empowerment that acceptance gives you. It helps for when the roller coaster begins.

How to Be More Assertive Around Medical Care

Seeking information and education around the medical-care aspect of HIV gives the PWA empowerment to partake in her own medical decisions.

It is important for the PWA to be assertive (as opposed to being passive, a victim) in doctor/patient consultations. By showing the PWA that she should be assertive, we are pointing to the direction she needs to take to reach empowerment in adequate care:

1. Know what tests should be taken and what the results mean—for example, T-cell subsets, CBC, toxo. Early indication of change in any blood results must be understood to the fullest. (Don't just think, "Oh, this means nothing.")
2. It is important for the PWA to know what her actual diagnosis is—what stage she is in, according to the CDC definition. This helps the individual come to terms with her illness and gives her better insight for what direction she needs to go in and what steps need to be taken.
3. Taking control in a doctor/patient relationship begins with being informed as to "where I am." This will enable the individual to make demands and not feel intimidated by the doctor in the decision around treatment. If conflict arises, the individual should take the initiative to go elsewhere to seek her treatment of choice.
4. People should evaluate media coverage of drugs (trial or approved) and not feel overwhelmed by conflicting views. What is good for another is not necessarily good for you. If you feel strong and good about your choice of treatment, do not feel influenced by outside pressures.

GET TO KNOW YOUR BODY

To get to know your body is to understand yourself emotionally, physically, mentally, and spiritually. No matter what stage the PWA is in—HIV-positive, HIV-symptomatic, or AIDS—there will be limitations that she may experience. Play out those limitations: accept *only* what you are capable of doing (don't hype yourself up—it's okay that you are limited for today).

a. *Nutrition:* Eat properly: fresh vegetables, fruits, grains, balanced diet. It is very important for PWAs not to eat uncooked red meat (it can harbor toxoplasmosis).
b. *Exercise:* Walking, stretching, calisthenics, even aerobics. *But* within limits, according to how you are feeling. Don't overexert

yourself; accept that today I can't do so much. Tomorrow is another day.

c. *Relaxation:* Learn the proper techniques. Try to incorporate a relaxation period (twenty minutes to a half hour) at least once, if not twice, a day. Yoga, meditation, short naps, massage—all are beneficial.

d. *Stress reduction:* Life is stressful, so it is impossible to avoid stress altogether. But one can learn to reduce stress by either using some relaxation techniques and/or by being aware of and addressing the problems that are causing stress.

We don't create controversy in the workshop by saying such things as "Don't smoke," "No recreational drugs," "No caffeine." We all know that these substances have long-term negative effects on the body. But we *cannot* tell anyone what not to do. Practices that may seem destructive or life-threatening to one individual may be helpful to others. It is an individual choice. Just get the facts, and realize some of those may be cofactors (possibly leading to faster progression of the disease).

The individual has to do what is necessary for her to keep sane. Stopping smoking for some can create more stress; elimination of some recreational drugs can create depression. So one has to do what is necessary for one to survive and thrive.

How to Cope Mentally and Have a Positive Outlook

a. Don't give up on hope. Hope is the only thing a PWA has to keep her from feeling defeated. Hope will carry you through many rough days.

b. Learn to love oneself and others again. Some PWAs feel that this happened to them because they no longer cared about themselves or what happened to them. You must first realize that even though some people's behavior exposed them to the HIV, and some others' behavior did not, no one purposely wanted to get exposed.

It is very important to love yourself regardless of what the circumstances are. Without love of self, you cannot love others. When you love yourself, you make sure to surround yourself with things crucial for your survival.

c. Learn to let go of anger and fear. These are two dangerous emotions. Negative emotions can harm you. It is most important to feel good about oneself in order to want/demand good from others. Negative emotions can only make one susceptible to a whole lot of harm. Also, anger and fear can create stress.

d. Make a commitment to health. It is up to you, the individual who is infected, to make sure that you take the best care of yourself. No one is going to do it for you.

e. Keep a sense of humor. It is quoted that humor can bring up one's immune system. Everyone enjoys laughter. It is healthy. Besides, feeling sad can only bring on depression.

f. Forgive yourself and others. Again, no one chose to contract this illness. Don't blame yourself or others. Learn to accept the reality and move on. The quicker you accept the reality, the longer you have to live a *life of quality*.

g. Learn to accept that we cannot always have control but never give up. No one who is human is in control of everything 100 percent of the time, but strive for self-control. Yes, it is going to be very difficult when we begin to lose control (that is, get ill), and the only thing we can do is to realize that any illness is ultimately beyond anyone's control. But hope will carry you through these rough times.

Voices: Living with AIDS

Living with AIDS has different meanings to the different women in ACE. In the last workshop, many women "testify" about their experience living with AIDS. It is not uncommon for someone to "come out" as a PWA or reveal something about a family member in this setting. What follows are some examples of these statements and writings.

* * *

What I Leave Behind: "Treasure Chest"

I've become a chest of treasures.
The jewels and gems I possess are
made of
Wisdom and experience of living.

They have become invaluable,
through the years of my being.
They're no duplicates, these are original.
They've been made by my personal
teachers, and molded by me.
You can open my chest and gaze
on the pearl of tears,
the diamonds of love, the ruby of joy,
the emerald of shame, the sapphire, my
soul, the opal, my dreams.
These are just to mention a few of my
favorites.
When you look you will see
a display of all my secrets.
You cannot remove anything from the chest.
They'll lose their luster.
They must remain together, I've had them since birth.

—DORIS MOICES

* * *

I lost two sisters-in-law to AIDS, one as late as November 1987. I had no knowledge of what this disease was all about. I knew for certain that I, Renee Scott, could not possibly have this virus, disease, this word that was not spoken even in the most sacred of places or amongst the closest of friends. Why should I worry, after all. I was gay, and I stopped using drugs two years prior to my arrest, so that in itself excluded me from that category, or so I thought.

Before coming to Bedford, I read in the Sunday *Daily News Magazine* how some people were being buddies to PWAs, and I said to myself, that's what I want to do. After arriving at Bedford, I soon found out that the word "AIDS" was also taboo up here. Then D.G. told me she was going to a meeting to try to form a group to do something about the AIDS epidemic up here in Bedford. I jumped at the chance and practically begged her to let me go with her.

D. let me go with her to the meeting, and I was amazed at the impact that AIDS had on "our community," so to speak. I mean people were talking about the treatment they were receiving from staff members and peers alike, not to mention the medical treatment, which I might add was the bottomless pit.

At this meeting and many others, we discussed everything that a person could think of pertaining to the AIDS virus, and more. I learned about how the virus can be dormant in your system for so many years, without you even knowing that it's there. I learned that people were being treated unjustly because they were, or were suspected of, carrying this horrid virus in their bodies. And most of all I learned about Empathy — you know the word, sounds like "sympathy," but that's where the alikeness ends.

After I learned so much about this disease I started hating myself for being so nosy. What I learned was that my past behaviors had endangered me to the point that I was a prime candidate for this virus.

At this time, I was a full-fledged member of ACE and loved the work I was doing with a passion. But I still hated myself for being so curious; I was so sure, so positive — would have bet my life on it — that I did not have these horrendous antibodies in my body.

What ACE has taught me — I know that there could never be a college course, degrees, or any certification given, because ACE in itself is what love is all about, and love for your fellow man can't be taught. It's something that is innate.

When I learned that I had put myself at risk because of past behavior, I was a prime candidate for "Marcy" (a facility for the criminally insane), but ACE walked with me every step of the way, from being tested, accepting my positive status, accepting that I had to take the AZT for my own benefit, and just being there for me, regardless of what it was that I needed or what time of day, evening, or night it was. ACE was there for me, as it is there for other women in this facility.

I am glad I took the time to become involved in an organization such as ACE. It saved my life.

—RENEE

* * *

I entered this prison system February 10, 1984, and at that time AIDS was not even a thought, let alone an issue. By the end of 1985, AIDS was being whispered about in the yard, in the gym, in the mess hall, and above all, in the hospital building. People would look at the call-out and come back with a list of names, said to have had AIDS, and even though I didn't run to get the call-outs, I did point fingers at people because of what I was told.

In the beginning, I didn't feel as if there was a need for me to know anything internally about AIDS. All I needed to know was who had it so I could keep my distance. I did not want to be in the same room with an AIDS person, as if one could have gotten it like that. I was told that I was more dangerous to a person with AIDS than them to me. So I figured, "Why not put them in a building by themselves away from regular population. That way no one would make anyone sick." In a word, I *stigmatized* PWAs. I didn't want to be bothered with anyone who was said to have had AIDS.

The turning point for me was my peers in college—one in particular. We were sitting in class, "Death and Dying," when she disclosed to the class her health status. What she said didn't surprise me because it was pointed out to me that she had the virus, but it was something about the way in which she worded it. She said she was HIV-positive asymptomatic. I had absolutely no idea what that meant. I spent the rest of that hour trying to figure out the right way to approach her with what was puzzling me. We (Mercy College students) had a ten-minute smoke break and I took total advantage of that time. She gave me the basic information in about five minutes.

Through that conversation, something happened that made me want to look into my past, something that made me want to remember where I had come from and what I had done. It was at that moment that AIDS became an internal feeling for me.

I joined ACE through a series of workshops and a strong sense of need. I am now an ACE member, and through my interaction with people I realize all I need is a need to learn, a need to live, and a need to love.

—PEARL

KATRINA AND KATHY TALKING ABOUT LIVING WITH AIDS:

KATHY: Katrina and I were very close friends. We used to jog together and cook together. We shared feelings about love and religion, we talked about children, and we worked together in ACE. Katrina used to tell me how, if she were ever HIV-positive, she would never tell anybody, 'cause she would not want anyone to change a single bit about how they were being her friend. I was her friend, and I'm still her friend. Then, one night she said she had taken the test, and she was positive. All I could remember was that she did not want me to change, or have any feelings of sadness, or worry. She wanted me to treat her as if nothing was different. As I was sitting on the floor of her cell, listening to music, I remember how many times she had said to me, "Don't act any differently." So I sat there with this new information, trying to be the friend that she wanted me to be, and finding it hard. Because inside of me I wanted to cry, I wanted to hug her, I wanted to scream. But she had said she wanted me to treat her no differently. This was one of my first moments experiencing what trying to be a friend of a PWA is, dealing with what they want from you, and what you yourself want and need, and trying to fit all of that together.

KATRINA: I guess I knew this information would have an impact on you, but there was my own need for you not to display that impact. I don't know why, I guess it would allow me not to be more vulnerable. I felt like I would be sharing it with you but we wouldn't be vulnerable about it. I guess I felt as if in sharing it, we could be intellectual about it. Yet I wanted you to play an emotional role. It's contradictory. It's funny now, but then I just wanted you to digest this information and for us to move on. And although moving on meant you living with me with AIDS on a daily basis, we were just going to deal with the reality of the diagnosis now and nothing else. And by that, in my mind, I knew it was just AIDS, without emotion, without sentiment, without the reality of our relationship or connection with each other, just with saying "AIDS," and saying it to someone.

And then after that I just kind of wanted you to know that I had said it and that I had shared it with you and to forget about feeling right then and to somewhat put it in the back of our heads and to come back to it later. Part of me needed me to react emotionally, but I wanted it stifled because I was burned out myself being emotional about it. I thought I was regrouping emotionally, but I didn't know that there was a lot more to come. I just wanted to tell you and I guess grow to a place where together we would play it out together. Even if I wasn't sure we would, but that maybe we would have some neat little structure where we could play it out together—part of me knowing that it wouldn't get worked out like that but needing to feel like I was in control. Because I couldn't control the illness, I thought at least I could control how we responded to it. But that was contradictory too, because you'd walk away feeling fucked up and I'd feel fucked up. But as my friend I was dictating how you should play it out. Even though we both knew we were both suppressing.

KATHY: I knew that I felt like crying and like holding you and I also knew you well enough to know you had lots of feelings, but I felt I had to control myself emotionally, because that's what you had said to me month after month—you just didn't want any sympathy or tenderness. But it wasn't long after that that you came to me and said, "Kathy, what's this on my body?" and I knew that you were going to share with me your freakouts at everything that changed physically, and that was very emotional. I also remember soon after that saying, "Let's go jogging," and on the one hand it was a way of saying, nothing has changed, but as we jogged I kept saying, "Are you tired, are you okay?" and you didn't seem to mind my concern. So our emotions were connecting slowly.

KATRINA: And I think I was glad that we had come to that place, still not having redefined the roles that we were to play. Still sometimes I ask, "What do I want from her?" I know that then and now I want you to be there to talk to me about issues that may be new, I want you to encourage me to continue struggling with it, to give advice when I need it, to just listen and stare perplexedly when I need it, and to know when I need a hug when I need it. It really is just like guesswork, but you're learning the patterns—even from that it is like figuring out what is needed.

And even though it is still unclear what roles I want you to play and when, you are playing that ambiguity out, and I guess that's the sum, I want you to just be there. And it's a big demand, I know. But you've taken it on and after each phase we laugh about it and try to learn about it, and after each phase we learn, and that too is part of the friendship of living with AIDS.

KATHY: I think we've been lucky because we know each other. When you feel very healthy and strong and when something has happened to you like T-cell drop or really bad headaches, then it throws me emotionally into an intense state of worry and anxiety, and then, because I know you're going home, I feel that sense of wanting to be able to be with you if you do get sick and need a friend and knowing that I won't be there with you.

KATRINA: At any time of playing this out, did you feel helpless in terms of being there? And if so, what did that to you?

KATHY: I guess when you were suffering so much from those headaches and I was both scared and also helpless in the face of your pain, and I knew you were both really worried about whether they meant a severe deterioration physically and also that the pain was terrible.

KATRINA: Did you think, That could be the reality, and in light of that, how do I help her deal with that? Or did you just feel helpless about eliminating the pain?

KATHY: I really didn't know, without your having the tests done, whether it was very serious or not. So while I worried, I put my energy into trying to work with you around getting the necessary tests. But the pain I felt was as much as anyone who isn't experiencing it directly might feel.

KATRINA: Part of me felt like it was just another crisis and that together we would get over it, but part of me also felt like the plot thickens, and I know like I felt like I was in a race with time. The race was to leave physically well.

KATHY: Definitely—because your time is so short. And being able to leave healthy, to go out feeling self-reliant, to have that time out there to fulfill your dreams of giving back to your people and community through doing work around AIDS—something you speak of all the time—sure I've internalized your dreams, and for a moment there, suddenly I was afraid that they might not come true. So I felt that race for time very strongly.

KATRINA: I know that you have watched other friends go through a process of leaving and making plans. In this relationship, AIDS adds to it. How does it intensify this relationship? How do you prevent yourself from being totally engulfed in it? Or if you could stop yourself . . .

KATHY: It's funny, I think that the experience of working together and living with AIDS together builds a specially deep connection, so that in a way I feel more confident than usual that a friendship will continue when you leave because of what we share. It doesn't feel as much as usual like the possible end of a friendship. But like I said, that desire to be able to be there for you if and when you need a friend, it's very frustrating to know that I won't be able to in that way, but that's my problem.

KATRINA: Do you feel like I instill your leaving with some sort of burden or continued commitment to remember the friendship? Is that also a role I'm asking you to play?

KATHY: No I think that's a role that comes naturally to me with you because that's what it means to me to be friends. Before, when you were talking, you said it was in the PWA group, when significant others were invited, that you suddenly realized something about our role.

KATRINA: I suddenly realized that they have to be asked if they can play the role that you're asking them to play—do they feel comfortable playing it?—and they have to be able to say what they're capable of giving back. And I didn't really realize that until that meeting. And it put everything that we've been playing out right there in front of me. I never even asked if that was too much: Is this overwhelming? What are you going to need from me to be able to continue this? Then it was that I realized we all are indeed living with AIDS, you as much as me, because we are all having to live it daily. It was then that I saw that.

KATHY: For me, it has been a continual process of feeling that what would happen if we had more time is that I would feel freer to express my feelings—and would not always worry whether I was doing the right thing for you, but would know that sometimes even if my feelings were not what you wanted to hear, it was important for me and for you to play that out. So I think we started from a point of my trying to be who you wanted slowly but surely. As we really accept the idea that we're both living with AIDS but in different ways, then it makes it easier for me to say how I feel too. Which has brought us to a different place.

KATRINA: And I don't know if without that group I would have understood the impact of that.

* * *

The reason I joined ACE was I never knew anything about AIDS until I came here. People were pointing at people who had AIDS, and I felt it was very cruel. There was a lot of negative talk from women here. What I found was women were meeting with other women in the yard, discussing AIDS. They were opening up and sharing. I felt I wanted to learn much more in order to help others. All the negative talk drew me in closer, wanting to listen. By doing this I was learning so much from each person. I discovered that I could help others by sharing a friendship, a warm embrace, or even a hug, because these things were more important than all the material things.

I feel positive around the women, and I'm able to lend a helping hand, a listening ear, even a shoulder to cry on. I am there to share love with these people, who are important to us in every way. I also learned that material things only last for a while, but a smile goes a lifetime, even just one hug. I have learned that I fulfill myself more by helping someone other than myself. I feel strong inside by helping and caring for others. It brings me joy and happiness to be a friend to someone who is reaching out. I am there for them. AIDS is a big problem and we must live with it and face the truth of it, teach the children and adults that there are ways to prevent it, discussing it among our children or groups. I feel positive, and each day I hope to teach others around me. I'm there to help.

There is a word called "empathy," and it's not just a word. Empathy is a very profound experience. It is our taking someone else's pain into our hearts and feeling it without having to experience the same exact source of pain. I have felt this in speaking to the women, and I enjoy working to help others.

—JENNY

* * *

Living with AIDS, for me, is often about having to live with many secrets. Women confide in me about their HIV status. I'm glad that they can trust me and that I can be a haven for them; a friend to talk with, a peer counselor to work through feelings, choices, problems. But it's also painful to know that even though we've begun to create a supportive community, stigma still surrounds and haunts us and women still need the protection of confidentiality. So I walk around with secrets. And I'll see someone who I have spent time with, listening and sharing her pain, her struggles, her courage and determination to survive and thrive. And we will be in the yard, or school, or among others, and no one else knows what the sister is going through, and I have to act like that part of what we share doesn't exist. I have to tell my own heart to quiet down, to not show too much closeness and emotion. And I know that the sister is having to do the same thing, only more so, and more often. And this hurts.

I'm gay. For years after I came out within myself and among close friends, I didn't feel like I could be open about being gay to my family or on my job and in other situations. It was painful, because I felt like I wasn't genuine, that I couldn't be real about all of me, that in too much of my life I couldn't be whole. Eventually, I chose to come out in all the spheres of my life, because I needed to be a whole person. Even though I sometimes caught hell, it was less pressure than the burden of keeping who I was secret. I relate to this when I think of the burden of secrets that PWAs and all of us affected by HIV bear.

I've talked about some of the hard parts of living with AIDS. But the other side of it is the strength that I have gained by loving, being friends, and working with women who are PWAs in here. I am a long-termer; I have a life sentence. When I was brought to Bedford Hills, they said to me, "This is the end of the line; you will die here." They sent me here to die. But it is in me to want to continue to live, and live the best and fullest I can, no matter what. I've come to know women who are HIV-positive who have faced that moment when they are told they have a deadly disease. And yet they are not just dying. They are living and growing, taking each day fully. They give me strength and hope. We face different forms of a similar challenge: to overcome the fear, the walls, the odds, to keep on keeping on; to know that life is what we make it and freedom starts with our choice to live each day on our own terms—fully, responsibly, with love, compassion, and connection to others.

—JUDY

RUMINATIONS

Today is a good day to die; my life is worth shit. A pill today, a liquid tomorrow. The only thing worth living for is my three stars, Meeghen, Alexandra, Isidro. Help! Stop the world I want to lay down. I want to bury my head. Help my suffering, help my pain. Give me the will to fight. It's a good day to die. . . . Maybe it's just a stage that I'm going through. I feel so useless to myself, I feel so sick of being sick.

Wait, footsteps, maybe someone is coming to say hello to me. Wrong again, just the plumbers. Better luck next time. Maybe I can find someone to talk to, but everyone says they are busy.

Can't eat, can't sleep, shake like a leaf. The best part of my day is mail. I hope that I get some today. I feel lost in space. I look at t.v., can't make out what I'm watching. No radio, no newspaper, no touch with the outside world. I went to mental health. They can't even help me. They sit there asking me, "How can I help you?" When I tell them what's bothering me, they ask me, "What do you think you should do?" If I was able to think it out, I would not need to go and see them.

Wait, I hear footsteps, it's the doctor. "Walters, your blood sugar came back 245. It's still high. We are going to try a new medication." Like always, I was waiting for that, another pill, just as I thought. My body belongs to the state, my mind belongs to—I don't even know who. My inner body belongs to medicine. A pill here, a pill there. Maybe they will run out of pills.

I look out the window, it's a gray Wednesday. Cold ice on the ground, the geese are gone, and the trees are bare. Everything is gloomy. The peace of mind that I search for can only come in the form of happiness with my children. That is what I long for.

Oh, how I could use a hug, a squeeze to let me know everything will be all right. Wait, footsteps. It's just the officer making rounds; almost time for her to leave. They come and go, and before you know, it's time for bed. Thank God we don't lock in, no telling what I would do then.

Five P.M., here comes a pill. Dinner sucks, veal patties, mashed potatoes, and beets. It maybe sounds good but it tastes bad. I guess I will cook something later. Maybe I can just starve to death. With my luck I will gain weight. My goodness, I can't believe this is me. I am actually letting all this out rather than not saying anything. Maybe there is hope.

Now what? Mail. A letter from my sister and father. I am looking forward to writing my sister back, but I can't do it tonight. I am feeling very tired. The doctor said I have gotten better since I have been here. He is right about that. I can breathe a little better, but other things don't look so good. My body is doing things I don't understand—swollen face, they called it moon face, skin is tightening, comes from the medication. I am starting to think properly. I don't really want to die, but I am so tired of being sick. But I'm doing the best I can with what I got. The love of God will see me through.

Wait, footsteps. Just the nurse wanting to collect spit.

Don't want to talk, eat, or look at TV or read. Don't want to feel, but pain always makes its way through. Just when you think you are free of it, here comes Mr. Pain, calling your name so soft and sweet. Wolves in Sheeps' clothing. Just as I thought, he brought company today, he brought Mr. Depression. They must walk hand in hand. Mr. Pain, you take him back and you stay with him. If only it was that easy!

I am smoking like a chimney, my lungs are already rotten, but that is my happiness. Makes me feel like I have control. I can light it, put it out, and best of all, it's mine. The state did not give me that. But I suffer. Not very smart, but just like in life, things that are no good for you, you always love the most.

Going back to sleep. Maybe I'll have nice dreams. Dream that everything is lovely, carefree, no bad times. Got to get it together. My stars need me. Be strong, stand up, fight back. Life is worth more than I realize.

Wait, footsteps. Happy day, an ACE member. Ethel and Lisa. I hate to be mean, but I don't want any company, don't want to be bothered. More footsteps—Cathy, Carmen, still don't want to be bothered. I am allowed to feel like this, these are my feelings, and at least I can have that. Wait, someone coming again. Romeo. Thank God, she won't take no. She stuck it out with my rudeness, my saying I don't want to be bothered, she stayed till I got up. Guess I'll take a shower and eat something.

Today is the first day of my life. Tomorrow is the first day of my life. I will take one day at a time, live each day like I want to be here tomorrow. Then I know I can make it.

—LESLIE

* * *

My name is Joanne. I am HIV-positive. When I first found out, I wanted to die. I did not want to deal with it at all. I felt that I had nothing to live for, not even my children. I didn't know anything about this disease until one day a friend spoke to me about it. I went to ACE, and it was there that I met Yolanda, an ACE civilian counselor. She told me a lot of things I needed to know about AIDS. My T-cell count was 414 at the time. I still did not really care about myself and went around telling everyone that I was HIV-positive. As a result, they laughed at me and talked bad about me, which made me feel terrible. I then met Wendy and some others at the ACE office. They spoke with me and that helped a lot. Wendy took the time not only to talk to me, but she accompanied me to the doctors. I realized that I have two children that need me, so I decided to fight back. My T cells are now 738, and my overall health is good.

Thanks to the women at ACE, I'm interested in taking care of myself and being there for my children. ACE has given me a lot of love and support. The worst part of this ordeal was when my family found out I was HIV-positive. They stopped coming to see me and would no longer accept phone calls from me. This hurt, because it was at this time that I needed them more than ever. The women at ACE took the place of my friends and family and showed me a lot of love. I will always be grateful and will never forget all they've done for me.

* * *

THE POINTERS and BILLY

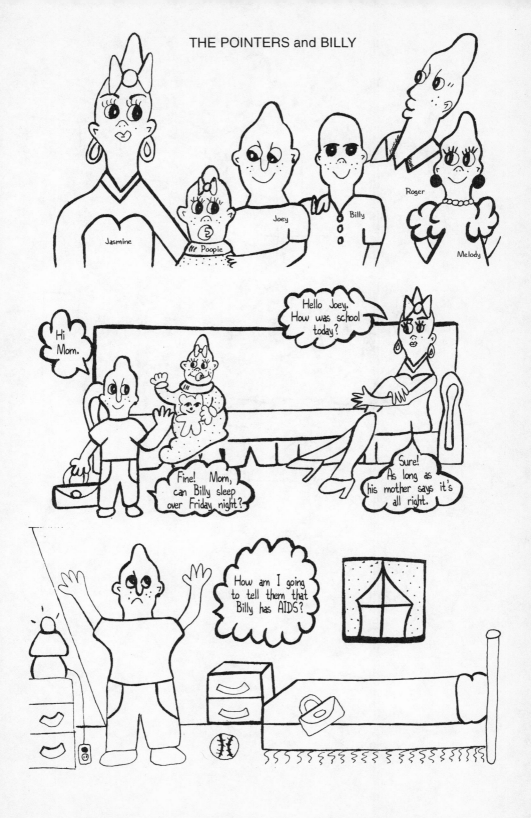

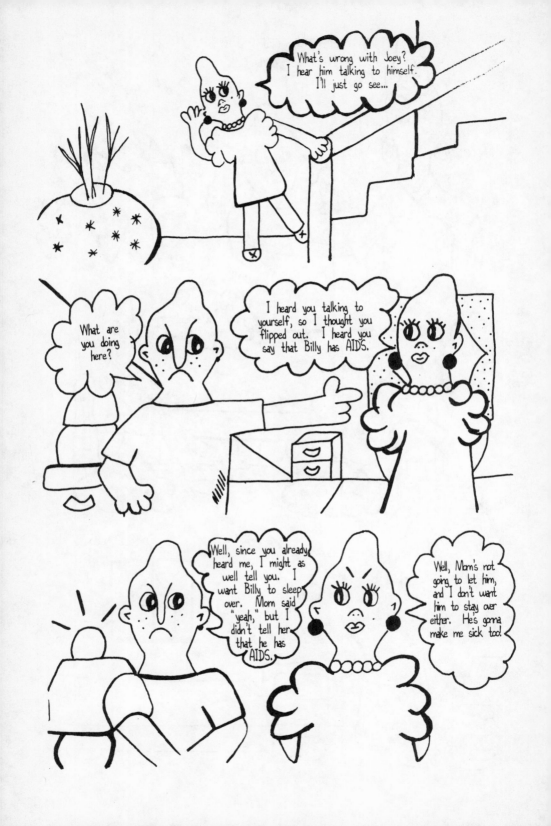

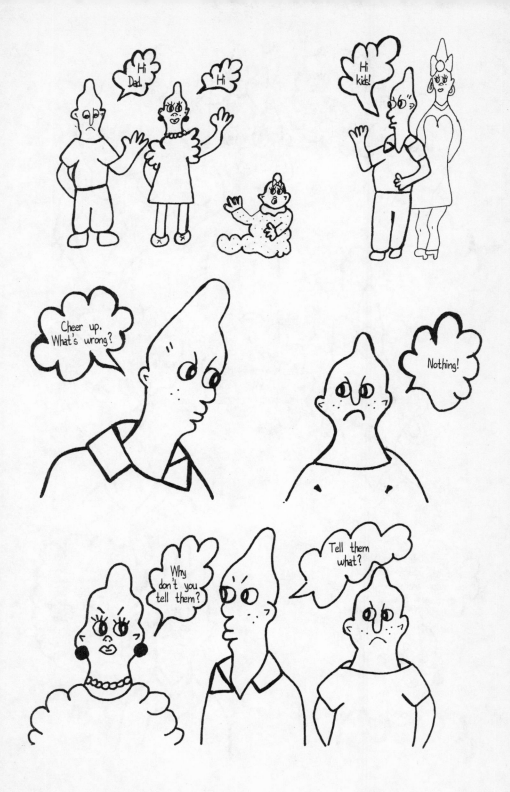

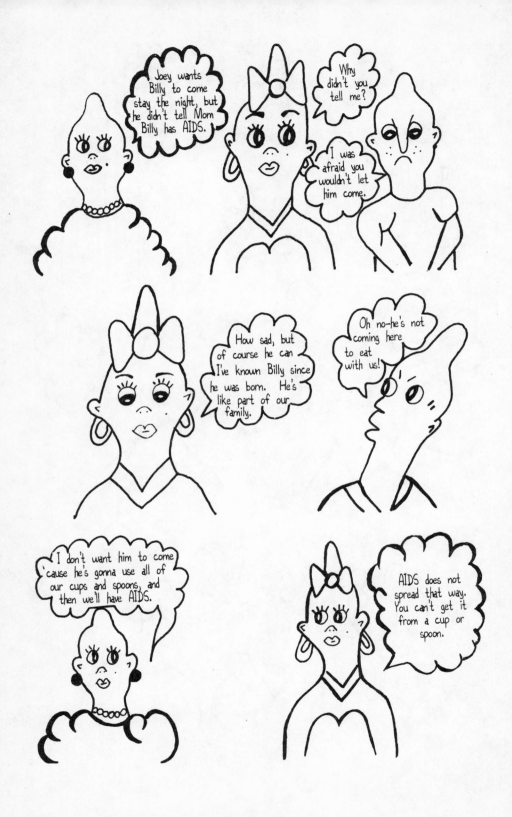

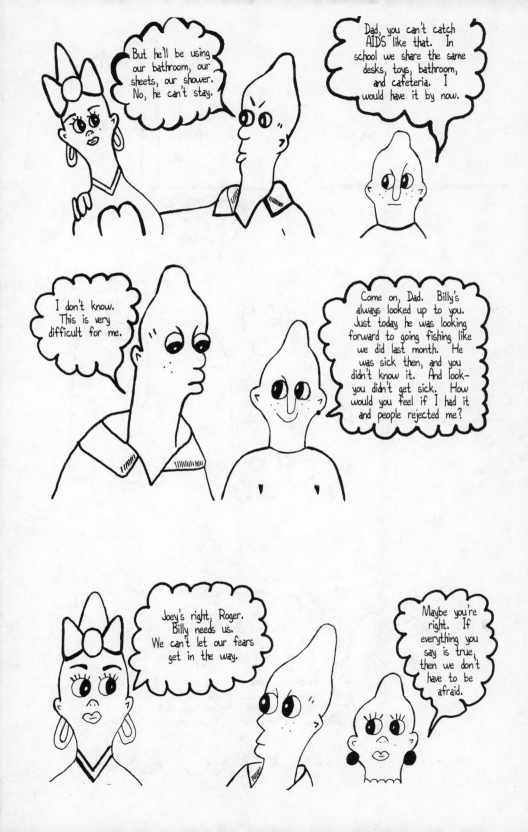

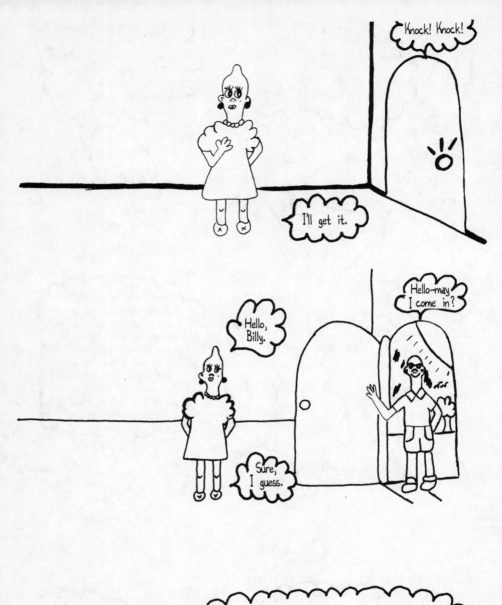
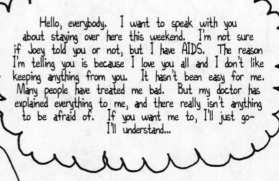

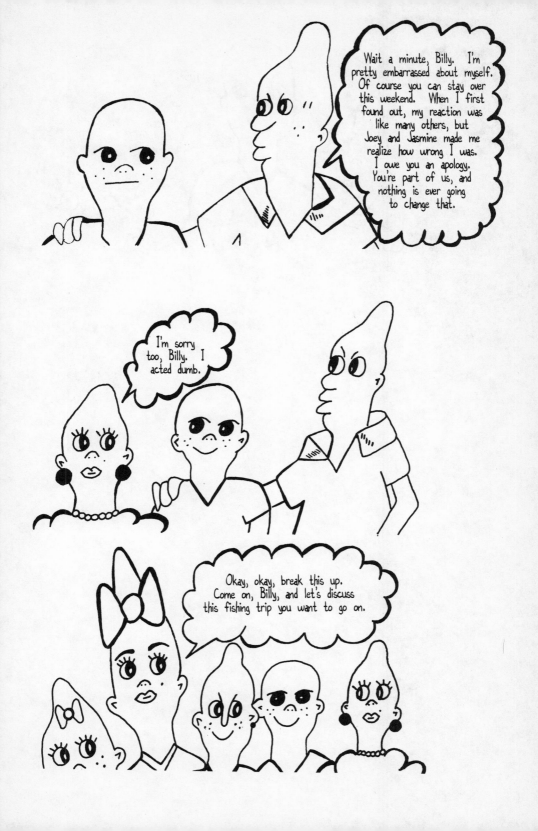

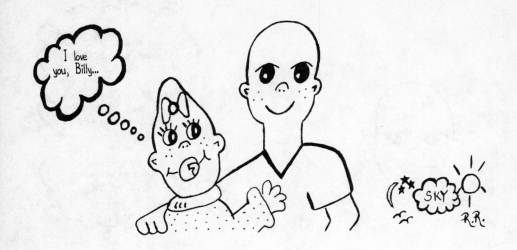

Appendixes

A
Sample Orientation

I am a member of ACE—AIDS Counseling and Education Program. I am here to share some things about AIDS and about ACE. Let me share with you something first about myself and what brought me to be standing before you today. [Give personal introduction.]

HIV/AIDS, as you probably know, is a very serious disease. At present there is no cure for it. So it is very important that you know how you can catch HIV/AIDS so that you can protect yourselves from getting it.

It is also very important to know how you *won't* catch HIV/AIDS, because a lot of unnecessary fear comes from not understanding this.

Fortunately, the HIV/AIDS virus is hard to catch:

- You cannot get HIV/AIDS by hugging, shaking hands, or simply being near a person who is infected with the virus.
- You cannot catch HIV/AIDS by sharing a shower, from eating next to someone in the cafeteria, from sharing a toilet seat, from watching TV with someone in the rec room, from sharing the kitchen, from sharing washing machines.

These are all things that we do in this facility, since we have to share a lot of things.

How do we know for sure that you cannot get HIV/AIDS from the kind of casual contact described in these examples? We know this because the HIV/AIDS disease has been carefully watched by scientists and doctors, and studies have been done and there is not a single case of casual contact that has been recorded.

There are three main ways in which you can get the HIV/AIDS virus:

1. Having sex with an infected person.
2. Sharing IV drug needles and syringes with IV drug users.
3. Babies can be born with the virus if the mother has been infected.

It is important to maintain personal hygiene to protect our health against many different infections. In an institutional setting such as this, where we live closely with many people, personal hygiene is especially important.

One of the issues on many people's minds is whether or not to take the HIV-antibody test, which tells you whether or not you are infected with the virus. The test is available here at Bedford Hills and at other correctional facilities in New York. Deciding whether or not to take the test is a very personal issue, and you should have counseling before you take that test. Both counseling and confidentiality about test results are part of the facility policy. If you want the test, you go to a nurse's screening as the first step and request it. From there you will see a doctor, who will discuss it with you. If you are going to take it, then you will have counseling before any further steps are taken.

What we have said is only a brief introduction to the many issues surrounding HIV/AIDS. There are different kinds of issues that women here face related to HIV/AIDS, in addition to how to protect ourselves from getting HIV/AIDS.

Some women are HIV-positive HIV symptomatic or have AIDS and need ongoing support. They want to discuss issues such as sexual relations, talking to children and families, and the effect of being HIV-positive on future pregnancies. Many women here are in the high-risk category for HIV/AIDS because of IV drug use, and they are trying to decide whether or not to take the HIV-antibody test. Women are feeling the impact of HIV/AIDS on their loved ones. Women need comfort themselves and need advice on how to give comfort to others.

Over the coming months, there will be different opportunities in the facility to deal with these issues, and you will hear about them through announcements on your living units or through programs. Speakers come; videos are shown in different programs; HIV/AIDS community groups are interested in the facility. You can write to the Office of Mental Health (OMH) to see a psychologist.

ACE is an inmate organization that was formed to help work on HIV/AIDS-related issues. Some of our work up to this time has included:

1. Going through an education process ourselves with doctors, nurses, and social workers on how to help others and ourselves deal with the HIV/AIDS epidemic.
2. Sharing this information and supporting people through informal discussions wherever we see you: on the units, in the yard, in school, on the café lines, and so on.
3. Putting on seminars in the classrooms and in other programs about HIV/AIDS-related issues; we run a nine-session workshop series for people who want to learn more about HIV/AIDS.
4. Spending time in the hospital unit with women who are sick.

If you have personal questions that you would like to talk about with an ACE member, put your name on this form and give it back to us and one of us will call you to the ACE Center to speak with you privately.

In addition to the above orientation, we usually show a video that relates to AIDS.

B
Outline of Seminar

1. *Introduction to the seminar*

We are here from ACE, HIV/AIDS Counseling and Education. We are a group of inmates who are dedicated to doing something about the crisis of HIV/AIDS in our community. And we want to talk with you about this crisis, share information, do role-plays with you, and talk about what it means to be living with HIV/AIDS, which in different ways we all are.

HIV/AIDS is a new disease. Scientists are still learning about it; statistics are still being gathered to understand it. A lot is still not known. Yet some things are known. We want to try to be clear with you about what is known for sure and also to be clear about where the doctors and scientists are not sure. As we will see, there are areas of uncertainty. This means that each of us is faced with difficult choices. We hope that this seminar will clarify what these choices are and begin to give you the tools for making choices.

Finally, who are we? We are not experts. We have been through a training and learning process with professionals about HIV/AIDS, and we have studied. However, we are committed to being able to say to your questions, "I don't know the answer to that, but I'll try to find out the answer." And that way we will be maintaining a spirit of accuracy and honesty as we all learn together through this process. We are prisoners, like yourselves. It has taken a long process to get to the point of being able to stand here and do this work, and yet there is so much to do if we are going to save the lives of ourselves and families and friends and give comfort to those who are already suffering. What we want to do today is work together to deal with the problems that HIV/AIDS has brought on us.

2. *Personal introductions*
Each of the ACE members then gives a short personal statement about what it is in her own life that brought her to want to do work around HIV/AIDS.

3. *How you don't get HIV/AIDS: Discussion on casual contact*
Present information through questions, answers, and discussion. Use role-play on casual contact and stigma.

a. Joni is cooking broccoli on the living unit and her friends Anna and Sue come over. Anna says that the food looks great. Sue pulls Anna aside and tells her not to eat that food because Joni has HIV/AIDS. Anna and Sue and Joni struggle over whether or not you can get HIV from food and discuss stigma.

b. Janis sees her shirt on her friend Doris. She is irritated that Doris is wearing her shirt. Even though they are good friends and Janis accepts the fact that Doris is HIV-positive, she calls Doris "an AIDS-ridden bitch." Wanda hears it and gets into the discussion, and struggles about stigma.

4. *Sexual transmission: Woman and man*
- Open with a role-play by presenters: Mona is talking to her friend Judy and tells her she finally has a date with a guy she has liked. Judy tries to raise the issue of using a condom. Mona says that he looks fine, he couldn't have HIV/AIDS, and raising the issue of a condom will end their relationship before it starts. It ends unresolved.
- Present information about sexual transmission.
- Do role-play in which you ask for audience participation:
    Sylvia is home after being in prison for five years. She and her man, Eddie, are alone at night getting ready to go to bed. Sylvia has attended discussions on HIV/AIDS in prison and tries to get Eddie to use a condom. Eddie doesn't want to.
- Brainstorm discussion: What are the reasons that men don't want to use condoms or that it is difficult for a woman to ask a man to use a condom?

5. *Sexual transmission: Woman and woman*
- Present information about woman-to-woman transmission through questions, presentation, and information.
- Do role-play on negotiating safe sex between two women.

    a. Juana and Marie have been in a relationship and Juana has just found out that she is HIV-positive. She tells Marie. Marie says she wants to end the relationship. Juana struggles with her to explore possibilities of safe sex.

    b. An alternative is: Marie says she doesn't believe that women can get the virus from another woman and doesn't want to discuss safe sex, and Juana struggles with her to talk about changing their behavior.

6. *Drugs and HIV transmission*
- Present information on IV drugs and HIV transmission.
- Present information on how crack, coke, and other non-IV drugs impair judgment and affect HIV transmission.
- Do a role-play in which two people are getting high and one is cleaning the works with bleach and water and the other is telling her to forget it.
- Brainstorm: Will people using drugs really take the time to do safety measures when using IV drugs?

7. *Testing*
- Present information about the HIV-antibody test, including the process by which people get the test in this facility.
- Brainstorm: What are the reasons people might want to take the test and what are the reasons people might not want to take the test?

8. *Living with HIV/AIDS: A PWA talks about living with HIV/AIDS*

9. *Singing the song "Sister"*
As a group we stand and hold hands and sing. After singing we hand out a form for people to sign if they want to be called to talk at a later time about personal questions.

C
Four Teaching Plans for Women and Our Bodies Workshops

WORKSHOP #1: KNOWING OUR BODIES

I. Introduction to Workshop: Role-Play

A woman visits her GYN doctor, who talks to her about problems located either on her cervix or in her ovarian tubes. She listens to the doctor, but when she goes back to tell a friend about the visit, it is clear that she doesn't understand what those words refer to or what is wrong with her.

Ask participants if they have ever had such an experience and, if they have, if they would like to describe it.

II. Learning About the Anatomy of Women

A. Discussion: Put up large-scale drawings of the sexual parts of a woman's body. Ask participants what names they use for each part. Write these down on newsprint.

B. Presentation:

1. The outside and inside sexual parts of a woman's body.

2. The reproductive parts of a woman's body.

Discuss the scientific names of each part; show where they are located; discuss what the function of each part is.

III. Discussion on Attitudes and Feelings Toward Our Bodies, Focusing on the Following Issues:

- Where did we learn about our bodies? When? From whom, if ever?
- What did we know before the workshop?

- How do we feel about knowing? Would we rather not know?
- Why do so many of us not know about our bodies, or even feel uncomfortable talking about them?
- Our children: Should we be teaching them? What should we be teaching them and at what ages?

WORKSHOP #2: THE MENSTRUAL CYCLE

I. A Scientific Presentation of the Menstrual Cycle
   A. Ask participants what they know about menstruation.

- Why do we bleed?
- When does the egg come out?
- When is the best time to get pregnant?
- Where does the egg get fertilized by the sperm?

B. Build from the information that the participants contribute. Fill in the missing or incorrect information. Use large pictures of the ovaries and fallopian tubes.

II. Discussion of Our Personal Experiences in First Getting Our Menstruation

- When did we first get it?
- Do we feel inadequate because someone else got it first?
- What are early experiences with it (embarrassing situations, feelings, etc.)?
- Who told us about it (friends, family, advertising, lovers, books, films, teachers, nurses, doctors)?
- What did we know about our period before we got it
- How did other people react when we got our period (mother, father, boys, teacher, etc.)?
- Were we afraid of the blood?

III. Discussion: What Are the Main Symptoms that Women Get from Their Period?
Discuss each symptom and any others that the participants name.

IV. Home Remedies

- Ask if women have home remedies for different symptoms.
- Present home remedies.

V. Discussion: Explore Feelings About Our Menstruation

- What words do we use for it?
- Do we know jokes about it?
- How do we feel about our menstruation (for example, we hate it, it makes us feel like a woman, other feelings)?

VI. Discussion: Different Social or Cultural Attitudes Toward Menstruation

- Ask participants how their family or culture views women who are menstruating.
- Describe how some cultures have isolated women entirely or put them only in the company of other women during their menstruation because people have thought menstrual blood is "unclean." Other cultures have thought menstruation gives women supernatural powers, which are sometimes good but more often destructive.
- Society frequently views women as less stable than men, using the menstrual cycle as evidence. What do you think about that?

VII. Menopause
A. Presentation: The biological process of menopause
B. Discussion: How do participants feel about menopause?

WORKSHOP #3: SEXUALLY TRANSMITTED DISEASES (STDS)

I. Role-Plays
   1. Showing Stigma: Two women are talking *sympathetically* about someone who got hurt while cutting food with a can top. A third woman comes and begins talking with *disgust* about a person with herpes, and all three of them act very disgusted.
   2. Showing Embarrassment: A man and woman accuse each other of having sex with someone else because both of them have a discharge, but the woman does not want to go to the doctor—she is ashamed.

Ask participants if they identify with either role-play and, if so, with which person. Ask if they want to share their experience.

II. General Discussion of STDs
1. Presentation of General Characteristics of STDs:
a. Definition of STD.
b. How STDs are spread.
c. How STDs are *not* spread.
d. How widespread is the problem?

III. Presentation of Main STDs
(Presented in related groupings)

IV. Prevention

V. Experiences
a. What are your experiences with STDS?
b. How did you feel about yourself?
c. Did you go to a doctor right away, or did you wait before going?
d. Have you ever tried to talk to a partner about an STD, and what was it like?
e. Have you ever discovered that your partner had a discharge, and how did you react?

WORKSHOP #4: CHOICES

I. Introduction: Define the issues that the workshop will cover: the focus is contraception options and related issues. The topic of birth control also relates to issues of protection against sexually transmitted diseases, HIV/AIDS, issues of decision making, and power in relationships between men and women.

II. Review the Process of Conception
Ask participants to describe what they know about the process of conception. Use large drawings to fill in their descriptions.

III. Discussion: Ask participants the following questions to explore their personal experiences with different types of contraception.

1. What type(s) of birth control did you use?
2. For what reasons did you use that particular type?
3. How did you feel about it—its pros and cons?

4. How effective was it?
5. Where did you learn about it?

IV. Presentation: Review each type of birth control method, discussing its effectiveness in terms of pregnancy and STDs and HIV/AIDS; also discuss its strengths and weaknesses in terms of sex and interpersonal dynamics between men and women.

V. Final Discussion: What are some of the factors that make it difficult for us as women to use or to determine birth control types that we use? Ask participants if they identify with any of the following reactions:

- We are embarrassed by, ashamed of, or confused about our own sexuality.
- We cannot admit we might have or are having intercourse because we feel (or someone told us) it is wrong.
- We are unrealistically romantic about sex; sex has to be spontaneous, and birth control takes that away.
- Birth control is too messy.
- We feel we might displease our partner.
- We don't recognize how much we don't like using the method we are using and we begin to use it carelessly.
- We feel tempted to become pregnant in order to prove we are fertile or to hold together a shaky relationship, or we want a baby so that we will have someone to care for.

D
Medical Advocacy Forms

AUTHORIZATION TO RELEASE
MEDICAL INFORMATION

On this _____ day of _____, 19_____, I, _____,
authorize _____ to be present during my medical interview (or
visit). I also authorize Dr. _____ to discuss my medical status in
front of this person. There will _____ will not _____ be limitations on
information allowed to be disclosed (specify below if limitations exist.)

I am requesting:

_____
SIGNATURE   DIN #

_____
PEER SUPPORT PERSON   DATE

_____
PHYSICIAN

Comment: _____

_____

_____

_____

DATE _____

PERMISSION TO UTILIZE THE ACE BUDDY SYSTEM

I, _____, wish to use ACE's Buddy System while I wait for my HIV-antibody test result.

NAME _____   # _____

UNIT _____   DATE _____

Please send to: ACE Coordinator

The Buddy System will aid the individual by providing the following:

- Ongoing confidential counseling (if desired).
- Up-to-date AIDS information.
- HIV/AIDS education materials (brochures, books, videos).
- A buddy that will be there to talk to you, to listen to your fears, and to answer your questions.
- A buddy who will accompany you, if you wish, to receive your test results.
- A buddy to help you get through the period between the actual test and the test results.
- A buddy who can remain your buddy regardless of your results, for as long as you wish.

E
Our Most Commonly Asked Questions

1. Q. Do you have to die if you're HIV-infected?

A. To say you will definitely live or definitely die would be misleading you. It would be an inaccurate answer to this question. As we know, many people have died from this virus, but there are also many people who are still living after ten years of infection. It is a fact that taking care of yourself—taking medication, eating properly, and feeling mentally secure—will help your immune system stay strong and able to fight off infections longer. If we're infected with the HIV virus, we must have *hope,* that a vaccine or other medicines will be discovered. And that *hope* will enable us to live longer.

2. Q. Where did AIDS come from?

A. No one knows where AIDS came from. Just as still no one knows where syphilis came from. However, there are a few theories. One theory is that the virus existed in an isolated ethnic group that had a natural protection against it. When some of the people moved to different areas, the virus spread either through sex or blood transfusions. People who were not immune to the virus became infected, and the virus began to spread. A second theory is that AIDS came from animals and perhaps the virus mutated when it infected human beings. A third theory is that HIV is a manmade virus, perhaps from a germ warfare laboratory. There are also people who believe that it was a punishment by God for homosexual behavior.

3. Q. Can someone be exposed to the virus and not get infected?

A. Yes! You can be exposed and not get infected, just as you can be exposed to other germs or viruses and not get sick.

4. Q. Can a person with no symptoms transmit the HIV virus?

A. Initially, most HIV-infected people have no symptoms and are not even aware they are infected. Any infected person can transmit the virus to another person through sexual contact or sharing drug-injection equipment.

5. Q. How soon after becoming infected with the HIV virus do antibodies develop?

A. Most people infected with the HIV develop antibodies to the virus within three to six months, but it has also been known to take up to several years for antibodies to develop. And in some exceptional cases, they never develop. However, there is a test that looks for the virus instead of the antibodies to determine if someone has HIV, but it is not entirely accurate and it is extremely expensive. It is called the PCR (polymerase chain reaction) test.

6. Q. How will I feel if I have the virus in me?

A. When someone gets infected with the HIV virus, it depends on each individual's immune system what the length of time is until symptoms appear. It has been known for someone who is infected with the virus to have no symptoms for up to ten years. On the other hand, someone else may get symptoms within six months of infection. Some of the symptoms that someone can look for include fatigue, swollen glands, unexplained weight loss, fever, diarrhea that lasts for many weeks, night sweats, continuing vaginal infections. But each of these symptoms could also be due to other illnesses. If they persist for weeks, you should see your doctor.

7. Q. Can a woman pass the HIV virus by having sexual contact with another woman?

A. It is a possibility, because the virus is in the woman's sexual fluids and in her menstrual blood. The fact is, there are not many studies done on woman-to-woman transmission, and therefore we do not know how often it has occurred and how likely it is to happen.

8. Q. Can HIV be transmitted through oral/genital sex?

A. A few people have become infected with HIV through oral sex. Infected semen, blood, or vaginal secretions in the mouth could transmit HIV through small cuts, canker sores, blisters, STDs (sexually transmitted diseases), or microscopic cuts that come from toothbrushing.

9. Q. How do children get AIDS?

A. The majority of HIV-infected children got the virus from their HIV-infected mother, presumably through blood exchange in the uterus or during birth. Studies indicate that in the United States, 20 to 30 percent of mothers who are HIV-positive pass the virus to their babies. An infected mother can transmit the virus even if she herself has no symptoms. HIV antibodies have been detected in breast milk. There have been a few cases of AIDS that may have been transmitted to infants through their mother's milk.

* * *

Your group may want to develop its own list of most commonly asked questions and answers, to help you reach out to your community.[1]

---

1. The background material for each of these workshops can be found in *The New Our Bodies, Ourselves,* by the Boston Women's Health Book Collective (New York: Simon & Schuster, 1992).

Glossary

MEDICAL TERMS

Attends Incontinence pads (like diapers) for adults.

M/11/Q A medical form needed for HIV-positive people to receive benefits. A history of the illnesses that a woman may have while HIV-positive. It accompanies them when they go home, so that they will have fewer difficulties when they go to get medical help after their release.

PAWA (Person Affected With Aids) A person who is affected by AIDS in some shape, form, or fashion. The person doesn't necessarily have to be HIV-positive.

PWA A person living with HIV/AIDS. Many people who are HIV-positive have preferred to define themselves with this term, because it has come to convey dignity and initiative, as opposed to terms such as "AIDS victim" or "AIDS carrier," which convey either passivity or a negative attitude.

ROM Range-of-movement exercises, done as physical therapy for patients on bed rest to maintain muscle tone.

Sputum test A test on the saliva or mucus in the mouth to detect active TB.

PRISON TERMS

Administration The "Executive Body," which is in charge of the overall running of the facility. This is made up of the superintendent and several deputy superintendents.

Back buildings Two dormitory buildings situated in the back of the facility, usually housing women who are in transition from one facility to another.

Board Parole Board—the committee that after an interview and review of all records concerning an inmate will decide whether or not to release the individual to parole status.

Bubble An elevated platform with Plexiglas partitions. It is the station where the correctional officer is posted on a living unit, from which the officer can view the entire living unit.

Call-out A daily listing of doctor appointments and other appointments and activities within the facility, distributed to all living units and program areas within the prison.

Civilian A person who works in the facility who is neither a uniformed officer nor an inmate (for example, teacher, volunteer, or counselor).

C.O. Correctional officer/prison guard—one who is responsible for ensuring the care, custody, and control of inmates.

Disbursement The financial system that handles inmate funds, similar in operation to a checking account. Through disbursements inmates can purchase things from the outside or inside the facility or send money out to relatives. This is used because inmates are not allowed to handle money and to do so would result in punishment.

DOCS Department of Correctional Services.

Draft The transfer of a prisoner from one facility to another. Drafts usually take place on short notice—for example, an inmate is told she is leaving the day before she is put on the bus.

East Wing A living unit that houses women who are unable to live in general population, either because of a chronic prolonged illness, a handicap, a disability, or an advanced pregnancy.

Furlough A temporary release from the facility for three to seven days to seek employment, or to help reconstruct and strengthen family ties.

Hospital 1 The Bedford Hill Correctional Facility medical clinic and infirmary. Outpatient medical service unit.

Inmate A person confined to a county jail or state or federal prison.

Inmate Liaison Committee (ILC) A group of inmates elected by general population to be representatives for inmate needs and concerns. It meets regularly with the administration.

Inside pharmacy Disburses the medication that is sent from the outside pharmacy to the women.

IPC (In-Patient-Care unit) The infirmary at Bedford for those who are ill or have come from the outside hospital and need observation for twenty-four to seventy-two hours.

Keeplock Confinement to one's cell, as punishment, for twenty-three hours a day. An hour is allotted the inmate for a shower, phone calls, and recreation.

Misbehavior Report/Charge Sheet/Ticket A form charging an inmate with breaking a facility rule, usually filled out by a corrections officer, and leading to a disciplinary hearing. If a finding of guilt is made, a punishment is imposed.

Module/Program A work or educational assignment that one is assigned to go to, lasting approximately three hours. Once assigned, one must go or a misbehavior report will be written. An inmate's day is divided into four modules: morning (8:30 to 11:00), early afternoon (1:00 to 3:30), late afternoon (3:30 to 5:00), and evening (6:00 to 9:30).

Nursery The living unit where the women who have children are allowed to live with their children as a privilege. It is a program for inmates who will give birth while incarcerated. Pregnant women can apply and, if accepted, can live on the nursery with their infants until the baby is a year old.

Nurse's Screening (Sick-Call clinic) A prerequisite to seeing the doctor. A person signs up to see a nurse and tells her/him what the medical problem is, and she/he schedules a time to see the doctor.

On the chow "Meal is called."

On the floor On the living unit.

On the street In the community as opposed to being incarcerated (is usually used when talking about someone who was released from prison or about life as it was lived outside of a prison).

Outside hospital The community hospital outside of the prison that the women go to when they are seriously ill or need hospitalization.

Outside pharmacy The pharmaceutical company that fills the prescriptions for the women in the facility.

Parole Release from prison before the completion of one's maximum sentence, with the requirement that the former prisoner report to a parole officer. For example, in New York State, if a prisoner has a sentence of 8-½ to twenty-five years, she *must* do at least 8-½ years and then she can be paroled. But she will have to report to her parole officer for a period of up to 25 years, unless her parole time is cut short.

Population (General Population) Where the majority of the inmate population is, where one can interact with others—the regular housing units of the prison (as opposed to East Wing, West Wing, SHU, etc.).

Role-Play A play that is very short that usually depicts a realistic situation. A skit.

Satellite The Crisis Observation Unit in Mental Health where one would go if one suffered from a short-term mental problem (severe depression, suicidal thoughts).

Security The personnel responsible for the security operations in the facility. Uniformed DOCS employees, consisting of corrections officers, sergeants, lieutenants, captains, and the deputy superintendent for security.

SHU (Special Housing Unit) A solitary-confinement unit where all of the individuals are keeplocked for more than a few days. Being confined to this unit is thought of as the ultimate of all punishments and is usually for those who are thought of as disciplinary problems.

Sign-up sheet A sheet that one would sign to participate in an activity.

Superintendent The warden of the prison.

TRC (Temporary Release Committee) A committee that reviews records and interviews inmates, that decides whether or not to allow the inmate to participate on work release or furloughs.

Tunnel A ground-floor corridor that links the three main housing units. The mess hall and many programs are located along the tunnel areas.

Violate To break a rule in the facility.

West Wing A housing unit for those who are unable to live in general population because of chronic mental illness.

Work Release A program where one can go to work during the day and return to the facility at night. Work release operates out of medium- and minimum-security facilities and is not available at Bedford Hills. The participants in the program are allowed to go on furloughs as well to help strengthen family ties.

WPA (Women's Prison Association) A not-for-profit agency founded in 1844 that provides direct services and advocacy for women in the criminal justice system from arrest through release, and is active in matters of public policy at the local, state, and national levels.

Afterword

The creation of ACE Home came out of the need for a bridge for women going home who are PWAs. The need for support for HIV-positive women who are coming out of prison is greater than ever. In the last decade, the prison population has doubled; the number of incarcerated women has multiplied by *five* times! It is overwhelming to contemplate the suffering that the data suggests: 80 percent of these women are mothers, 80 percent have drug problems, 80 percent have been victims of family violence, at least 30 percent are homeless, and over 25 percent are HIV-positive.

Behind these grim statistics is a tragically familiar pattern. Women use drugs and alcohol to escape the feelings of pain, rage, and helplessness that result from the abuse and violence that they experience. Their lifestyle puts them at a high risk of becoming infected with the HIV virus. They get into trouble for behavior associated with substance abuse or in response to family violence. Meanwhile, the children end up being raised by relatives or in the foster care system. The cycle goes on.

It seems to be a law of the universe, however, that people are remarkably resilient and resourceful. It is this transformational spirit that finds expression in ACE and ACE Home. There, women are discovering themselves and their power through service to others.

When this manuscript went to the publisher, the Women's Prison Association (WPA) celebrated a year of collaboration with the women of ACE. We are proud to have been able to help with the birthing of ACE Home, the community chapter of ACE, and the publication of this book.

WPA has a 150-year tradition of serving women in the criminal justice system. From our origin in 1844, WPA emphasized housing and transitional services, establishing the first halfway house and vocational training program for women in the country. We now work with women in prison to help them prepare for their release. When they are released, we aid in the transition to independent living. We also strive to keep women out of prison in the first place.

It is a privilege for me, as someone who has worked in criminal justice for twenty years, to be in a partnership with the women we seek to serve. I learn much more than I teach. I am honored by my evolving relationships with so many committed women. I am moved by their vitality, courage, and vision.

And sometimes the collaboration is very hard. I never get used to being inside correctional facilities. I am always glad to leave. I am also sad to leave the women behind. It is similarly hard to hear realities of the women living in the community. Few have adequate food and clothing, shelter, and, rewarding work. They struggle getting through each day.

I see the struggle with their own health, and together we watch the deterioration of some of our sisters. Sometimes a woman dies. I don't know what to say or how to be supportive. I worry that they will not be able to maintain the momentum of their work—even that working hard may kill them sooner.

And I watch *them* worry. Sometimes they question whether they can deliver on their promises. They periodically get on each other's nerves. It looks as if they will self-destruct. And then, the breakdown leads to breakthrough. They end up making a quantum leap. That's where we are now. Both ACE and ACE Home can take great pride and satisfaction in what they've accomplished and in the future work that they have outlined for themselves.

Besides thanking the women of ACE and ACE Home for their partnership, I would like to acknowledge some of the others who have contributed to our collaboration: Terri Wurmser, for first introducing ACE and WPA; Superintendent Elaine Lord, for everything she did to enable WPA and ACE to work together; Deb Levine, for her considerable talents and for her commitment that this book would get published; and the Daniel and Florence Guggenheim Foundation and New York Women's Foundation for their generous support of parts of the work.

—ANN L. JACOBS
Executive Director
Women's Prison Association
New York, New York
1996

A c k n o w l e d g m e n t s

Breaking the Walls of Silence is the story of women and their commitment to cope with the AIDS epidemic. This story includes many women who are living with HIV/AIDS and many who have died. And it is a story which was written by the day-to-day caring of women who have been at the Bedford Hills Correctional Facility. Hundreds of women have been a part of ACE—and many hundred others have been a part of the broader community of caring for their sisters, either through helping programs of ACE or acting individually to support those in need. We want to acknowledge you.

There is no single list. Our collective memory cannot possibly remember each person in order to acknowledge each by name; nor are we able to get the necessary permission to publish your names. We are going to acknowledge some of the women who have been part of this effort and whose commitment and work give life to the pages of this book. Those of you whose names are not written on these pages, know that you have also written in real life the story of a community of women who took care of one another when faced by the AIDS epidemic. We acknowledge all of you.

The founding collective that brought ACE into existence: January, 1988:

Rosa Barbot; Kathy Boudin; Judith Clark; Diane Gooch; Arlene Mohammed; Marilyn T.J. Rivera.

The following women came forward to create the ACE organization in March of 1988 out of their commitment to break the silence in the Bedford Hills Correctional Facility:

Lori Addante; Rosa Barbot; Giovanni Baez; Blackie; Kathy Boudin; Michelle Colon; Jane Davis; Francis Caro Franco; Diane Gooch; Katrina Haslip; Rachel Luna; Joanne (Jay) Minor; Arlene Mohammed; Sylvia Nadal; Sonia Perez; Maria Ramos; Aida Rivera; Marilyn T.J. Rivera; Ruth Rodriguez; Carmen Royster; Mary Robinson; Tiffany Robinson; Gloria Rubero, Cathy Salce; Renee Scott; Shorty; Linda Smith; Sheryl Sohn; Janice Watkins.

The core group that acted as steering committee from March 1988 to March 1990 until ACE had an office and an inmate staff

Kathy Boudin; Judith Clark; Katrina Haslip; Aida Rivera; Mary Robinson; Carmen Royster.

ACE has been driven by an empowerment process of women, prisoners and, in particular, PWA's—prisoners with HIV/AIDS. We want to acknowledge those PWA's who, through their willingness to break the silence, moved—and continue to move—all of us forward.

Sonia Perez	Pat C.	Vanessa Morgan
Carmen Royster	Vivian M.	Fayetta G.
Blackie	Carmen A.	Luz
Jane Davis	Tiffany Robinson	Linda J.
Rosa Barbot	Mary Robinson	Wilma
Katrina Haslip	Xiomara Rubin	Terry Krum
Black	Angelina S.	Jeweline
Cynthia Rhodes	Nancy Ayala	Frenchie Laugier
Renee Scott	Priscilla Gittens	Joanne Brown
Doris Moices	Lee	Migna
Deborah Denardo	Laura Sudol	Nancy P.
Gloria Boyd	Denise Huggins	Sonia Diaz (Scooby)
Scottie	Viniece Walker	Francine Rodriguez
Bessie Mejias	Diane Smith	
Joanne Taubenkraut	Amina	

ACE Staff Workers: 1990-1997

Marleny Agero; Nancy Ayala; Kathy Boudin; Denise Bush; Pamela J. Chase; Judith Clark; Tiffany Collins; Loyda Diaz; Gloria Edwards; Rosa Filipe; Lisa Gail Finkle; Bonnie Forant; Frenchie Laugier; Awilda Gonzalez; Mona Graves; Priscilla Gittens; Fayetta G.; Katrina Haslip; Maria Hernandez; Carol Jones; Debra Irving; Rachel Luna; Sherri Martindale; Migdalia Martinez; Dory Medina; Arlene Mohammed; Doris Romeo; Doris Moices; Lisa Osborne; Sandra Ospina; Judy Perez; Sonia Perez; Sharon Richardson; Ruthie Rodriguez; Xiomara Rubin; Cathy Salce; Angelina S.; Ethel Scarpulla; Jenny Serrano; Diane Smith; Betty Tyson, Pearl Ward, Viniece Walker; Patricia Zimmerman.

Past and present members of the ACE organization who are currently at the Bedford Hills Correctional Facility

Violeta Acevedo, Esperanza Acosta; Lori Addante; Marleny Agero; Adelaide Alvarez; Yerly Andrade; Ana; Fatimah Basir; Precious Bedell; Donna Bell; June Benson; Yuly Blanco; Kathy Boudin; Leah Bundy; Toni Bundy; Gloria Burns; Milanesa Cardenes; Martha Carillo; Wendy Centeno; Elsa Cuadrado; Donna Charles; Cheryl Christenson, Judith Clark; Juanita Cotto; Rosalie Cutting; Donna; Karen T. Ely; Urbelina Emiliano; Rosa Felipe; Lisa Gail Finkle; Joan Fiumfreddo; Elisia (Lisa) Fomines; Cherie Gallipoli-Alzate; Paula Germano; Debra Gore; Maria Grana; Mona Graves; Rebecca Groom; Tashaunia Guillary; Darlena Harris; Shirelle Howard; Donna Hylton; Patsy Kelly Jarrett; Marie La Pinta; Lena Leonor; Nancy Lopez; Amy Mackson; Sherri Martindale; Migdalia Martinez; Cathy Migliore; Claude Millery; Joanne (Jay) Minor; Arlene Mohammed; Alyda Montoya; Sara Munoz; Virginia Lasooki-Nepa; Iris Nerys; Susan O'Connell.; Melita Oliveira; Elice Orichello; Reyna Ortega; Sandra Ospina; Melba Padilla; Nicole 'Nikki' Pappas; Esperanza Patino; Carol Patterson; Frances Perez; Miriam Polanco; Selma Price; Maria Ramos; Sharon Richardson; Diana Rodriguez; Francine Rodriguez; Linda Rodriguez; Doris Romeo; Gloria Rubero; Maria Ruiz; Kym Rusk; Mildred Santiago; Sheryl; Shorty; Diane Smith; Roslyn Smith; Wendy Bummer Smythe; Sheryl Sohn; Denise Solla; Speed; Carol Taylor; Ann Marie Truscio; Joann Tulko; Betty Tyson; Valerie; Ada Velasquez; Gina Velasquez; Elena Vento; Viniece Walker; Jan Warren; Joy Wosu.

We want to also acknowledge

The following ACE Coordinators who have given of themselves to ACE: Marie St. Cyr; Suzanne Kessler; Jacquelyn McDonald; Sylvia Samilton-Baker; Liz Mastroieni; and the civilian advisers who volunteered to work with ACE before the formal contract existed: Dr. Keats; Rose Palladino.

The following civilian counselors who have counseled and helped to heal: Agnes Alvarez; Dee Holmes; Linda Malmberg; Yolanda Rosado; Maria Cerletti; Marcy Feltman; Dora Lisa Goitia; Kiesha Simon; Mindy Venetek.

The New York State Department of Health AIDS Institute, which made a decision to support the ACE Program in 1989 and has continued to do so.

The organizations in the outside community which have been our formal contract liaison with the AIDS Institute: Columbia University School of Public Health; WARN; ARCS; Women's Prison Association.

The Women's Prison Association, our current contractual agency, Executive Director Ann Jacobs and Transitional Service Unit staff of Sam Rivera; Yvonne Soto and our present ACE Coordinator who has given four years of her life to be with us, Liz Mastroieni.

From the Division of Parole, Terry Wurmser who made it possible to create the program ACE-HOME, in which inmates on parole could have contact with one another in order to give each other very much needed support.

To those of you who work at Bedford Hills Correctional Facility: So many people employed at different Jobs in Bedford Hills have helped—either through supporting an individual or in their relationship to ACE as a program. We thank those of you who have made a special effort ...

> ...The Executive teams, Captains, Lieutenants, Sergeants, whose policy and individual decisions have supported individuals and allowed ACE to function;
> ...The medical directors and nurse administrators who worked with ACE;
> ...The medical staff and dental staff who have cared for the sick and dying in our facility;
> ...C.O.'s who from day-to-day make things happen here; the numerous C.O.'s who supported individuals with HIV/AIDS and supported ACE to be able to do the work, gave us respect, and allowed us to have responsibility;
> ...The Chaplains who have helped people mourn and honor those who pass;
> ...The Children's Center which first set the tradition of an inmate-centered program and has interacted with ACE to help women and their children bond with one another;
> ...The academic and vocational teachers and their supervisors who encourage and support our educational outreach in their classrooms;
> ...The print shop personnel who have helped ACE design and print materials;
> ...Civilians throughout the many programs in the facility who counsel and support those in need;
> ...The Mercy College personnel who supported those with HIV as they struggled to get their degrees against the pressure of illness and encroaching death;
> ...The Family Violence Program who helped us to realize the connection between HIV/AIDS and Family Violence and who support women coping with both issues;
> ...The Office of Mental Health, which gives necessary support to those women who are struggling with both mental health issues and HIV/AIDS;
> ...The ASAT Program with whom we developed programs that address the combined problems of HIV/AIDS and drug use;
> ...The Food Service Administration and its staff who have supported all of our special events.

We thank those of you on the present Executive Team of Bedford Hills Correction Facility:

> Superintendent Elaine A. Lord; Deputy Superintendent of Programs Joseph Smith; Deputy Superintendent of Administration Susan Schultz; Deputy Superintendent of Security William Fenton; Deputy Superintendent of Health Saundra Johnson

Looking back to the beginning: We want to acknowledge some of the individuals and groups that ten years ago—in the very beginning—helped us to break new ground and create ACE. It was a difficult period and one which required vision, risk-taking and commitment:

> Superintendent Elaine A. Lord; Deputy Superintendent of Programs K. Pearlman; Deputy Superintendent of Administration Susan Schultz; First Deputy Superintendent V. Herbert; Captain V. Palmer; former DOCS Medical Director R. Greifinger; Linda Loffredo; Gloria Cuccurullo; Lynne McArthur; Joyce Hughes; Sally Perryman, Cathy Potler; Sister Elaine Roulet; Sharon Smolick; Marcy May; Dr. Keats; Rose Palladino; Dr. Nereida Ferran; Dr. Gary Wormser; Nurse Administrator Wycke; Nurse Administrator Rosado; Dr. Frank Rundel; Prisoners Rights Project; Prisoners Legal Services; Father Gorman; Monnie Callen and the team from Montefiore Hospital; Joan Koch-Devereaux; Norma Hill; John King; Millie Kaplan; ACT-UP Womens Caucus; Nurse Steiner.

To those of you beyond the prison walls... We acknowledge and thank you who have come into the prison from outside, given of your time, your information and your commitment. We are unable to go back over the almost ten years since the founding of ACE and remember each of you who has supported and educated women at Bedford Hills Correctional Facility, either while they were here or when they left. We decided not to create an incomplete list, thereby omitting individual names by an error. Therefore, we are listing as many of the groups that we currently work with or who have worked with us in the past which we remember. We acknowledge all of the agencies who have been supportive of us, with the many different speakers, advice, and support for the women inside and out. We thank all of you as individuals who have given of your time to work with the women of Bedford Hills and ACE. You have shared your commitment with us and thereby strengthened all of us inside in our struggle to cope with the epidemic.

> PWAC; PWA NEWSLINE; Cicatelli Associates Inc.; My Sisters Place; WomenCare; Open Door Health Facility; Division of Parole; EARS; St. Clare's Hospital and Spellman Clinic; Division of H.I.V. Services/Albert Einstein College of Medicine; Memorial Sloan Kettering Hospital; New Jersey Women and AIDS Network; Columbia University School of Public Health; Bronx AIDS Services; Incarnation Children's Center; Life Force; Bronx AIDS Services; WARN; Columbia University School of Public Health; Camp VIVA; Gay Mens Health Crisis, ARCS; Beth Israel Hospital; Montefiore Hospital and Department of Social Medicine; Brooklyn AIDS Task Force; Manhattan AIDS Task Force; Prisoners Legal Services; Prisoners Rights Project; World Magazine; Osborne Association; Correctional Association; Women's Prison Association; Community Health Commission; Stand UP Harlem; Community Health Project; Poz; Beta; Human Rights Division; Housing Works; Mid-Hudson AIDS Task Force; Lesbian AIDS Project; the Names Project; Upper Manhattan AIDS Task Force; Minority AIDS Task Force; Hispanic AIDS Forum; New York State AIDS Institute; Philliber Research Association; Project Jeraco; Hunter College; Women's Equality Day; NOW; Haitian Coalition on AIDS; AIDS Treatment Registry; PEPA; ACT-UP and ACT-UP Women's Caucus; HELP-AYUDA; Women in Crisis; Hyacinth AIDS Foundation; Center for Community Alternatives; Rivington House; Highbridge-Woodycrest Center; Turning Point; Samaritan House; The Boston Women's Health Book Collective; Latino Commission on AIDS; The Osborne Association; The Correctional Association; SAID Program; REACH; Passage Homes; Open Society; Columbia University College of Physicians and Surgeons; visitors from many correctional facilities throughout the United States as well as from other countries including Sweden, Canada, South Africa, Scotland, England, and Australia.